Student Workbook for use with

Clinical Procedures for Medical Assisting

Fourth Edition

Kathryn A. Booth RN, RMA (AMT), RPT, CPhT, MS
Total Care Programming, Inc.

Leesa G. Whicker, BA, CMA (AAMA)
Central Piedmont Community College

Terri D. Wyman, CPC, CMRS
Wing Memorial Hospital

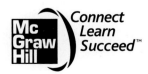
Connect
Learn
Succeed™

The McGraw-Hill Companies

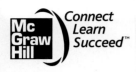

STUDENT WORKBOOK FOR USE WITH
CLINICAL PROCEDURES FOR MEDICAL ASSISTING, FOURTH EDITION
Kathryn A. Booth, Leesa G. Whicker, and Terri D. Wyman

Published by McGraw-Hill, a business unit of The McGraw-Hill Companies, Inc., 1221 Avenue of the
Americas, New York, NY 10020. Copyright © 2011 by The McGraw-Hill Companies, Inc.

1 2 3 4 5 6 7 8 9 0 WDQ/WDQ 1 0 9 8 7 6 5 4 3 2 1 0

ISBN 978-0-07-735827-3
MHID 0-07-735827-9

www.mhhe.com

Contents

Procedures

Preface

The *Student Workbook* provides you with an opportunity to review and master the concepts and skills introduced in your student textbook, *Clinical Procedures for Medical Assisting,* Fourth Edition. Chapter by chapter, the workbook provides the following:

Vocabulary Review, which tests your knowledge of key terms introduced in the chapter. Formats for these exercises include Matching, True or False, and Passage Completion.

Content Review, which tests your knowledge of key concepts introduced in the chapter. Formats for these exercises include Multiple Choice, Sentence Completion, and Short Answer.

Critical Thinking, which tests your understanding of key concepts introduced in the chapter. These questions require you to use higher-level thinking skills, such as comprehension, analysis, synthesis, and evaluation.

Applications, which provide opportunities to apply the concepts and skills introduced in the chapter. For example, using role play, you will perform such activities as developing a personal career plan and interviewing a medical specialist.

Case Studies, which provide opportunities to apply the concepts introduced in the chapter to lifelike situations you will encounter as a medical assistant. For example, you may be asked to decide how to respond to a patient who calls the doctor's office to say that she is having difficulty breathing or you may be requested to give information about the thyroid gland to a patient who has just been referred for thyroid testing.

Procedure Competency Checklists, which enable you to monitor your mastery of the steps in the procedure(s) introduced in a chapter, such as Preparing a Patient Medical Record/Chart and Performing a Surgical Scrub. Each procedure is correlated with the CAAHEP and ABHES competencies you will need to know to become a medical assistant. Answers to the material in the *Student Workbook* are found in the *Instructor's Resource Binder.*

Procedure Work Product Forms, are provided in a separate new section. These forms can be used when practicing and testing your skills. Make extra copies since you may use them more than once.

Application Activity Forms, are used to complete the application activities found in your student textbook and this workbook. This new section helps tie together the learning between the textbook and workbook.

Ask your instructor for permission to check your work against these answers.

Together, your student textbook and the *Student Workbook* form a complete learning package. *Clinical Procedures for Medical Assisting,* Fourth Edition will prepare you to enter the medical assisting field with the knowledge and skills necessary to become a useful resource to patients and a valued asset to employers and to the medical assisting profession.

Medical Assisting Reviewers

In addition, many people and organizations provided invaluable assistance in the process of illustrating the highly technical and detailed topics covered in the text. Their contributions helped ensure the accuracy, timelines, and authenticity of the illustrations in the book.

We would like to thank the following organizations for providing source materials and technical advice: the American Association of Medical Assistants, Chicago, Illinois; Becton Dickinson Microbiology Systems, Sparks, Maryland; Becton Dickinson Vacutainer® Systems, Franklin Lakes, New Jersey; Bibbero Systems, Petaluma, California; Burdick, Schaumberg, Illinois; the Corel Corporation, Ottawa, Ontario, Canada; Hamilton Media, Hamilton, New Jersey; Nassau Ear, Nose, and Throat, Princeton, New Jersey; Princeton Allergy and Asthma Associates, Princeton, New Jersey; Richmond International, Boca Raton, Florida; and Winfield Medical, San Diego, California.

We would like to express our appreciation to the following New Jersey physicians and medical facilities for allowing us to photograph a variety of procedures and procedural settings at their facilities: the Eric B. Chandler Medical Center, New Brunswick; Helene Fuld School of Nursing of New Jersey, Trenton; Mercer Medical Center, Trenton; Mercer County Vocational-Technical Health Occupations Center, Trenton; Plainfield Health Center, Plainfield; Princeton Allergy and Asthma Associates, Princeton; the Princeton Medical Group, Princeton; Robert Wood Johnson University Hospital, New Brunswick; Robert Wood Johnson University Hospital at Hamilton, Hamilton; St. Francis Medical Center, Trenton; St. Peters Medical Center, New Brunswick; Dr. Edward von der Schmidt, neurosurgeon, Princeton; Wound Care Center/Curative Network, New Brunswick.

We would also like to thank the following facilities and educational institutions for graciously allowing us to photograph procedures and other technical aspects related to the profession of medical assisting: Total Care Programming, Palm Coast, Florida; Wildwood Medical Clinic, Henrico, North Carolina; Central Piedmont Community College, Charlotte, North Carolina; Daytona Beach Community College, Daytona Beach, Florida; Roanoke Rapids Clinic, Roanoke Rapids, Virginia; and Everest University, Jacksonville, Florida.

Thanks also to Lynn Egler and Susan Findley for their assistance with various aspects of the project. A special thank you to Tiffany Heath for her content review.

Reviewers

Every area of the text was reviewed by practitioners and educators in the field. Their insights helped shape the direction of the book.

Medical Advisory Board

Gerry A. Brasin, AS, CMA (AAMA), CPC
Premier Education Group

Dr. Marina Klebanov, BDS, MSPH
Mandl College of Allied Health

Tabitha L Lyons, NCMA, AS
Corporate Program Manager–Medical Assisting
Anthem Education Group

Barry Newman, MD
PC Tech

Diane Peavy
Fortis Colleges

Adrienne Predko, M.A. Ed.
National Director of Education
MedVance Institute

Dr. Gary Zuckerman
Washington University School of Medicine

Connect Contributors

Dolly R. Horton, CMA(AAMA), BS, M.Ed.
Asheville Buncombe Technical Community College

Sepanta Jalali, M.D.
Columbus State

Merideth Sellars, M.S.
Columbus State Community College

Sherry Stanfield, RN, BSN, MSHPE
Miller-Motte Technical College

Nerissa Tucker, MHA, CPC
Kaplan University School of Health Sciences

Dr. Wendy Vermillion, DVM
Columbus State Community College

Mindy Wray, BS, CMA(AAMA), RMA
ECPI College of Technology

Byron Hamilton, BA, MA
Australian College of Advanced Education

Digital Symposium Attendees

Courtney M. Conrad, MBA, MPH, CMA
Robert Morris University Illinois

Bonnie J. Crist, BS, CMA, AAS (AAMA)
Harrison College

Patrick J. Debold
Vice President of Academic Affairs
Concorde Career Colleges, Inc.

Robert Delaney
Chair, Allied Health
Brookline College

Alice Macomber, RN, RMA, AHI, RPT, CPI, BXO
Keiser University, Port Saint Lucie Campus

Barry Newman, MD
PC Tech

Kathleen Olewinski, MS, RHIA, NHA, FACHE
Medical Assisting Program Director
Bryant & Stratton College - Milwaukee Market

Mickie Roy, LPN, CCMA
Delta College of Arts & Technology

Lisa M. Smith, B.S., RMA(AMT), BXMO
Medical Assisting Program & Externship Coordinator
Keiser University

Michael Weinand
Kaplan Higher Education

Dr. Barbara Worley, DPM, BS, RMA
Program Manager, Medical Assisting
King's College

Patti Zint, M.A., N.C.H.I.
Apollo College

Reviewers

Hooshiyar Ahmadi, MD, DC
Remington College

Diana Alagna, RN, RMA (AMT)
Branford Hall Career Institute

Yvonne Beth Alles, MBA
Davenport University

Ramona Atiles, LPN
Allied Health Program Chair
Career Institute of Health and Technology

Vanessa J. Austin, RMA (AMT), CAHI, BS
Clarian Health Sciences Education Center

Dr. Joseph H. Balatbat, MD
Sanford-Brown Institute

Katie Barton, BA, LPN
Savannah River College

Suzanne Bitters, RMA (AMT)-NCPT/NCICS
Harris Business School

Alecia C. Blake, MD
Medical Careers Institute at ECPI College of Technology

Kathleen Bode, MS
Flint Hills Technical College

Cynthia Boles, CMA (AAMA)
Bradford School

Cindi Brassington, MS, CMA (AAMA)
Quinebaug Valley Community College

Robin K. Choate, LPN, CHI
Pennsylvania Institute of Technology

Stephen M. Coleman, NCMA
Central Florida Institute

Sheronda Cooper, BSD, BSN, MSFN, RMA (AMT), NRCPT(NAHP)
Director of Medical Assisting
Bradford School of Business

Janet H. Davis, BSN, MS, MBA, PhD
Robert Morris College

Linda Demain, LPN, BS, MS
Wichita Technical Institute

Carol Dew, MAT, CMA-AC (AAMA)
Baker College

CHAPTER 1

Principles of Asepsis

REVIEW

Vocabulary Review

Matching

Match the key terms in the right column with the definitions in the left column by placing the letter of each correct answer in the space provided.

_____ **1.** An inanimate object that may be contaminated with infectious organisms and therefore transmit disease

_____ **2.** A highly specific protein that attaches itself to a foreign substance

_____ **3.** Harmless or beneficial microorganisms that have taken up residence in the body

_____ **4.** An infection that occurs when there is a malfunction or abnormality in a routine body process, causing normally beneficial microorganisms to become pathogenic

_____ **5.** An infection caused by introduction of a pathogen from outside the body

_____ **6.** A foreign substance that invades the body

_____ **7.** A simple form of life commonly made up of a single cell that can be seen only through a microscope

_____ **8.** Phagocytes found in lymph nodes, liver, spleen, lungs, and bone marrow

_____ **9.** The condition of being resistant to pathogens and the diseases they cause

_____ **10.** A manifestation of an infection that is so slight as to be unnoticeable

a. antibody
b. antigen
c. macrophage
d. immunity
e. exogenous infection
f. resident normal flora
g. fomite
h. microorganism
i. subclinical case
j. endogenous infection

True or False

Decide whether each statement is true or false. In the space at the left, write T for true or F for false. On the lines provided, rewrite the false statements to make them true.

_____ **11.** Pathogens are microorganisms that do not cause disease.

_____

_____ **12.** *Mycobacterium tuberculosis* is spread through droplet transmission.

_____

_____ **13.** Monocytes are a type of T cell.

_____

_____ **14.** Infections by microorganisms that can cause disease only when a host's resistance is low are called opportunistic infections.

_____

_____ **15.** Another name for the disease diphtheria is whooping cough.

_____

_____ **16.** Phagocytes are special white blood cells that engulf and digest normal flora.

_____

_____ **17.** Macrophages are phagocytes found in the lymph nodes, liver, spleen, lungs, bone marrow, and connective tissue.

_____

_____ **18.** A carrier is a reservoir host who is unaware of the presence of the pathogen and so spreads the disease.

_____

_____ **19.** An endogenous infection is an infection in a reservoir host caused by the introduction of a pathogen from outside the body.

_____

_____ **20.** A fomite is a living organism, such as an insect, that carries microorganisms from an infected person to another person.

_____

_____ **21.** A susceptible host is a person who has little or no immunity to infection by a transmitted pathogen.

_____

_____ **22.** The scientist who discovered how to use chemical antiseptics to control surgery-related infection by microorganisms was Hippocrates.

_____

_____ **23.** Antigens are part of the body's natural defenses against infection.

_____

_____ **24.** When a person receives an immunization or vaccine with killed or weakened organisms, the result is natural active immunity.

_____

_____ **25.** B cells are a group of proteins always present in the body to help white blood cells ingest microorganisms.

_____

_____ **26.** Viruses are the smallest known infectious agents.

_____

Content Review

Multiple Choice

In the space provided, write the letter of the choice that best completes each statement or answers each question.

_____ 1. The chain of infection consists of a(n)
   A. infectious agent.
   B. reservoir host.
   C. mode of transmission.
   D. portal of entry.
   E. All of the above.

_____ 2. A microorganism's disease-producing power is called
   A. a pathogen.
   B. convalescence.
   C. immunity.
   D. virulence.
   E. resistance.

_____ 3. Beneficial microorganisms found in the body that help create a barrier against pathogens are known as
   A. resident normal flora.
   B. carriers.
   C. endogens.
   D. fomites.

_____ 4. A reservoir host who is unaware of the presence of a pathogen and therefore spreads disease is called
   A. transmission.
   B. a portal of exit.
   C. a portal of entry.
   D. a susceptible host.
   E. a carrier.

_____ 5. The condition of being resistant to pathogens and the diseases they cause is called
   A. virulence.
   B. immunity.
   C. resistance.
   D. nonspecific.

_____ 6. An animal, insect, or human whose body is capable of sustaining the growth of a pathogen is known as
   A. a reservoir host.
   B. a susceptible host.
   C. a pathogen.
   D. flora.
   E. an environmental factor.

_____ 7. An insect that carries microorganisms from one infected person to another is a
   A. fomite.
   B. pathogen.
   C. host.
   D. vector.
   E. droplet.

_____ 8. An infection in a reservoir host in which an abnormality or malfunction in routine body process has caused normally beneficial or harmless microorganisms to become pathogenic is called a(n)
   A. endogenous infection.
   B. subclinical case.
   C. exogenous infection.
   D. carrier state.

_____ 9. The process by which phagocytes destroy pathogens is known as
   A. digestion.
   B. engulfment.
   C. protection.
   D. humoral response.
   E. phagocytosis.

_____ 10. Cells that produce antibodies are called
   A. T cells.
   B. B cells.
   C. lymphocytes.
   D. antigens.
   E. phagocytes.

_____ 11. Administration of an immunization or a vaccine results in which type of immunity?
   A. Natural active
   B. Natural passive
   C. Artificial active
   D. Artificial passive

_____ 12. Exposure to a disease-causing organism results in which type of immunity?
   A. Natural active
   B. Natural passive
   C. Artificial active
   D. Artificial passive
   E. Complement

_____ 13. Which of the following are phagocytes that are formed in bone marrow and circulate throughout the blood for a short period of time?
   A. Antibodies
   B. Macrophages
   C. Neutrophils
   D. Monocytes

Short Answer

Write the answer to each question on the lines provided.

14. What are four ways in which microorganisms can damage the body?

_____

_____

_____

15. How does resident normal flora protect the body against pathogens?

_____

_____

_____

16. What is the process by which phagocytes destroy a pathogen?

_____

_____

_____

17. Describe how the body achieves active immunity to a particular disease.

_____

_____

_____

18. How does cell-mediated immunity function to protect the body?

_____

_____

_____

19. What are monocytes and how do they protect the body?

_____

_____

_____

20. What are the five means by which pathogens may be transmitted?

_____

_____

_____

21. List ways to contain tuberculosis bacteria at their source and prevent their entrance into another host.

_____

_____

_____

22. Describe the body's first lines of defense.

_____

_____

_____

23. What are the CDC's four strategies for reducing the incidence of antibiotic-resistant microorganisms?

_____

_____

_____

Critical Thinking

Write the answer to each question on the lines provided.

1. How will understanding the cycle of infection help you maintain an aseptic environment?

_____

_____

_____

2. How could a common cold be spread by shaking hands with someone?

_____

_____

_____

3. What instructions would you give a patient suspected of having tuberculosis?

_____

_____

_____

4. What information can you give a patient who is insistent he receive a prescription for antibiotics to treat his common cold?

_____

_____

_____

APPLICATION

Follow the directions for the application.

Signs and Symptoms of Diseases

Listed below are signs and symptoms of contagious diseases you may encounter as a medical assistant. Write the name of each disease on the line provided and identify its cause.

a. Patient has fluid-filled blisters that began as a rash of tiny red bumps.

b. Patient has a harsh, barking cough, with difficulty breathing, hoarseness, and a low-grade fever.

c. Patient experiences fever and an itchy rash.

d. Patient has fever and painful swelling near the back of the jaw.

e. Patient has fever, sore throat, swollen lymph nodes, and occasionally spleen and liver involvement.

f. Patient experiences the symptoms of strep throat, as well as nausea and vomiting, and has tiny, bright-red spots on his trunk, neck, face, and extremities.

CASE STUDIES

Write your response to each case study on the lines provided.

Case 1

A patient tells you she heard there was a vaccine for tuberculosis. She wants to know if she can receive the vaccine. What information about the tuberculosis vaccine will you give her?

_____

_____

_____

Case 2

You are the clinical supervisor in a pediatric office. You notice that a coworker does not wash her hands after taking a child's temperature. You know the child has chickenpox. After mentioning to the medical assistant that she did not wash her hands, she states, "I will be fine. I had the chickenpox when I was a child." Based on what you have learned about the cycle of infection, why is this statement unacceptable? What should you tell the medical assistant? What part of the cycle of infection does the patient represent? The medical assistant?

_____

_____

_____

Case 3

Imagine that you are a preformed, immune protein that has been injected into the body of a person recently exposed to a disease. What are you? What work will you do in the body? What disease or diseases are you being sent to treat?

_____

_____

_____

Case 4

Maria had measles as a child. She is now immune to the disease. What type of immunity does this represent?

_____

_____

_____

Case 5

Sam received a tetanus booster at the time of his last physical exam. What type of immunity did Sam produce to the vaccine?

_____

_____

_____

CHAPTER 2

Infection Control Techniques

REVIEW

Vocabulary Review

True or False

Decide whether each statement is true or false. In the space at the left, write T for true or F for false. On the lines provided, rewrite the false statements to make them true.

_____ 1. The three methods of infection control are sanitization, disinfection, and sterilization.

_____

_____ 2. Sanitization is a scrubbing process used to remove the microorganisms that cause disease.

_____

_____ 3. Bleach is an effective means of immunization.

_____

_____ 4. Asepsis is the condition in which pathogens are absent or controlled.

_____

_____ 5. After sterilization, items wrapped in a sterile pack have a shelf life of 30 days.

_____

_____ 6. Sanitization involves raising the number of microorganisms on an object or a surface to a fairly safe level.

_____

_____ 7. Sterilization is the destruction of all microorganisms, including bacterial spores, by specific means.

_____

_____ 8. Hospitals now use Standard Precautions, which are a combination of Universal Precautions and rules to reduce the risk of disease transmission by means of moist body substances.

_____

_____ 9. According to OSHA guidelines, an example of a Category I task is giving mouth-to-mouth resuscitation.

_____

_____ 10. The penalty for a violation of OSHA's infectious waste disposal regulations is a fine from $5000 to $70,000.

_____

_____ **11.** Preventing the spread of microorganisms in the medical environment through maintaining cleanliness is known as septic technique.

_____

_____ **12.** According to OSHA requirements, all health-care workers who have occupational exposure to blood or other potentially infectious materials must be provided with the hepatitis B vaccine, a procedure that is to be billed to their insurance company.

_____

Content Review

Multiple Choice

In the space provided, write the letter of the choice that best completes each statement or answers each question.

_____ **1.** The processes of sterilization include dry heat, chemicals, and
  A. sanitization.
  B. disinfection.
  C. autoclaving.
  D. scrubbing.
  E. None of the above.

_____ **2.** A chemical agent that leaves an instrument clean but not sterile is a(n)
  A. cold sterilizer.
  B. antiseptic.
  C. chemical sterilizer.
  D. detergent.
  E. disinfectant.

_____ **3.** Which of these methods would be the most effective in loosening debris from sharp instruments while also reducing the risk of injury?
  A. Submersion in water and detergent
  B. Ultrasound
  C. Autoclaving
  D. Chemical disinfecting

_____ **4.** Sterilization tape that is used to secure autoclave wrap is also used to
  A. identify and date the contents.
  B. prove that the sterility of the items has taken place.
  C. indicate that the pack has been exposed to the autoclave process.
  D. *A* and *C* only.
  E. All of the above.

_____ **5.** The proof that an instrument pack has been sterilized is achieved by using a
  A. chemical indicator strip placed under the instruments.
  B. chemical indicator strip placed in the center of the pack.
  C. chemical indicator tape around the outside of the pack.
  D. biological monitor placed next to a pack.
  E. biological monitor placed in the load with the packs.

_____ 6. The critical step of the autoclave cycle when the microorganisms are destroyed is when
  A. the greatest temperature is reached.
  B. the water is changed into pressurized steam.
  C. heat is transferred to the items in the chamber.
  D. the steam saturates items in the chamber.

_____ 7. While using an autoclave, the medical assistant must monitor
  A. temperature-pressure combinations.
  B. time-temperature combinations.
  C. pressure-time combinations.
  D. All of the above.
  E. None of the above.

_____ 8. When storing items removed from an autoclave, the major factor contributing to the integrity of the sterility is
  A. preventing dust accumulation.
  B. maintaining the temperature of the environment.
  C. the state of dryness when the pack is stored.
  D. the shelf-life expectancy.

_____ 9. The use of alcohol is an effective means of
  A. sterilization.
  B. immunization.
  C. disinfection.
  D. sanitization.
  E. All of the above.

_____ 10. Instruments that do not require sterilization can safely be prepared for their next use by
  A. washing them until they are visibly clean and free from stains and tissues.
  B. wiping them off with a paper towel.
  C. rinsing them under extremely hot water.
  D. visually inspecting them and storing them if nothing is seen on their surface.
  E. Any of the above.

_____ 11. The method that most hospitals use to reduce the risk of disease transmission by means of moist body substances is
  A. Standard Precautions.
  B. Universal Precautions.
  C. personal protective equipment.
  D. isolation.

_____ 12. The cleansing process to decrease the number of microorganisms before disinfection or sterilization is called
  A. sanitization.
  B. hand washing.
  C. asepsis.
  D. biohazardous waste.
  E. All of the above.

Name _____ Class _____ Date _____

Short Answer

Write the answer to each question on the lines provided.

13. What are three medical instruments you can sanitize and reuse without further disinfection or sterilization?

_____

_____

_____

14. List three factors that can have an impact on the effectiveness of a disinfectant.

_____

_____

_____

15. What are the disadvantages of using acid products to disinfect instruments and equipment?

_____

_____

_____

16. What are the three leading factors that cause incomplete autoclave sterilization?

_____

_____

_____

17. What aseptic technique should be used when administering tablet or capsule medications and why?

_____

_____

_____

18. Explain how vaccines protect the body against infectious diseases.

_____

_____

_____

19. Describe possible duties and responsibilities of medical assistants in providing immunizations.

_____

_____

_____

20. Describe the process you would use to sanitize surgical instruments.

_____

_____

_____

21. When is it important to wear protective eyewear or face shields? Give an example.

_____

_____

_____

Critical Thinking

Write the answer to each question on the lines provided.

1. What should you do with a curette that a coworker says has "probably been sterilized"?

_____

_____

_____

2. Would you use transfer forceps during a procedure if you were wearing sterile gloves to handle instruments in a sterile field? Explain.

_____

_____

_____

3. Why should you know your own HIV and HBV status if you are participating in high-risk procedures?

_____

_____

_____

4. Why is informed consent important in the immunization of adults and children?

_____

_____

_____

5. How might less-invasive techniques for delivering medications help hospital patients avoid nosocomial infection?

_____

_____

_____

APPLICATION

Follow the directions for each application.

1. Sanitizing Instruments and Equipment

Work with one partner and sanitize a group of instruments. One person should sanitize the instruments and equipment. The second should act as an evaluator and should refer to the detailed description provided in the text while observing the procedure. Assume that a surgical procedure has just been completed.

a. Collect all the instruments from the procedure; place them in a sink or container filled with water and an appropriate neutral-pH detergent solution.

b. Put on utility gloves and separate the sharp instruments from all other equipment.

c. Rinse each piece of equipment in hot running water. Scrub the instruments and equipment with hot, soapy water and a plastic scrub brush. Then rinse the instruments and dry them properly.

d. Rinse and sanitize syringes following appropriate procedures for these items.

e. When the sanitizing process is complete, the observer should present a critique of the procedure, pointing out any errors in the procedure and offering suggestions for improved technique.

f. Exchange roles so that each of you has the opportunity to practice the procedure while the other observes and offers comments and suggestions.

g. When each of you has completed the sanitization procedure, follow the same process to practice and develop skill in disinfection and sterilization.

2. **Making a Biohazardous Materials Checklist**

Work with two partners. The chief physician wants to make sure her staff is aware of the guidelines for managing different types of biohazardous materials. She has asked your team to prepare a Biohazardous Materials Checklist.

a. As a team, decide which biohazardous materials should be included in the checklist. Have one partner make a list.

b. Each team member should choose one type of biohazardous material from the list and write guidelines for managing that particular material. Guidelines should include information about handling and disposing of the biohazardous material. Use medical journals, textbooks, or other sources as references.

c. Team members should evaluate each other's guidelines. The critique should answer these questions: Are the guidelines described in enough detail? Will the guidelines prevent potentially infectious waste materials from endangering people or the environment? Is the writing clear and concise?

d. The team should discuss the critique, noting the accuracy and completeness of the guidelines as written. Revise the guidelines as needed.

e. Members of the team should take turns choosing a different biohazardous material from the list until the checklist is complete.

f. As a team, review your Biohazardous Materials Checklist. Discuss these questions with your partners: Have all the various biohazardous materials in the medical office been accounted for? Are the guidelines as complete as they need to be?

g. Compare your Biohazardous Materials Checklist with another team's checklist. Evaluate each other's checklists. Revise your checklist to make it as complete and accurate as possible.

3. **Educating Patients**

Work with two partners. Have one partner play the role of a patient recovering from an infection. Have the second partner act as a medical assistant. Let the third partner act as an observer and evaluator.

a. Have the student playing the medical assistant prepare a presentation about the basic principles of hygiene and disease prevention. The aim of the presentation is to help educate patients about general ways to protect themselves from disease. It may include charts, diagrams, drawings, or other visual aids.

b. Have the medical assistant talk to the patient about ways to protect herself and her family from disease. Have the patient ask questions to clarify or expand upon the information.

c. Have the observer provide a critique of the medical assistant's patient education techniques. The critique should examine the content of the presentation as well as the medical assistant's attitude, tone, accuracy, and clarity. Comments should include both positive feedback and suggestions for improvement.

d. Exchange roles and repeat the role-playing exercise.

e. Exchange roles again so that each member of the group has an opportunity to play the role of the medical assistant in this scenario.

f. As a group, discuss the strengths and weaknesses of each group member's ability to educate a patient about hygiene and disease prevention.

CASE STUDIES

Write your response to each case study on the lines provided.

Case 1

You have been asked to check the autoclave to make sure it is sterilizing instruments. How will you accomplish this task?

_____

_____

_____

Case 2

The receptionist at your medical office arrives at work coughing and sneezing. She appears to have the signs and symptoms of a common cold. What, if anything, should you do?

_____

_____

_____

Case 3

A patient enters your reception area with a severe laceration on his arm. The blood is dripping from his arm onto the carpet and the front desk area. What actions should you take?

_____

_____

_____

Case 4

You need to take the vital signs of a patient who is suspected of having scabies. What personal protective equipment should you wear?

_____

_____

_____

Case 5

You are assisting the doctor during a minor surgical procedure. You are wearing sterile gloves and handling sterile items directly. The doctor knocks an instrument to the floor and needs a replacement. The instruments are in a supply cabinet next to you. What should you do?

_____

_____

_____

CHAPTER 3

HIV, Hepatitis, and Other Bloodborne Pathogens

REVIEW

Vocabulary Review

True or False

Decide whether each statement is true or false. In the space at the left, write T for true or F for false. On the lines provided, rewrite the false statements to make them true.

_____ 1. A person who is unable to react to a TB skin test because he is immunocompromised is said to be allergic.

_____

_____ 2. HIV, hepatitis B virus, and hepatitis C virus are the bloodborne pathogens posing the greatest risks.

_____

_____ 3. Hepatitis B is spread mainly through the fecal-oral route.

_____

_____ 4. Shingles is caused by the reactivation of the virus that causes chickenpox.

_____

_____ 5. A bloodborne infection that may be contracted by handling cat litter is erythema infectiosum.

_____

_____ 6. The Federal Drug Administration (FDA) regulates the safety of health-care workers.

_____

_____ 7. White blood cells that are a key component of the body's immune system and that work in coordination with other white blood cells to combat infection are known as helper B cells.

_____

_____ 8. The Centers for Disease Control and Prevention (CDC) are provided with timely reports on the incidence of infectious diseases from state health departments.

_____

Content Review

Multiple Choice

In the space provided, write the letter of the choice that best completes each statement or answers each question.

_____ 1. The disease that is transmitted by handling cat feces is known as
A. syphilis.
B. malaria.
C. toxoplasmosis.
D. *Pneumocystis carinii.*
E. hairy leukoplakia.

_____ 2. The vaccine against hepatitis B provides immunity for at least
A. 3 years.
B. 4 years.
C. 5 years.
D. 6 years.
E. 7 years.

_____ 3. Which of the following is the only readily available method to detect evidence of HIV infection?
A. Patient history
B. Signs and symptoms
C. Serologic test(s)
D. Urinalysis

_____ 4. Hepatitis D occurs only in people who are infected with
A. hepatitis A.
B. hepatitis B.
C. hepatitis C.
D. hepatitis E.
E. HIV.

_____ 5. Erythema infectiosum, a childhood disease, is also known as
A. fifth disease.
B. red measles.
C. chickenpox.
D. listeriosis.

_____ 6. Which of the following is a possible means of transmission of HIV?
A. Tears
B. Intact skin
C. Saliva
D. Blood

_____ 7. Hepatitis primarily affects the
A. lungs.
B. liver.
C. brain.
D. skin.
E. intestines.

_____ **8.** An immunization for protection against the HIV virus may be acquired by

    A. vaccination.

    B. contracting the disease.

    C. taking a protease inhibitor.

    D. a blood transfusion.

    E. None of the above.

Short Answer

Write the answer to each question on the lines provided.

9. What are the five different types of hepatitis?

_____

_____

_____

10. Describe the three stages of hepatitis infection.

_____

_____

_____

11. What are four symptoms of hepatitis?

_____

_____

_____

12. List three ways that HIV infection can be passed from person to person.

_____

_____

_____

13. List five symptoms of AIDS.

_____

_____

_____

14. What are five chronic disorders commonly experienced by a patient with AIDS?

_____

_____

_____

15. Name the four classes of drugs used to treat AIDS.

_____

_____

_____

16. List four symptoms of *Mycobacterium avium* complex (MAC) infection.

_____

_____

_____

17. What are two disadvantages of early HIV treatment?

_____

_____

_____

18. List three ways that you can help patients who are terminally ill come to terms with death.

_____

_____

_____

Critical Thinking

Write the answer to each question on the lines provided.

1. Why are law enforcement officers and firefighters at increased risk for infection by bloodborne pathogens?

_____

_____

_____

2. Why does living with a partner infected with hepatitis B or hepatitis C increase one's risk for the disease?

_____

_____

_____

3. Why might it be more important for health-care workers to have the hepatitis B vaccine than the hepatitis A vaccine?

_____

_____

_____

4. What are the advantages of delaying HIV treatment?

_____

_____

_____

5. Why is it important for AIDS patients with symptoms of tuberculosis to have a Mantoux skin test and a chest x-ray?

_____

_____

_____

APPLICATION

Follow the directions for each application.

1. Completing a Communicable Disease Form

Complete a communicable disease form to report the outbreak of hepatitis B in your community.

a. Make a photocopy of side A of the form.

b. Create a fictitious patient profile, including the patient's name, date of birth, sex, and race. Record this information on the lines provided.

c. Determine and record the patient's full name, phone number, and address. Provide information on the patient's occupation. If the patient is younger than age 18, give the name and address of the school he attends. Indicate whether the patient is in a high-risk occupation by circling Y or N.

d. Provide a physician's name and address or phone number. Indicate whether the patient was hospitalized and, if so, provide the name of the hospital and dates of hospitalization.

e. Record the date of the onset of the infection and the date of recovery. Describe the symptoms.

f. Complete the chart for members of the patient's household who may be at risk for infection.

g. Record your name and title of "Medical Assistant" and the county in which you work. Record the source of your information (the patient, patient's mother, or so on), and indicate the method by which the information was gathered.

h. Check to be sure you have completed all portions of the form and that your writing is legible.

2. Educating the Patient with HIV Infection

Work with two partners. One partner should take the role of a medical assistant, the second should take the role of a patient with HIV infection, and the third should take the role of an observer and evaluator. The patient has just learned she has HIV infection. The doctor has asked the medical assistant to explain the disease and answer the patient's questions.

a. Before starting, the medical assistant should prepare for the discussion by reviewing the symptoms and causes of HIV infection. The patient should think of questions she would like answered about the disease and how she can avoid transmitting it to her family. The observer should review the discussion of HIV in the text and should refer to the text during the interview.

b. The medical assistant should explain the symptoms of HIV infection and the stages of the disease to the patient. The patient should feel free to interrupt with questions about her disease and to express her concerns. The medical assistant should answer all questions to the best of his ability.

c. The medical assistant should explain how HIV can be transmitted. He might ask the patient questions to pinpoint possible sources of the patient's infection.

d. The medical assistant should explain how the patient can avoid transmitting the disease to her family. The patient should ask pertinent questions.

e. The observer should evaluate the interview on the basis of the accuracy of the medical assistant's explanation of HIV infection and skill in educating and reassuring the patient.

f. Exchange roles and role-play an interview with a patient who has been diagnosed with another bloodborne infectious disease.

CASE STUDIES

Write your response to each case study on the lines provided.

Case 1

A patient complains of fatigue, nausea and vomiting, stomach pain, diminished appetite, and joint pain. His skin and mucous membranes appear yellowish. What questions might you ask to determine whether he has contracted hepatitis?

_____

_____

_____

Case 2

A patient with HIV tests negative for tuberculosis according to the Mantoux skin test but exhibits many of the symptoms of the disease. Is it still possible that she has tuberculosis? If so, how can you find out?

_____

_____

_____

Case 3

A patient tells you of syphilis-like symptoms she experienced several years ago. At that time, she did not seek medical attention because the symptoms disappeared, but she is concerned that they may recur. Is she correct? What would you advise her to do?

_____

_____

_____

Case 4

A patient who is terminally ill becomes angry when he learns that he must take a new medication three times a day, which will disrupt his schedule to a greater degree than the once-a-day dose he has become accustomed to. Is this a normal reaction? How do you respond?

_____

_____

_____

CHAPTER 4

Preparing the Exam and Treatment Area

REVIEW

Vocabulary Review

True or False

Decide whether each statement is true or false. In the space at the left, write T for true or F for false. On the lines provided, rewrite the false statements to make them true.

_____ 1. Absorption of a substance through a cut or crack in the skin is known as ingestion.

_____

_____ 2. In order to assist a patient in getting onto the examining table, you should provide him or her with a rolling stool.

_____

_____ 3. Putting an exam room in order is not the medical assistant's responsibility.

_____

_____ 4. The thermostat in an exam room should be set at 55°F to discourage the growth of bacteria.

_____

_____ 5. A glass slide is an example of a consumable supply.

_____

_____ 6. After washing your hands, you should use a clean paper towel to handle doorknobs.

_____

_____ 7. ADA accessibility guidelines require doorways to be trimmed in metal casing.

_____

_____ 8. Toys in a medical office waiting room should be sanitized frequently because of their contact with sick children.

_____

_____ 9. An instrument used to examine the external ear canal and tympanic membrane is a tuning fork.

_____

_____ 10. Examples of risk management in the office include closing drawers and cabinet doors, keeping electrical cords out of walking areas, and picking up toys or other objects that could cause tripping.

_____

Content Review

Multiple Choice

In the space provided, write the letter of the choice that best completes each statement or answers each question.

_____ 1. Ideally, how many exam rooms should a doctor have reserved for exclusive use?
    A. 0
    B. 1
    C. 2
    D. 3

_____ 2. An instrument used to examine the external ear canal and tympanic membrane is a(n)
    A. anoscope.
    B. tuning fork.
    C. reflex hammer.
    D. ophthalmoscope.
    E. otoscope.

_____ 3. A common disinfectant used in exam areas and on surfaces is
    A. ammonia.
    B. dish detergent.
    C. a 10% bleach solution.
    D. window cleaner.

_____ 4. The ADA requires that doorways be at least
    A. 22 inches wide.
    B. 30 inches wide.
    C. 36 inches wide.
    D. 60 inches tall.
    E. 96 inches tall.

_____ 5. An instrument used to check pupil response in the eye is a(n)
    A. otoscope.
    B. exam light.
    C. stethoscope.
    D. penlight.

_____ 6. The ease with which a person can move in and out of a space is known as
    A. accessibility.
    B. ADA.
    C. clearance.
    D. stability.
    E. accommodations.

_____ 7. If a medical assistant accidentally brings a patient into a room before it is cleaned, which of the following would be the most appropriate action to take?
    A. Have the patient wait in the room while it is cleaned.
    B. Simply put a clean sheet on the examining table and ignore the rest of it.
    C. Ignore the whole situation.
    D. Clean the table, have the patient sit on the table, and then remove the waste.
    E. Ask the patient to wait outside just for a moment while the room is prepared.

_____ 8. Which of the following terms is used to describe supplies that are used once and discarded?
   A. Disposable
   B. Consumable
   C. Fixed
   D. Restockable

_____ 9. An instrument used to measure size or development of a body part is a
   A. thermometer.
   B. tuning fork.
   C. tape measure.
   D. speculum.

_____ 10. An instrument used to measure blood pressure is a(n)
   A. stethoscope.
   B. anoscope.
   C. ophthalmoscope.
   D. tuning fork.
   E. sphygmomanometer.

_____ 11. The first step in preventing infection transmission in the exam room is
   A. disinfecting work surfaces.
   B. handwashing.
   C. arranging supplies.
   D. keeping the examining table clean.
   E. maintaining proper room temperature.

_____ 12. Which of the following items is a chemical spray used for preserving a specimen?
   A. Isopropyl alcohol
   B. Lubricant
   C. Fixative
   D. Curette

Short Answer

Write the answer to each question on the lines provided.

13. Where in the exam room should the examining table be placed?

_____

_____

_____

14. Why is it important to maintain proper ventilation in an exam room?

_____

_____

_____

15. List four general cleaning tasks a janitorial service might perform in a medical office.

_____

_____

_____

16. When must you disinfect surfaces in the exam room?

_____

_____

_____

17. Good lighting serves many purposes in an exam room. Name three.

_____

_____

_____

18. The illustrations show a variety of instruments used during a general physical exam. On the lines provided, write the name of each instrument and briefly explain its use.

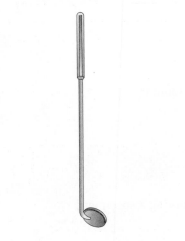

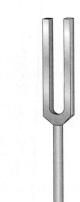

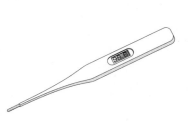

A. _____

_____

_____

B. _____

_____

_____

C. _____

_____

_____

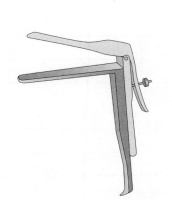

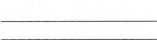

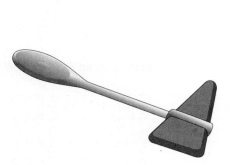

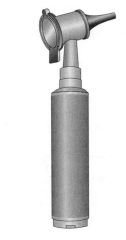

D. _____

_____

_____

E. _____

_____

_____

F. _____

_____

_____

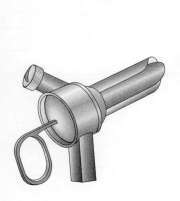

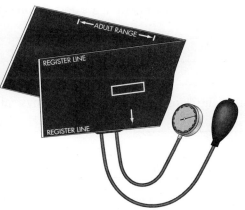

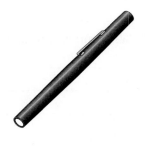

G. _____

H. _____

I. _____

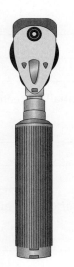

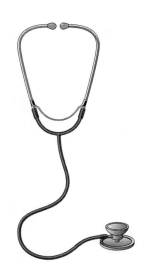

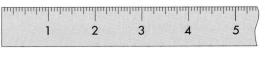

L. _____

J. _____

K. _____

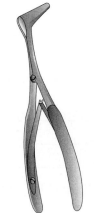

M. _____

N. _____

19. What tasks are involved in maintaining the instruments and supplies needed in the exam room?

_____

_____

_____

20. What can you do to ensure that the floor of an exam room is physically safe?

_____

_____

_____

Critical Thinking

Write the answer to each question on the lines provided.

1. What tasks in the preparation of the exam and treatment area can influence a patient's perception of a medical practice?

_____

_____

_____

2. Why do you think OSHA regulations prohibit applying cosmetics in a room where potentially infectious materials are present?

_____

_____

_____

3. What tasks in preparing the exam and treatment area are done to aid the physician in performing his work?

_____

_____

_____

4. Why is it important to maintain proper temperature in the laboratory refrigerator? How will you accomplish this?

_____

_____

_____

5. What steps will you take to ensure the otoscope and ophthalmoscope are in good working order?

_____

_____

_____

APPLICATION

Follow the directions for each application.

1. Cleaning Instruments

Indicate the proper method of cleaning for each instrument—sanitization, disinfection, or sterilization. Then, in the space provided, give the basic guidelines for performing each cleaning method.

a. Otoscope: _____

b. Anoscope: _____

c. Sphygmomanometer: _____

d. Nasal speculum: _____

e. Syringe: _____

Guidelines

f. Sanitization: _____

_____

g. Disinfection: _____

_____

h. Sterilization: _____

_____

2. Inspecting the Medical Office

Suppose you are a health and safety inspector for your state. Describe the things you would look for, in each area listed below, when inspecting a medical office.

a. Compliance with the Americans with Disabilities Act of 1990

_____

_____

_____

b. Infection control

_____

_____

_____

c. Fire prevention

_____

_____

_____

CASE STUDIES

Write your response to each case study on the lines provided.

Case 1

While reviewing the patient list for the next day, you notice that the patient for Dr. Tejada's 10:00 AM appointment is in a wheelchair. What "reasonable accommodations" have already been made for this patient?

_____

_____

_____

Case 2

You have been asked to train Sam, a newly hired medical assistant. Sam's main responsibility will be to keep the exam rooms in proper order. What information will you give Sam?

_____

_____

_____

Case 3

At a weekly staff meeting, a coworker announces her intention of cutting overhead costs by turning thermostats down to 65°F and using only under-cabinet lights rather than overhead lights. She then asks the group for feedback on these ideas. What would you say?

_____

_____

_____

Case 4

Hearing a shout, you run into the hallway and see smoke pouring from a storage closet. Sue, a nurse, is running toward the closet with a fire extinguisher. What should you do?

_____

_____

_____

CHAPTER 5

Interviewing the Patient, Taking a History, and Documentation

REVIEW

Vocabulary Review

Matching

Match the key terms in the right column with the definitions in the left column by placing the letter of each correct answer in the space provided.

_____ 1. Stating what you think has been suggested

_____ 2. Formed as a result of deeper thought

_____ 3. Restating what is said in your own words

_____ 4. Term that describes the patient's most significant symptoms

_____ 5. Using agents in a way that is not medically approved

_____ 6. A physical or psychological dependence

_____ 7. Asking questions that provide an increase in understanding of a problem

_____ 8. Thoughts, feelings, and perceptions

_____ 9. Apparent and measurable

_____ 10. A way of organizing information so that the most recent information is featured on top

_____ 11. Repeating something back to a patient in your own words

a. addiction
b. chief complaint
c. substance abuse
d. reverse chronological
e. subjective
f. objective
g. mirroring
h. verbalizing
i. restatement
j. reflection
k. clarification

True or False

Decide whether each statement is true or false. In the space at the left, write T *for true or* F *for false. On the lines provided, rewrite the false statements to make them true.*

_____ 12. The chief complaint is the physician's diagnosis of a patient's problem.

_____

_____ 13. The Health Insurance Portability and Accountability Act (HIPAA) is part of the patient's responsibilities when receiving health care.

_____

_____ 14. Sitting back and just hearing the patient is part of active listening.

_____

_____ 15. The patient's tone of voice, facial expression, and body language are signs of nonverbal communication.

_____

_____ **16.** The statement "I think you probably just have the flu" is an example of making a diagnosis and should be said by the medical assistant.

_____

_____ **17.** A patient who has white-coat syndrome is anxious about visiting the physician.

_____

_____ **18.** If a patient is using the drug Ecstasy, you may notice an increase in her heart rate and blood pressure.

_____

Content Review

Multiple Choice

In the space provided, write the letter of the choice that best completes each statement or answers each question.

_____ **1.** During a patient interview, repeating in your own words what the patient has said is an important part of
    A. effective questioning.
    B. being aware of nonverbal clues.
    C. using a broad knowledge base.
    D. summarizing to form a general picture.
    E. effective listening.

_____ **2.** "Have you had this pain long?" is an example of a(n)
    A. hypothetical question.
    B. open-ended question.
    C. encouragement for the patient to take the lead.
    D. closed-ended question.

_____ **3.** "This pain seems to be causing you more problems than it did last week" is an example of which of the following interviewing skills?
    A. Verbalizing the implied
    B. Asking a hypothetical question
    C. Challenging the patient
    D. Asking a closed-ended question
    E. Being aware of nonverbal clues

_____ **4.** "What activities seem to make the pain worse?" is an example of which of the following interviewing skills?
    A. Asking a hypothetical question
    B. Encouraging the patient to provide more information
    C. Mirroring the patient's responses
    D. Asking a leading question

_____ **5.** Where would you look on the patient's chart for information about a previous hospitalization?
    A. Laboratory report
    B. Discharge summary
    C. Patient registration form
    D. Consent form
    E. Physician's treatment plan

_____ **6.** Which of the following is an example of *subjective* data?
  A. Pain in the right arm
  B. A blood pressure reading of 138/88
  C. A height measurement of 5'6" and a weight measure of 138 lbs.
  D. A reddened rash on the left arm

_____ **7.** Which of the following is an example of *objective* data?
  A. Dizziness
  B. Pain
  C. Swollen feet
  D. Weakness
  E. Tiredness

Sentence Completion

In the space provided, write the word or phrase that best completes each sentence.

8. An elderly patient who seems to be senile may actually be _____.

9. Abuse can be physical, _____, or both.

10. _____ combine SOMR and POMR and are easily accessible to health-care workers.

11. _____ are used more extensively in medical offices than any other type of medical record.

12. The _____ is the reason the patient came to the health-care facility.

13. The _____ includes information about the level of stress, exposure to hazardous substances, and heavy lifting.

14. The _____ includes information about allergies.

15. A medical assistant should obtain information about the parents, siblings, and grandparents to complete the _____.

8. _____

9. _____

10. _____

11. _____

12. _____

13. _____

14. _____

15. _____

Short Answer

Write the answer to each question on the lines provided.

16. What are the six Cs of charting?

_____

_____

_____

17. Name seven kinds of standard information that should appear in a patient's chart.

_____

_____

_____

18. To what does the acronym SOAP refer? What does each letter represent?

_____

_____

_____

19. Why might depression be called a hidden illness?

_____

_____

_____

20. What are six signs of possible physical or psychological abuse?

_____

_____

_____

_____

Critical Thinking

Write the answer to each question on the lines provided.

1. What are important guidelines to consider when using progress notes?

_____

_____

_____

2. Why is it important to consider a patient's polypharmacy when obtaining a chief complaint or medical history?

_____

_____

_____

3. Name two general kinds of errors in taking a patient's history that could affect a physician's ability to care for the patient.

_____

_____

_____

4. Which of the following is a definite sign of depression in an adolescent patient: problems in sleeping, problems in eating, sudden mood changes, or illogical thought patterns?

_____

_____

_____

5. Name two abbreviations that have been banned by the JCAHO. Why are these abbreviations banned from patient charting?

_____

_____

_____

APPLICATION

Follow the directions for each application.

1. Conducting a Patient Interview

a. In groups of three or four, discuss and record on index cards appropriate open-ended questions for the following chief complaints:
   1. Low back pain
   2. Diabetes follow-up
   3. Insomnia

b. As a class, discuss the questions each group prepared. Formulate a list of interview questions for each of the patient complaints.

c. In pairs or groups of three, role-play each scenario, interviewing and documenting the chief complaint on the progress note provided in the documentation section in the back of the workbook.

2. Charting Patient Data

a. You have collected the following information during a client interview. Use a progress note example in the documentation section in the back of the workbook on page 591.

   A 14-year-old girl comes to the client because she has had a sore throat and fever for the past 2 days. Her vital signs are TPR 99.8-88-24, BP 110/70. She describes the pain as burning and says she has just not felt like eating lately.

b. You have collected the following information during a client interview. Use the example encounter form in the documentation section in the back of the workbook on page 428 or 581.

   A 70-year-old male arrives at the client for a blood pressure checkup. He denies pain. His vital signs are TPR 97.4-66-20, BP 158/90, O_2 Sat 96%. He is 69¾ inches tall and 165 lbs. His previous records indicate he is allergic to "sulfa drugs." He states that he is currently taking Lipitor, 20 milligrams, one every day; Atenolol, 50 milligrams, one every day; and 81 milligrams of aspirin daily. He denies using alcohol, tobacco, and recreational drugs and does not know when he had his last tetanus shot.

CASE STUDIES

Write your response to each case study on the lines provided.

Case 1

As you interview a patient before he sees the physician, he points out a mysterious rash that developed during the night. He asks what you think it is. You explain that he needs to talk to the doctor about it. The patient insists that you know him because you were assisting the physician during his last visit. He is sure you can tell him what caused his rash. You know this patient has many allergies and probably touched something that caused his rash. What should you tell the patient?

_____

_____

_____

Case 2

A 17-year-old girl arrives alone for an appointment with the doctor. She seems tense and stiff; she avoids looking at you. When you ask why she has come to the doctor's office today, she whispers that she will tell the doctor. What should you do?

_____

_____

_____

CHAPTER 6

Obtaining Vital Signs and Measurements

REVIEW

Vocabulary Review

Matching

Match the key terms in the right column with the definitions in the left column by placing the letter of each correct answer in the space provided.

_____	**1.** Difficult or painful breathing
_____	**2.** An exceptionally high fever
_____	**3.** A slow heart rate of less than 60 beats per minute
_____	**4.** A fast heart rate of more than 100 beats per minute
_____	**5.** Having a body temperature within the normal range
_____	**6.** Curve in the surface of mercury in a mercury sphygmomanometer
_____	**7.** Instrument that amplifies body sounds
_____	**8.** A measure of blood pressure taken when the heart relaxes
_____	**9.** A measure of blood pressure taken when the left ventricle contracts
_____	**10.** Deep, rapid breathing
_____	**11.** Pulse at the lower left corner of the heart
_____	**12.** Temperature scale on which a healthy adult's temperature would be 98.6°
_____	**13.** High blood pressure
_____	**14.** Low blood pressure
_____	**15.** To make sure an instrument is measuring correctly
_____	**16.** The bend of the elbow
_____	**17.** The lower left corner of the heart, where the strongest heart sounds can be heard
_____	**18.** Having a body temperature above the normal range
_____	**19.** A breathing pattern that includes shallow and deep breaths and apnea
_____	**20.** A device used to measure the temperature on the forehead

a. Fahrenheit
b. hypotension
c. meniscus
d. diastolic pressure
e. febrile
f. systolic pressure
g. stethoscope
h. dyspnea
i. hypertension
j. apical
k. hyperpnea
l. calibrate
m. antecubital space
n. apex
o. afebrile
p. hyperpyrexia
q. Cheyne-Stokes respirations
r. temporal scanner
s. bradycardia
t. tachycardia

True or False

Decide whether each statement is true or false. In the space at the left, write T for true or F for false. On the lines provided, rewrite the false statements to make them true.

_____ **21.** An adult will have his weight, head circumference, and height measured once a year.

_____

_____ 22. A patient is febrile if her body temperature is above normal.

_____ 23. On a Fahrenheit scale, the normal oral temperature in a healthy adult is about 98.6°.

_____ 24. A patient with tachypnea breathes slowly.

_____ 25. A tympanic temperature is taken in the ear canal.

_____ 26. A tympanic thermometer measures the temperature of a patient's inner ear.

_____ 27. You should measure an adult's pulse at the radial artery.

_____ 28. The temporal artery is located at the side of the neck.

_____ 29. A sphygmomanometer is used to measure blood pressure.

_____ 30. Using the palpatory method, a medical assistant can take an estimate of a patient's systolic blood pressure before measuring it exactly.

_____ 31. The axilla is the armpit.

_____ 32. Auscultated blood pressure is determined by palpation.

_____ 33. Hypertension is also known as low blood pressure.

_____ 34. Body temperature is affected by numerous factors including the patient's weight.

Content Review

Multiple Choice

In the space provided, write the letter of the choice that best completes each statement or answers each question.

_____ 1. A crying, fussy infant needs his respirations counted. What should you do?
   A. Count the respirations and report them to the physician immediately as ordered
   B. Attempt to quiet the infant or wait until later in the visit to count the respirations
   C. Do not worry about counting the respirations; the physician will need to see the infant as soon as possible
   D. Using an electronic sphygmomanometer, you should be able to obtain the correct respiration count
   E. Have the parents attempt to count the respirations while you do the other vital signs

_____ 2. An adult patient has started taking a medication for hypertension since his last visit. Which of the following would you most likely expect at this visit?
   A. A blood pressure within the normal range
   B. A blood pressure result higher than normal
   C. A blood pressure result lower than normal
   D. A blood pressure result lower than the results from the previous visit

_____ 3. Review the following vital sign results for an adult patient older than age 65 and determine which set is considered out of the normal range.
   A. BP 120/80, T 98.6°F, P 98, R 20
   B. BP 150/90, T 98.6°F, P 98, R 20
   C. BP 108/78, T 37°C, P 88, R 18
   D. BP 120/80, T 98.2°F, P 106, R 20
   E. BP 120/80, T 97.2°F, P 98, R 20

_____ 4. A patient enters the facility with open lesions on his arms and hands. What *special* OSHA precautions should you take while measuring his vital signs?
   A. Wear a mask and gown
   B. Wear gloves and wash your hands
   C. Clean the exam area before the patient arrives
   D. Take a rectal temperature to ensure accurate results

_____ 5. Which of the following would most likely cause rales?
   A. Congestive heart failure
   B. Head injury
   C. Asthma
   D. Brain tumor
   E. Influenza

_____ 6. What are the preferred methods for taking the temperature of a child younger than 2 years of age?
   A. Oral
   B. Axillary and tympanic
   C. Oral, rectal, and temporal
   D. Rectal, temporal, and axillary

_____ 7. Which of the following is generally *not* a health problem?
   A. Apnea
   B. Hypertension
   C. Dyspnea
   D. Hyperpnea
   E. Hypotension

_____ 8. Which of the following is the best way to weigh a toddler?
   A. Ask the toddler to stand very still on the scale
   B. Weigh the parent and the toddler together, and then subtract the weight of the parent from the result
   C. Lay the toddler on the infant scale
   D. Have the toddler hold the height bar during the weighing process to encourage him to stand still

_____ 9. Which of the following is an internal factor that affects the blood pressure?
   A. Papilledema
   B. Blood viscosity
   C. Malignant hypertension
   D. Hyperpyrexis

Sentence Completion

In the space provided, write the word or phrase that best completes each sentence.

10. On the top moveable bar of the height scale, the numbers _____ as you go down the bar.

11. To ensure the proper size cuff when taking the blood pressure, the bladder inside the cuff should encircle _____ to _____ of the distance around the arm or leg being used.

12. Deep and rapid respirations associated with hysteria or excitement are called _____.

13. Abnormal changes in height or weight can indicate a disorder of a person's _____.

14. A person's axillary temperature is usually about 1° lower than her _____ temperature.

15. The eardrum was selected as a location to measure body temperature because it has the same blood supply as the _____.

16. If a patient's pulse rate is high, his _____ rate is also likely to be high.

17. Electronic sphygmomanometers are _____ likely to provide more accurate readings than other types of sphygmomanometers.

10. _____

11. _____

12. _____

13. _____

14. _____

15. _____

16. _____

17. _____

Short Answer

Write the answer to each question on the lines provided.

18. Name the five vital signs.

_____

_____

_____

19. Name and describe the parts of a stethoscope.

_____

_____

_____

20. Explain why pulse and respirations should be taken together.

_____

_____

_____

21. Name five methods for taking temperature, and discuss the circumstances under which each method might be used.

_____

_____

_____

22. How can you ensure that a tympanic temperature is accurate?

_____

_____

_____

23. Why is it necessary to hold the thermometer in place when taking a rectal temperature?

_____

_____

_____

24. When you are taking a blood pressure measurement, how do you determine that patient's proper inflation amount in mm Hg?

_____

_____

_____

25. Identify the blood pressure values on the illustration of aneroid gauges below. Write your answers on the lines in the figure.

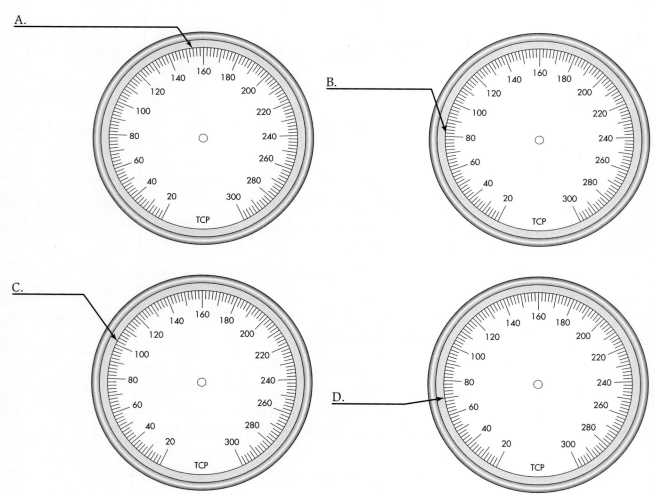

26. Explain why is it important for a physician to keep a record of how much a patient weighs.

_____

_____

_____

27. The following illustrations show sites for taking a patient's pulse rate. Identify and label the artery used for each measurement.

A. _____   B. _____   C. _____   D. _____

E. _____   F. _____   G. _____   H. _____

28. Name and describe the five phases of Korotkoff sounds.

_____

_____

_____

_____

_____

Critical Thinking

Write the answer to each question on the lines provided.

1. Discuss at least three ways that you can ensure accuracy when performing vital signs and measurements.

_____

_____

_____

2. When performing a head circumference on a 6-month-old infant, you note that the measurement is the same as it was when the infant was 3 months old. What should you do?

_____

_____

_____

3. Explain why you should not take a blood pressure in a patient who has lessened circulation in his or her arm.

_____

_____

_____

4. What would you do if a patient has just had a cup of coffee and you need to take his temperature?

_____

_____

_____

5. Why is the measurement of the length of a 3-month-old infant likely to be less accurate than the measurement of the height of a 3-year-old child?

_____

_____

_____

APPLICATION

1. Using Procedure Checklist 6-1, Measuring and Recording Temperature, review and practice taking temperatures. Use the following circumstances during your practice:

    a. Taking turns as the patient, role-play the sequence of taking a temperature. Be certain to use proper communication with the patient and document your results.

    b. Obtain various types of thermometers—electronic, tympanic, temporal, and disposable—and compare the results of the temperatures among them, and then document your results.

2. Using Procedure Checklist 6-2, Measuring and Recording Pulse and Respirations and the form on page 583 of this workbook, review and practice taking pulse and respirations.

Use the following circumstances during your practice:

    a. On yourself, find and count each of the pulse sites found in the figure on page 39. Determine if the results are the same.

    b. Find and count each of the pulse sites on a partner. Compare your results.

    c. Count a classmate's respirations while she is not aware that you are doing so. Then count the respirations when she is aware. Is there a difference?

    d. Obtain and record the radial pulse on five different classmates. Keep your results confidential. Once completed, compare your results with other classmates. If the difference in one person's rate is greater than 5 beats per minute, recheck the pulse of that classmate at the same time that the classmate himself does to ensure an accurate measurement.

3. Using Procedure Checklist 6-3, Taking the Blood Pressure of Adults and Older Children and the form on page 583 of this workbook, review and practice taking blood pressure.

Use the following circumstances during your practice:

a. In groups of three, practice taking blood pressure readings. With one student as the patient, the other two students should take the blood pressure and record the results without telling them to the other students. Each student should have her blood pressure taken by the other two team members. Once all the blood pressure readings have been taken, compare your results. Repeat the blood pressure readings until all the results on one student are within 10 mm Hg for the systolic measure and 4 mm Hg for the diastolic measure.

4. Using Procedure Checklists 6-4, Measuring Adults and Children, and 6-5, Measuring Infants, review and practice measuring adults, children, and infants.

Use the following circumstances during your practice:

a. Obtain the height, weight, and head circumference of at least three other students. Record your results on the form on page 585 of this workbook. Do not disclose your results while measuring. Compare your results with other classmates who have measured the same students. If the results are different, retake the measurements until they are the same.

b. Visit a daycare center or bring infants and children to class to measure. Practice on at least one child, one toddler, and one infant. Check your results with another student.

5. Take at least one complete set of vital signs and record them correctly on the medical record example found on page 583.

6. On his first visit to your clinic, an 18-month-old male infant was 33 inches in length and weighed 33 pounds. His head circumference was 19 inches. Plot these results on the growth charts, examples on page 569, and note the percentiles for the following:

a. Length for Age _____

b. Weight for Age _____

c. Head Circumference for Age _____

d. Weight for Length _____

CASE STUDIES

Write your response to each case study on the lines provided.

Case 1

A female patient arrives at the clinic and you must take her blood pressure. During the patient interview, you discover that she has had a double mastectomy. What should you do when taking her blood pressure?

_____

_____

_____

Case 2

A parent brings her infant to the clinic for a routine checkup. You complete the infant's weight and length measurements and the parent asks you the results. When you provide her with the measurements, she says, "That can't be right!" Should you have given the parent the measurement results? What should you do now?

_____

_____

_____

Case 3

An adult patient who uses a wheelchair comes in for his annual checkup. How would you weigh him? How would you check his height?

_____

_____

_____

Case 4

An overweight 13-year-old girl comes in for an annual checkup. Her mother waits for her in the reception area. The patient seems nervous and she refuses to get on the scales when it is time to weigh her. She says she does not want anyone to know how much she weighs, not even you. You and the patient both know that another girl from her school was in the office last week and you are sure the other patient weighed much more than this patient does. The patient asks you how much the other girl weighed. Maybe telling the patient would make her feel better and she would let you weigh her. What should you do?

_____

_____

_____

CHAPTER 7

Assisting with a General Physical Examination

REVIEW

Vocabulary Review

True or False

Decide whether each statement is true or false. In the space at the left, write T *for true or* F *for false. On the lines provided, rewrite the false statements to make them true.*

_____ 1. A clinical diagnosis is based on the signs and symptoms of a disease.

_____

_____ 2. Before any laboratory or diagnostic testing is ordered, a differential diagnosis may be recorded.

_____

_____ 3. Symmetry is when one side of the body is different from the other side.

_____

_____ 4. Culture is based on a person's race.

_____

_____ 5. Nasal mucosa is the lining of the nose.

_____

_____ 6. Hyperventilation is shallow breaths caused by the loss of carbon monoxide in the blood.

_____

_____ 7. The four equal sections of the abdomen are referred to as quadrants.

_____

_____ 8. An example of a digital exam is palpating for breast lumps.

_____

_____ 9. A lateral curvature of the spine is referred to as kyphosis.

_____

_____ 10. Following the physician's orders is referred to as patient compliance.

_____

_____ 11. A drape with a special opening for easier access during an exam is called a fenestrated drape.

_____

_____ 12. The proper medical term for earwax is cerumen.

_____

_____ **13.** A prognosis is the probable course or outcome of a disease.

_____

_____ **14.** Scoliosis is a forward curvature of the spine.

_____

_____ **15.** Patients should be instructed on proper respiratory hygiene and cough etiquette.

_____

Content Review

Multiple Choice

In the space provided, write the letter of the choice that best completes each statement or answers each question.

_____ **1.** Which of the following is *not* an example of a safety measure you would take while assisting a physician with a patient's general physical exam?
   A. Performing a thorough hand washing before and after each procedure
   B. Cleaning and disinfecting the exam room after the exam
   C. Consulting the list of OSHA safety rules
   D. Wearing gloves whenever there is a possibility of contact with blood or body fluids

_____ **2.** When you prepare a patient for a physical exam, you will
   A. give the patient the opportunity to empty his bladder or bowels.
   B. explain to the patient what will occur during the exam.
   C. ask the patient to disrobe and put on an exam gown.
   D. All of the above.
   E. None of the above.

_____ **3.** One of the six methods for examining a patient during a general physical exam is
   A. palpation.
   B. supination.
   C. positioning.
   D. draping.

_____ **4.** Most physicians perform the general physical exam in the same order, starting with an exam of the patient's
   A. chest and lungs.
   B. head.
   C. overall appearance and the condition of the skin.
   D. abdomen.
   E. musculoskeletal system.

_____ **5.** Which of the following is a common problem of elderly patients that frequently goes undiagnosed?
   A. Depression
   B. Scoliosis
   C. Incontinence
   D. Lack of compliance when taking medications

_____ 6. Which of the following assists the physician in developing a prognosis?
   A. Laboratory test results
   B. An MRI report
   C. Physical therapy reports
   D. All of the above
   E. None of the above

_____ 7. In which of the following positions does the patient lie flat on his back during a procedure?
   A. Prone
   B. Sims'
   C. Trendelenburg's
   D. Fowlers
   E. Supine

_____ 8. Which of the following positions is used for gynecological exam procedures?
   A. Knee-chest
   B. Sims'
   C. Proctologic
   D. Lithotomy

_____ 9. Which of the following is the exam method in which the physician assesses characteristics such as texture, temperature, shape, and the presence of vibrations or movements by touching the skin surface and pressing against underlying tissues?
   A. Inspection
   B. Manipulation
   C. Palpation
   D. Auscultation
   E. Percussion

_____ 10. Which of the following is the exam method in which the physician is able to determine the location, size, and density of organs?
   A. Percussion
   B. Inspection
   C. Mensuration
   D. Auscultation

Sentence Completion

In the space provided, write the word or phrase that best completes each sentence.

11. One of the best positions for examining patients who are experiencing shortness of breath, _____ position has the patient on his back with his head elevated.

11. _____

12. When checking a patient's general appearance, a physician looks at the patient's skin, hair, and _____.

12. _____

13. By using a(n) _____, the doctor can view a patient's retinas and other internal structures of the eyes.

13. _____

14. _____

14. The physician uses a(n) _____, an instrument that allows her to auscultate the heart sounds.

15. _____

15. You should pay special attention to educating patients about _____ for disease.

Short Answer

Write the answer to each question on the lines provided.

16. What are the two reasons why physicians perform general physical exams?

_____

_____

_____

17. Why do physicians use six different exam methods during a general physical exam?

_____

_____

_____

18. Write the name of the exam position on the line below each illustration.

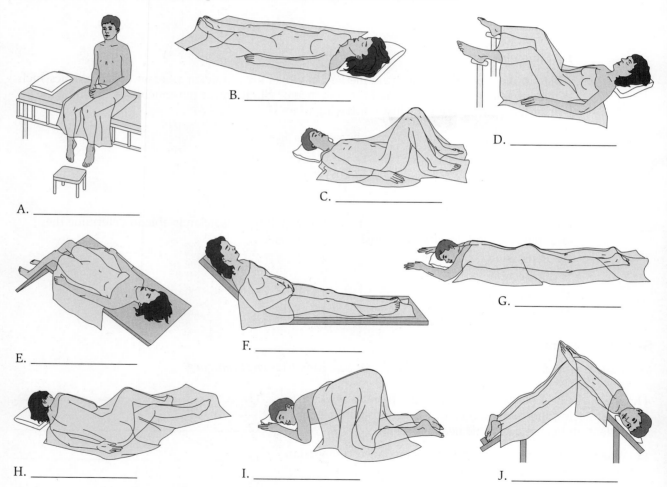

A. _____

B. _____

C. _____

D. _____

E. _____

F. _____

G. _____

H. _____

I. _____

J. _____

19. Label the instruments and supplies used for the general physical exam and identify what component of the exam each is used for.

A. _____

B. _____

C. _____

D. _____

E. _____

F. _____

G. _____

H. _____

I. _____

J. _____

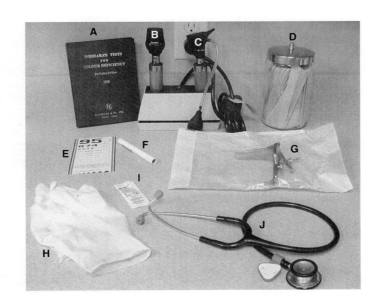

20. What are the six methods of examining a patient during a general physical exam?

_____

_____

_____

21. During an exam of the lungs, what does the stethoscope allow the physician to do?

_____

_____

_____

22. Label the nine parts of the abdomen on the illustration below.

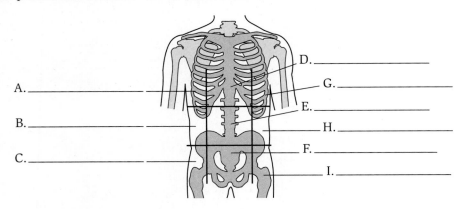

A. _____

B. _____

C. _____

D. _____

G. _____

E. _____

H. _____

F. _____

I. _____

23. What are examples of tests and procedures the doctor might order following a general physical exam?

_____

_____

_____

24. What can you do to ensure that patients understand the instructions you give them?

_____

_____

_____

25. Give three examples of patient follow-up that might be done after a physical exam.

_____

_____

_____

26. Give two behaviors that a medical assistant should observe when screening for visual acuity.

_____

_____

_____

Critical Thinking

Write the answer to each question on the lines provided.

1. Why is it particularly important to prepare children emotionally for a physical exam?

_____

_____

_____

2. Why is it important to avoid making any assumptions about patients from other cultures?

_____

_____

_____

3. Why is it necessary to assist patients into a variety of positions during a physical exam?

_____

_____

_____

4. Why is it important to help patients with disabilities during a physical exam, and what are some ways this can be accomplished?

_____

_____

_____

5. How would you prepare a patient for a diabetes follow-up? What testing may be ordered?

_____

_____

_____

APPLICATION

Follow the directions for each application.

1. Assisting During a Physical Exam

Working with two partners, role-play the procedures for assisting with the eyes, ears, nose and sinuses, and mouth and throat portions of a general physical exam. One partner should take the role of the medical assistant, one that of the patient, and the third should act as observer and evaluator. Your instructor will play the role of the doctor.

a. The medical assistant should first prepare the instruments for the exam: penlight, ophthalmoscope, vision charts, color charts, otoscope, audiometer, nasal speculum, and tongue depressor. The instruments should be organized in the order of the exam: eyes, ears, nose and sinuses, mouth and throat.

b. The assistant should wash her hands thoroughly and observe appropriate safety precautions throughout.

c. The assistant should prepare the patient emotionally and physically by explaining the procedure, what the patient will feel, and so on. She should then direct the patient to take the appropriate sitting position on the examining table.

d. The assistant should put on gloves, protective clothing, and a face mask.

e. While the doctor conducts the exam, the assistant should hand the doctor the instruments as needed as well as provide assistance to the patient.

f. After the exam, the observer should critique the medical assistant's role in the exam. Comments should concern the emotional and physical preparation given the patient, the observance of all safety precautions, aid given to the physician, and assistance given to the patient during the exam. All three students should discuss the procedure and the observer's comments.

g. Exchange roles and have the new medical assistant assist with another portion of the exam, assembling equipment and supplies, preparing and positioning the patient, and assisting the physician. Critique and discuss the exam at its conclusion.

h. Exchange roles one more time so that each partner has the opportunity to play each role during one portion of the exam.

2. Educating the Patient

Work with a partner. One partner should take the role of a medical assistant, the other the role of a patient who is at risk for breast cancer.

a. The medical assistant should review the information on the patient's chart. This patient is 42 years old. Both a sister and her mother have had breast cancer. The patient began menstruating at age 12 and has never had children. The medical assistant knows that breast cancer is the most common cancer diagnosed in women. With early detection, however, breast cancer can be successfully managed. Regular, routine screening, which includes a clinical breast exam and a mammogram, is essential for early detection and prompt treatment.

b. The medical assistant should use the foregoing information to educate the patient about breast cancer. The medical assistant should explain to the patient that she is at risk for breast cancer and why and should explain the need for regular screening. The assistant should periodically assess the patient's understanding of what is being discussed by questioning her and should then clarify misunderstandings.

c. The medical assistant should carefully explain the mammography procedure. The patient should ask questions. The medical assistant should answer all questions as fully as possible. If the assistant does not know the answer, she should tell the patient she will check with the physician and provide the information later.

d. Following the educational discussion, assess the interview with your partner. Was all pertinent information covered? Was the mammography procedure accurately and completely explained? Check the textbook for details.

3. Vision Testing of Patients with Special Needs

Two clinical situations that require special considerations when conducting vision tests are described below. In the space provided, complete each sentence.

The father of a 4-year-old boy has brought his son to your medical office for vision testing.

a. Prepare the child for testing and encourage his cooperation by _____.

b. During the testing, help the child by _____.

c. While you are using a pictorial eye chart to test the child's vision, watch for signs that he is having difficulty seeing the chart, such as _____.

d. Enlist the father's help during the testing by having him _____.

The husband of a 73-year-old woman with Alzheimer's disease has brought his wife to the office for vision testing.

e. Before the test, make the patient feel more comfortable by _____.

f. When explaining procedures to the patient, _____.

g. During testing, help the patient by _____.

h. If the patient's memory and language skills are impaired, _____.

i. If the patient seems to have trouble with one part of the exam, _____.

CASE STUDIES

Write your response to each case study on the lines provided.

Case 1

You normally place patients in the prone position to allow the physician to examine the back, feet, and musculoskeletal system. The patient being examined is extremely obese and has had some respiratory difficulties. Would you place him in this position? If not, what position(s) would you recommend?

_____

_____

_____

Case 2

A patient presents with symptoms of low back pain. What questions should you ask about the symptoms when obtaining the chief complaint? What supplies will be needed by the physician? When asking the patient to disrobe, what do you tell the patient to remove? Per the style of the practice, what testing can you perform prior to the physician's examining the patient?

_____

_____

_____

Case 3

You are performing a Snellen visual acuity exam on a patient who is being seen for an occupational physical. You notice that the patient is beginning to read the lines before you ask him to. What is the probable reason for this?

_____

_____

_____

CHAPTER 8

Assisting with Examinations in the Basic Specialties

REVIEW

Vocabulary Review

Matching

Match the key terms in the right column with the definitions in the left column by placing the letter of each correct answer in the space provided.

_____ 1. An instrument that permits the viewing of the vagina and cervix by expanding the vagina

_____ 2. A disorder that may cause a hunched-over posture

_____ 3. Of rapid onset and progress

_____ 4. An accumulation of fatty deposits along the inner walls of arteries

_____ 5. The development of secondary sexual traits and reproductive functions

_____ 6. The first day of the last menstrual period.

_____ 7. A chemical placed on a Pap smear slide to hold the cells in place until microscopic evaluation

_____ 8. Lasting a long time and recurring frequently

_____ 9. The measurement of oxygen and carbon dioxide in the blood

_____ 10. A moving blood clot

_____ 11. An exam of the vagina and cervix to identify abnormal tissue

a. acute
b. arterial blood gases
c. atherosclerosis
d. chloric
e. colposcopy
f. embolism
g. osteoporosis
h. puberty
i. speculum
j. fixative
k. LMP

Content Review

Multiple Choice

In the space provided, write the letter of the choice that best completes each statement or answers each question.

_____ 1. Which of the following is a noninvasive test used to rule out DVT?
   A. Venogram
   B. Arterial blood gas analysis
   C. Venous ultrasound
   D. Electrocardiogram
   E. Arteriogram

_____ **2.** Lyme disease is carried by
    A. ticks.
    B. fleas.
    C. mosquitoes.
    D. dogs.
    E. deer.

_____ **3.** Which of the following is a risk factor for elder abuse?
    A. Isolation of the victim from family members and friends
    B. Presence of a child in the household
    C. History of divorce in the family
    D. History of heart disease in the family

_____ **4.** What is the best thing you can do to help a patient with high cholesterol?
    A. Prescribe medication
    B. Perform a biopsy
    C. Teach about healthful eating habits
    D. Not mention the condition to the patient but inform the doctor

_____ **5.** Which of the following measures is the most effective way to prevent sexually transmitted diseases?
    A. Latex condoms
    B. Spermicide
    C. Diaphragm
    D. Abstinence
    E. Monogamy

_____ **6.** When a parent reports a child with a high fever, what should you do?
    A. Recommend aspirin
    B. Tell the doctor
    C. Take a biopsy
    D. Send the patient literature about fevers

_____ **7.** An obstetrician
    A. treats bone disorders.
    B. cares for women during pregnancy and childbirth.
    C. cares for children.
    D. treats both men and women.

_____ **8.** After the age of 2, a child should have checkups
    A. every 6 months.
    B. yearly.
    C. every 18 months.
    D. every 2 years.
    E. every 3 years.

_____ **9.** A Pap smear is used to determine
    A. pregnancy.
    B. menopause.
    C. the presence of abnormal or precancerous cells.
    D. the presence of an embolism.

_____ **10.** A digital exam is done during the gynecological exam to
   A. check the position of the internal organs.
   B. test for cancer of the cervix.
   C. obtain a smear for cytologic exam.
   D. check for abnormalities in the cervix.

_____ **11.** During her pelvic exam, you notice that Sonya seems nervous and uncomfortable. To help her relax, you suggest that she
   A. move closer to the end of the table.
   B. pull her knees together.
   C. hold her breath.
   D. take her feet out of the stirrups.
   E. take several deep breaths.

_____ **12.** Reddening of the eyes, increased heart rate, heightened appetite, and muscular weakness are signs of which of the following types of abuse?
   A. Alcohol
   B. Cocaine
   C. Marijuana
   D. Narcotics
   E. Sedatives

Sentence Completion

In the space provided, write the word or phrase that best completes each sentence.

13. Internal medicine is the specialty of an internist, who diagnoses and treats disorders and diseases of the body's _____.

14. Gout is a metabolic disease of the joints caused by over-production or retention of _____.

15. When patients are prescribed antibiotics to treat strepto-coccal infection, it is important that they _____; other-wise, the bacteria will build up a tolerance to the drug.

16. Single parenthood and financial problems are among the risk factors for _____.

17. A physician may order an AFP test to rule out _____ defects.

18. During _____, a woman may experience irregular periods, hot flashes, and vaginal dryness.

13. _____

14. _____

15. _____

16. _____

17. _____

18. _____

Short Answer

Write the answer to each question on the lines provided.

19. What are three general guidelines to offer victims of domestic violence?

_____

_____

_____

20. There are several signs of neglect of an elderly patient. Name four.

_____

_____

_____

21. Describe the symptoms of viral gastroenteritis.

_____

_____

_____

22. What signs in a child might prompt you to alert the doctor to possible child abuse?

_____

_____

_____

23. Why is viral gastroenteritis of concern in young children?

_____

_____

_____

24. What test might a doctor order to confirm a negative rapid strep test?

_____

_____

_____

25. Describe the guidelines for breast cancer screening.

_____

_____

_____

26. Genital warts are caused by which organism?

_____

_____

_____

Critical Thinking

Write the answer to each question on the lines provided.

1. In what ways would you handle readying a child for a general physical exam differently than readying an adult for this exam?

_____

_____

_____

2. Why is it important for a patient to finish the complete course of an antibiotic?

_____

_____

3. Why might the isolation of an elderly person from family and friends lead to elder abuse?

_____

_____

4. Which method of birth control might be controversial? Why?

_____

_____

5. Two days after a cervical biopsy, a patient calls to tell you that she is experiencing some bleeding and does not know what she should do. What would you tell her?

_____

_____

6. Using Nagele's rule, estimate the delivery date of a pregnant woman whose last menstrual period was July 16, 2010.

_____

_____

_____

APPLICATION

Follow the directions for each application.

Assisting with Exams and Procedures

Describe how you would prepare the patient for and assist with each of these exams and procedures.

a. A pediatric physical exam

_____

_____

_____

b. An annual gynecological exam with follow-up

_____

_____

_____

_____

CASE STUDIES

Write your response to each case study on the lines provided.

Case 1

Austin, a 6-year-old male, is seen at the pediatrician's office today. He complains of a severe sore throat. His throat is red and he has a fever of 102.8°F. The doctor orders a rapid strep test, which is negative. Why might the doctor order a throat culture for Austin?

_____

_____

_____

Case 2

Mr. Mayer has recently been diagnosed with high cholesterol. What patient teaching would be helpful for Mr. Mayer?

_____

_____

_____

Case 3

An 18-year-old female patient has just been diagnosed with an STD. What general information should you ensure that the patient knows before she leaves the clinic? How would you go about telling her?

_____

_____

_____

Case 4

Jeanette Carson, a long-time patient at the OB/GYN practice where you work, is just past her eighth month of pregnancy. During her regular prenatal visit, Jeanette asks about classes she can take on breast-feeding. She then tells you that her sister lost her 4-month-old son to SIDS. Jeanette wants to know what she can do to avoid having the same thing happen to her baby. She wonders whether genetic factors play a role in SIDS cases. What can you tell Jeanette?

_____

_____

_____

Case 5

Megan Thomas's annual Pap smear is classified HSIL. How might the physician decide to proceed?

_____

_____

_____

CHAPTER 9

Assisting with Highly Specialized Examinations

REVIEW

Vocabulary Review

Matching

Match the key terms in the right column with the definitions in the left column by placing the letter of each correct answer in the space provided.

_____ 1. The transfer of abnormal cells to body sites far removed from an original tumor

_____ 2. A test used to diagnose contact dermatitis

_____ 3. A radiographic exam that produces a three-dimensional, cross-sectional view of the brain

_____ 4. An exam of the skin using an ultraviolet lamp

_____ 5. A technique for viewing areas inside the body without exposing patients to x-rays or surgery

_____ 6. An exam of the lower rectum

_____ 7. An x-ray exam of a blood vessel after the injection of a contrast medium

_____ 8. A metal mesh tube used to keep a vessel open

_____ 9. A test that measures a patient's response to a constant or increasing workload

_____ 10. Any procedure in which a scope is used to visually inspect a canal or cavity within the body

_____ 11. A life-threatening allergic reaction

_____ 12. A test used to detect neuromuscular disorders or nerve damage

_____ 13. A disorder characterized by an elevated level of glucose in the blood

_____ 14. A procedure in which an orthopedist examines inside a joint

a. anaphylaxis
b. angiography
c. stent
d. patch test
e. computed tomography
f. diabetes mellitus
g. arthroscopy
h. endoscopy
i. proctoscopy
j. magnetic resonance imaging
k. metastasis
l. Wood's light exam
m. stress test
n. electromyography

True or False

Decide whether each statement is true or false. In the space at the left, write T for true or F for false. On the lines provided, rewrite the false statements to make them true.

_____ 15. Another name for Holter monitoring is ambulatory cardiography.

_____

_____ **16.** An intradermal test is more sensitive than a scratch test.

_____

_____ **17.** A stress test is usually performed with the patient lying down.

_____

_____ **18.** Cardiac catheterization is a diagnostic method in which a catheter is inserted into a vein or artery in the arm or leg and passed through the blood vessels into the lungs.

_____

_____ **19.** During a whole-body skin exam, a doctor examines the visible top layer of the entire surface of the skin.

_____

_____ **20.** A macule is a small, flat, discolored spot on the skin.

_____

_____ **21.** A wheal is an elevation of the skin caused by a collection of pus.

_____

_____ **22.** Sigmoidoscopy is an exam of the S-shaped segment of the large intestine.

_____

_____ **23.** Myelography is an x-ray visualization of the spinal cord after injection of a contrast medium or air into the spinal subarachnoid space.

_____

_____ **24.** Neuromuscular disorders or nerve damage can be detected through a lumbar puncture.

_____

_____ **25.** An ophthalmoscope is a handheld instrument with a light used to view the inner ear structures.

_____

_____ **26.** An ophthalmologist uses a retinoscope or a Phoroptor to perform a refraction exam.

_____

_____ **27.** Arthroscopy enables an orthopedist to see inside a muscle.

_____

Content Review

Multiple Choice

In the space provided, write the letter of the choice that best completes each statement or answers each question.

_____ **1.** A test using sound waves to examine the structure and function of the heart is known as a(n)
   A. electrocardiogram.
   B. echocardiogram.
   C. ultrasound.
   D. angiogram.
   E. stress test.

_____ 2. A patient with a suspected hormonal imbalance is likely to be referred to a(n)
   A. urologist.
   B. otologist.
   C. endocrinologist.
   D. gastroenterologist.

_____ 3. An electroencephalogram can be used to detect
   A. brain injuries.
   B. bone injuries.
   C. cardiac abnormalities.
   D. neuromuscular disorders.

_____ 4. A medical assistant in an otologist's office might
   A. perform a radioallergosorbent test.
   B. collect urine specimens.
   C. assist with electromyography.
   D. help administer tympanometry.

_____ 5. The American Cancer Society recommends that men perform a testicular self-exam every
   A. day.
   B. week.
   C. month.
   D. year.

_____ 6. An allergy test performed by introducing suspected allergens into the layers of skin by raising a wheal is known as a(n)
   A. patch test.
   B. scratch test.
   C. RAST test.
   D. antibody test.
   E. intradermal test.

_____ 7. A raised or unraised brown, black, or tan spot on the skin is known as a(n)
   A. tinea.
   B. pustule.
   C. nevus.
   D. wheal.

_____ 8. The type of diabetes that is usually diagnosed between the 24th and 28th weeks of pregnancy is known as _____ diabetes.
   A. gestational
   B. postpartum
   C. type I
   D. type II
   E. temporary

_____ 9. Neuromuscular disorders or nerve damage can be detected through
   A. lumbar puncture.
   B. cerebral angiography.
   C. electroencephalography.
   D. electromyography.

_____ **10.** The entire area visible to the eye when the patient looks straight ahead is known as
    A. refraction.
    B. visual acuity.
    C. visual field.
    D. macular vision.
    E. peripheral vision.

_____ **11.** A diagnostic procedure that uses strong magnets and radio waves to produce images of the heart is known as
    A. PET scanning.
    B. heart CT.
    C. balloon angioplasty.
    D. heart MRI.

_____ **12.** During a scratch test, the skin should be scratched no more than how deep?
    A. 1/16 inch
    B. 1/8 inch
    C. 3/16 inch
    D. 1/4 inch
    E. 3/8 inch

_____ **13.** Two cardiology procedures often performed together are cardiac catheterization and
    A. angiography.
    B. stress test.
    C. CABG.
    D. ECG.

_____ **14.** Paralysis on one side of the body is known as
    A. paraplegia.
    B. hemiplegia.
    C. hemiparesis.
    D. quadriplegia.
    E. paraparesis.

_____ **15.** An instrument used to view inside a joint and guide surgical procedures is an
    A. arthroscope.
    B. arthrogram.
    C. arthroscopy.
    D. arthrography.
    E. arthrocentesis.

_____ **16.** The most common test ordered in a urology practice is a(n)
    A. cystogram.
    B. semen analysis.
    C. urinalysis.
    D. cystometry.
    E. pyelogram.

Sentence Completion

In the space provided, write the word or phrase that best completes each sentence.

17. Treatments for acne vulgaris can be topical or _____.

18. Some gastrointestinal exams involve spraying the patient's throat with a(n) _____ to inhibit the gag reflex.

19. Cataracts block the passage of _____ through the eye, resulting in a progressive loss of vision.

20. During a needle biopsy, a surgeon removes _____ with a needle inserted through the skin and into a growth.

17. _____

18. _____

19. _____

20. _____

Short Answer

Write the answer to each question on the lines provided.

21. List four categories of chemotherapy drugs and describe their mechanism of action.

_____

_____

_____

22. List three types of skin cancer, and identify the most dangerous type.

_____

_____

_____

23. Which specialties use imaging techniques (such as x-ray, CT scan, MRI) as diagnostic tests?

_____

_____

_____

24. What are the five categories of neurological function evaluated in a complete neurological exam?

_____

_____

_____

25. List four procedures used to detect and diagnose cancer.

_____

_____

_____

26. Describe myopia and hyperopia, and name the types of lenses that are used to correct each disorder.

_____

_____

_____

27. When might joint replacement surgery be indicated?

_____

_____

_____

28. Describe three symptoms of a ruptured eardrum. List two treatment methods an otologist might use for this condition.

_____

_____

_____

Critical Thinking

Write the answer to each question on the lines provided.

1. Why is the medical assistant's role in educating a cardiology patient about diet and exercise especially important?

_____

_____

_____

2. What advice might you give to a patient in her teens who has fair skin and hair and who is planning to work outdoors during the coming summer months?

_____

_____

_____

3. Compare and contrast an incisional biopsy and a needle biopsy.

_____

_____

_____

4. Write three questions you might ask when taking a patient's history for a urologist.

_____

_____

_____

5. How might the pretest instructions for an upper endoscopy be different from those for a colonoscopy? Why might they be different?

_____

_____

_____

6. Why are diagnostic urine and blood tests essential in endocrine exams?

_____

_____

_____

APPLICATION

Follow the directions for each application.

1. **Interviewing a Patient Before a Highly Specialized Exam**

   Work with two partners. While you assume the role of a medical assistant, have one partner play the role of a patient who is about to have an annual eye exam performed by an ophthalmologist. Have the second partner act as an observer and evaluator.

   a. Take the patient's history, recording your questions and the patient's responses. On the basis of the responses, ask appropriate follow-up questions.

   b. Explain to the patient what the doctor is likely to do and why. Allow the patient to interrupt at any time with questions, which you should answer to the best of your ability. Record your statements, the patient's questions, and your responses.

   c. Have the observer present a critique of your patient interview. The critique should involve your approach and attitude as well as the appropriateness and accuracy of your questions and responses. The observer should also evaluate the order in which you took the history and its completeness.

   d. You and your partners should then discuss the observer's critique, noting the strengths and weaknesses of your interview. Comments should include both positive feedback and suggestions for improvement.

   e. Exchange roles and repeat the exercise with a patient who has an appointment for a general neurological, orthopedic, or urology exam. The student playing the observer chooses the specialty exam for the patient.

   f. Exchange roles again so that each group member has the opportunity to play the medical assistant, the patient, and the observer once.

   g. Repeat this role-playing exercise with your partners, this time with a patient who has an appointment for treatment of a specific disease or disorder. The disease or disorder may be chosen by the student who is playing the observer.

2. **Educating Patients**

   Work with a partner to plan a health-awareness booth for a community health fair.

   a. You and your partner choose one disease or disorder (such as heart disease, cancer, a thyroid gland disfunction, or a common ear disorder) to educate the public about. Brainstorm to decide what information to provide in the booth. Ask yourselves these questions: What are some important issues associated with this disease or disorder? Can these issues be organized into general categories?

   b. Decide whether you will use printed materials, an oral presentation, audiovisual materials, or a combination of these. Discuss with your partner interesting and appealing ways to present the information. What resources might be available in the community to increase awareness of the causes, diagnosis, treatment, and management of this disease or disorder?

   c. Outline your plan for the booth. Gather information on resources available in your community about the disease or disorder. If your plan includes posters, brochures, or flyers, make a sketch of these to demonstrate the type of information that would appear on them. If your plan includes an oral presentation, write it on paper and record it. If your plan includes audiovisual material, make or procure a videotape that demonstrates how the information would be presented.

   d. You and your partner prepare your booth.

   e. Present your booth to the class. Have your classmates critique your presentation. The critique should focus on the appropriateness of the content as well as its accuracy and clarity. Comments should include both positive feedback and suggestions for improvement.

   f. Continue until all pairs of students have had the opportunity to present their booths to the class.

CASE STUDIES

Write your response to each case study on the lines provided.

Case 1

You are assisting a cardiologist in administering a treadmill stress test to a patient when the doctor is suddenly called out of the room. It becomes apparent that the doctor will not return for several minutes. What should you do? Why?

_____

_____

_____

Case 2

Mr. Eisner, a 78-year-old, is being seen today for post-influenza follow-up. He states that he is feeling fine. However, his wife states that he is not hearing her lately and sometimes responds to her questions in an odd way. What might be the cause of Mr. Eisner's hearing difficulty?

_____

_____

_____

Case 3

You are a medical assistant in an ophthalmologist's office. One morning you awaken to discover a crusty substance around your left eyelid. The eye is red and feels as though there is sand in it. Should you work with patients today? Why?

_____

_____

_____

Case 4

You are taking the medical history of a patient who complains of a ringing in her ears. You ask the patient about her exposure to loud noise or to toxins. What is another important question you would ask regarding this condition?

_____

_____

_____

Case 5

Marge is a patient in your office who has recently been diagnosed with type II diabetes. She asks you why it is so important for her to monitor her blood sugar and diet so carefully if she is feeling fine. What can you tell her about the long-term complications of diabetes?

_____

_____

_____

Case 6

You have just given Mr. Arturas instructions for performing a testicular self-exam. He questions you about having to do this monthly, stating that he doesn't think it is necessary to do it that often. What will you say to Mr. Arturas?

_____

_____

_____

CHAPTER 10

Assisting with Minor Surgery

REVIEW

Vocabulary Review

Matching

Match the key terms in the right column with the definitions in the left column by placing the letter of each correct answer in the space provided.

_____ 1. Applied directly to the skin

_____ 2. Initial phase of wound healing

_____ 3. During surgery

_____ 4. The removal of dead tissue

_____ 5. The elimination of all microorganisms

_____ 6. A sterile cloth with cutout section in the center

_____ 7. Suture materials

_____ 8. A collection of pus that forms as a result of infection

_____ 9. The use of extreme cold to destroy unwanted tissue

_____ 10. To bring the edges of a wound together

_____ 11. Surgical stitches used to close a wound

_____ 12. A dilute solution of formaldehyde

_____ 13. The third stage of wound healing, when scar tissue forms

_____ 14. After surgery

_____ 15. The process of removing fluid or tissue cells by aspiration with a needle and syringe

_____ 16. A jagged, open wound in the skin that can extend down into the underlying tissue

a. abscess
b. approximate
c. cryosurgery
d. debridement
e. fenestrated drape
f. formalin
g. intraoperative
h. inflammatory phase
i. laceration
j. ligature
k. maturation phase
l. needle biopsy
m. postoperative
n. surgical asepsis
o. sutures
p. topical

True or False

Decide whether each statement is true or false. In the space at the left, write T for true or F for false. On the lines provided, rewrite the false statements to make them true.

_____ 17. Surgical asepsis reduces the number of microorganisms but does not necessarily eliminate them.

_____

_____ 18. Anesthesia is a loss of sensation.

_____

_____ 19. A sterile scrub assistant assists during a procedure by handling sterile equipment.

_____ 20. During the maturation phase, scar tissue forms at the wound site.

_____ 21. A medical assistant may be responsible for closing a wound after a surgical procedure.

_____ 22. During debridement, a doctor surgically removes healthy tissue from a wound.

_____ 23. During the inflammatory phase of wound healing, bleeding is reduced by constriction of the blood vessels.

_____ 24. During a surgical procedure, a sterile field is used as a work area.

_____ 25. During the preoperative stage in a procedure, the surgical room is prepared for surgery.

_____ 26. A doctor may use a needle biopsy to aspirate fluid or tissue cells for examination.

_____ 27. A minor surgical procedure is usually performed without an anesthetic.

_____ 28. Bleeding from a blood vessel can be stopped by the use of a hemostat.

Content Review

Multiple Choice

In the space provided, write the letter of the choice that best completes each statement or answers each question.

_____ 1. One event that occurs during the inflammatory phase of wound healing is
  A. the formation of a scab.
  B. the clotting of the blood.
  C. the formation of scar tissue.
  D. the formation of new tissue.
  E. clot retraction.

_____ 2. When a patient's skin is prepared for surgery, how far should the prepped area extend beyond the surgical field?
  A. 1 inch
  B. 2 inches
  C. 3 inches
  D. 4 inches

_____ 3. Lidocaine is the most commonly used
   A. anesthetic.
   B. antiseptic.
   C. disinfectant.
   D. dressing.
   E. preservative.

_____ 4. The procedure using extreme cold to destroy tissues is known as
   A. electrocautery.
   B. laser surgery.
   C. cryosurgery.
   D. approximation.

_____ 5. A collection of pus that forms as a result of an infection is a(n)
   A. ligature.
   B. incision.
   C. wound.
   D. debris.
   E. abscess.

_____ 6. A surgical wound created when a doctor cuts into body tissue is a(n)
   A. laceration.
   B. incision.
   C. puncture.
   D. irrigation.
   E. biopsy.

_____ 7. A ligature is a(n)
   A. jagged, open wound.
   B. deep layer of tissue.
   C. absorbable suture material.
   D. surgical stitch used to close a wound.
   E. type of biopsy.

_____ 8. Using a probe or needle heated by electric current to destroy tissue is known as
   A. electrocauterization.
   B. cryosurgery.
   C. anesthesia.
   D. approximation.
   E. a needle biopsy.

_____ 9. A dilute solution of formaldehyde used to prevent tissue changes is
   A. normal saline.
   B. lidocaine.
   C. povidone iodine.
   D. formalin.

_____ **10.** Using a needle and syringe to withdraw tissue or fluid for examination is known as a(n)
  A. debridement.
  B. needle biopsy.
  C. puncture.
  D. biopsy specimen.
  E. incision.

_____ **11.** An instrument used to hold back the sides of an incision to provide greater access and a better view is a
  A. probe.
  B. curette.
  C. hemostat.
  D. dilator.
  E. retractor.

_____ **12.** A 0.9% solution of sodium chloride is also known as
  A. zephiran chloride.
  B. normal saline.
  C. chlorhexidine gluconate.
  D. formalin.

_____ **13.** A sterile solution sometimes injected along with an anesthetic to constrict blood vessels and reduce bleeding is known as
  A. lidocaine.
  B. tetracaine.
  C. zephiran chloride.
  D. epinephrine.
  E. normal saline.

Sentence Completion

In the space provided, write the word or phrase that best completes each sentence.

14. A small wound may be approximated by using a(n) _____ or sterile strip.

15. With certain electrocautery units, a(n) _____ plate or pad will be placed somewhere on the patient's body during the procedure.

16. If a patient is allergic to _____, Hibiclens should be used as a preoperative antiseptic to swab the skin.

17. During surgery, scissors and clamps should be held by the _____ when you pass them to a surgeon.

18. Typically, suture removal takes place _____ days after minor surgery.

14. _____

15. _____

16. _____

17. _____

18. _____

Short Answer

Write the answer to each question on the lines provided.

19. The following illustration shows a variety of cutting and dissecting instruments used to perform minor surgery. Write the names of the instruments on the lines provided. Then explain the instruments' use.

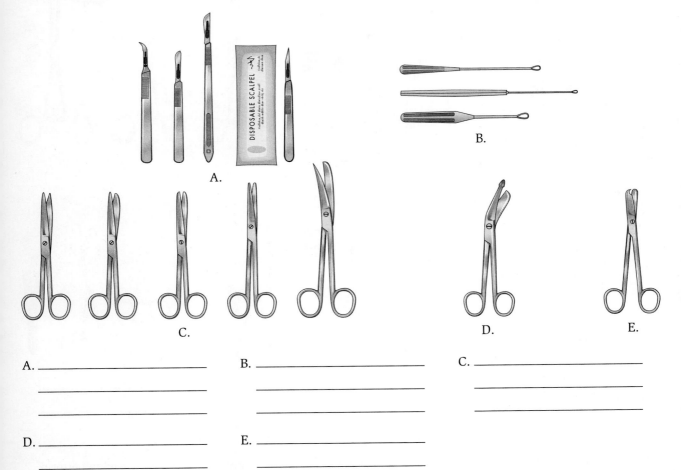

A.

B.

C.

D.

E.

A. _____

_____

_____

B. _____

_____

_____

C. _____

_____

_____

D. _____

_____

_____

E. _____

_____

_____

20. The following illustration shows a variety of grasping and clamping instruments used to perform minor surgery. Write the names of the instruments on the lines provided.

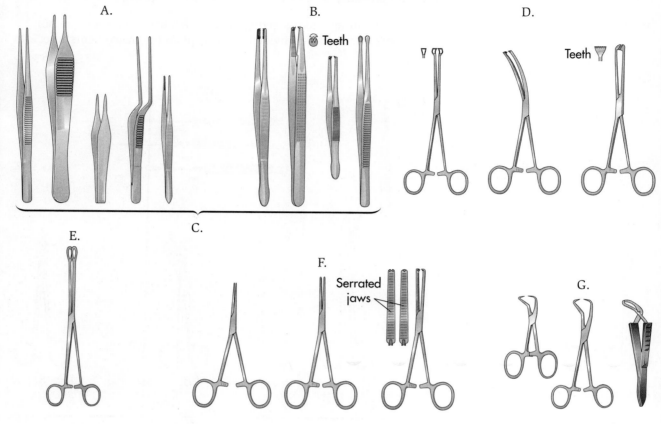

A. _____   B. _____   C. _____

D. _____   E. _____   F. _____

G. _____

21. The following illustration shows a variety of retracting, dilating, and probing instruments used to perform minor surgery. Write the names of the instruments on the lines provided. Then explain the instruments' use.

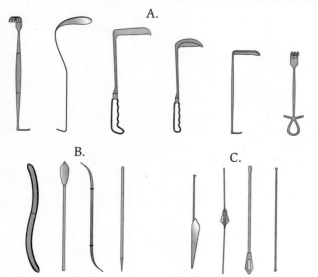

A. _____
_____
_____

B. _____
_____
_____

C. _____
_____
_____

22. The following illustration shows a variety of instruments and materials used to suture. Write the names of the instruments on the lines provided. Then explain the instruments' use.

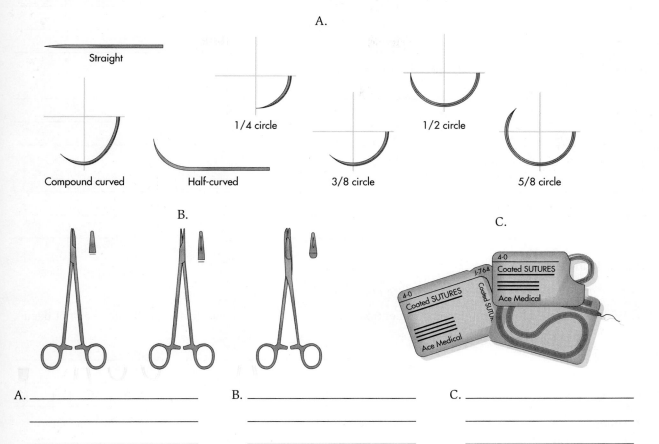

A.

Straight

1/4 circle

1/2 circle

Compound curved

Half-curved

3/8 circle

5/8 circle

B.

C.

4-0 Coated SUTURES
J-76A
4-0 Coated SUTURES
Ace Medical
Coated SUTUR
Ace Medical

A. _____

B. _____

C. _____

_____

_____

_____

_____

_____

_____

23. What are some potential side effects of local anesthetics?

_____

_____

_____

24. Instruments in a surgical tray should be arranged in the order in which they will be used. The following instruments are listed in random order. On the lines provided, rewrite the names of the instruments in the order the surgeon is *most likely* to use them.

Probes _____

Cutting instruments _____

Needle holders _____

Grasping instruments _____

Suture materials _____

Retractors _____

25. Why is epinephrine not used in areas such as the fingers, toes, or nose?

_____

_____

_____

26. Why is it important to place biopsy specimens in a formalin solution?

_____

_____

_____

27. Describe how a nonsurgical wound should be cleaned.

_____

_____

_____

Critical Thinking

Write the answer to each question on the lines provided.

1. While opening a sterile surgical instrument pack, you notice that the sterilization indicator has not been exposed. What should you do?

_____

_____

2. Following cryosurgery, a large, bloody, and painful blister often forms. Why is it important to avoid rupturing the blister?

_____

_____

_____

3. Why is a sterile field considered contaminated if you turn your back to the field?

_____

_____

_____

4. How does positioning the Mayo stand above waist height help prevent contamination?

_____

_____

_____

5. How can you avoid contaminating a sterile field when pouring liquids into a container on the field?

_____

_____

_____

6. How will you ease the fears of a patient who is about to have a minor surgical procedure?

_____

_____

_____

7. Describe how you should prepare the patient's skin before surgery.

_____

_____

_____

APPLICATION

Follow the directions for each application.

1. Interviewing Patients with Wounds

Work with two partners. One partner should assume the role of a patient with a wound. The second should play the role of a medical assistant and the third should act as an observer and evaluator. Assume the wound is an infected laceration.

a. The medical assistant should take a history, noting her questions and the patient's responses. A Progress Notes form is provided on page 591 of this workbook. On the basis of the responses, the medical assistant should ask appropriate follow-up questions.

b. The medical assistant should explain to the patient what the doctor is likely to do and why, allowing the patient to interrupt with questions, which the assistant should answer to the best of her ability. Again, the medical assistant should note her statements, the patient's questions, and her responses.

c. Have the observer present a critique of what the medical assistant has done. The critique should involve the assistant's attitude, or approach, as well as the appropriateness and accuracy of her questions and responses.

d. The three of you should then discuss the observer's critique, noting the strengths and weaknesses of the interview.

e. Exchange roles and reboot with a patient who has an appointment for another minor surgical procedure. The new observer should choose the procedure.

f. Exchange roles one final time so that each member of the team gets to play medical assistant, patient, and observer once.

2. Surgical Skin Preparation

You must prepare a patient's skin prior to any surgical procedure. This reduces the number of microorganisms and the risk of infection. Working with two partners, practice preparing a patient's skin prior to surgery. One student should act as the patient and one should observe and critique your performance.

a. Clean the area first with antiseptic soap and sterile water, using forceps and gauze sponges dipped in solution. Begin at the center of the site and work outward in a firm, circular motion. Discard the gauze sponge after each complete pass. Clean in concentric circles until you cover the full preparation area. Continue the process, repeating as necessary, for at least 2 minutes or the amount of time specified in the office's procedure manual. Cleaning takes more time if a wound is dirty or contains foreign materials. When procedures are performed on a hand or foot, clean the entire hand or foot.

b. Consider whether hair should be removed from the area and comment on the procedure used to remove the hair. *Do not remove the hair during this simulation.*

c. Apply antiseptic solution to the area. Swab an area 2 inches larger than the surgical field with the antiseptic solution in a circular outward motion, starting at the surgical site. For surgery on a hand or foot, swab the entire hand or foot. Allow the antiseptic to air-dry; do not pat it dry—that would remove some of the solution's antiseptic properties.

d. Cover the area with a sterile fenestrated drape, from front to back. Avoid reaching over the field. At this point, notify the physician that the patient is ready.

CASE STUDIES

Write your response to each case study on the lines provided.

Case 1

You are called away from the room while setting up a sterile surgical tray. What should you do?

_____

_____

_____

Case 2

A patient arrives at the office with a deep wound across the elbow. What type of suture should you make sure is at hand? Why?

_____

_____

_____

Case 3

You have just completed a surgical scrub and you are now donning sterile gloves. When lifting up the second glove, you think it touches the outer 1-inch margin of the sterile glove wrapper. What should you do?

_____

_____

_____

Case 4

Why is it important to use sterile solutions when irrigating a nonsurgical wound?

_____

_____

_____

CHAPTER 11

Assisting with Cold and Heat Therapy and Ambulation

REVIEW

Vocabulary Review

Matching

Match the key terms in the right column with the definitions in the left column by placing the letter of each correct answer in the space provided.

_____ 1. Applying cold to a patient's body for therapeutic reasons

_____ 2. A protractor device that measures the range of motion in degrees

_____ 3. Body position or alignment

_____ 4. Applying heat to a patient's body for therapeutic reasons

_____ 5. Redness of the skin

_____ 6. A type of heat therapy in which a machine produces high-frequency waves

_____ 7. A device designed to improve a patient's ability to move

a. cryotherapy
b. diathermy
c. erythema
d. goniometer
e. mobility aid
f. posture
g. thermotherapy

True or False

Decide whether each statement is true or false. In the space at the left, write T for true or F for false. On the lines provided, rewrite the false statements to make them true.

_____ 8. Art therapy provides treatment of musculoskeletal, nervous, and cardiovascular disorders.

_____

_____ 9. The most common form of diathermy is a hot pack.

_____

_____ 10. Cryotherapy causes blood vessels to constrict.

_____

_____ 11. Applying heat for therapeutic reasons is known as hydrotherapy.

_____

_____ 12. The degree to which a joint is able to move is known as gait.

_____

_____ 13. Posture is your body position and alignment.

_____

_____ **14.** During ROM exercises, the patient builds muscle strength.

_____

_____ **15.** Ultraviolet lamps are used to treat psoriasis.

_____

Content Review

Multiple Choice

In the space provided, write the letter of the choice that best completes each statement or answers each question.

_____ **1.** Which of the following is a mobility aid?
   A. Traction
   B. Cane
   C. ROM
   D. Diathermy

_____ **2.** Fluid accumulation in tissues is known as
   A. constriction.
   B. erythema.
   C. edema.
   D. inflammation.

_____ **3.** When using the three-point gait with crutches, the patient moves both the crutches and the affected leg forward from the tripod position and then
   A. moves the unaffected leg forward while weight is balanced on both crutches.
   B. moves the left crutch and the right foot forward at the same time.
   C. moves the right foot forward to level with the left crutch.
   D. swings both legs forward together.

_____ **4.** Redness of the skin is known as
   A. cyanosis.
   B. edema.
   C. diathermy.
   D. erythema.
   E. ROM.

_____ **5.** A treatment that uses heated wax and mineral oil is known as
   A. a paraffin bath.
   B. diathermy.
   C. fluidotherapy.
   D. a hot pack.

Sentence Completion

In the space provided, write the word or phrase that best completes each sentence.

6. Cold compresses and ice massages are types of _____ _____ applications used in cryotherapy.

6. _____

7. Static traction is also called _____ traction.

7. _____

8. _____ _____ exercises are self-directed exercises that the patient does without help.

9. During _____ traction, a physical therapist pulls gently on a patient's limb or head.

10. During _____ _____ exercises, the physical therapist moves a patient's body part.

11. _____ _____ stimulate muscles by delivering controlled amounts of low-voltage electric current to motor and sensory nerves.

8. _____

9. _____

10. _____

11. _____

Short Answer

Write the answer to each question on the lines provided.

12. What are four benefits of physical therapy?

_____

_____

_____

13. Why is it important to ask a patient how a hot pack feels?

_____

_____

14. What are four beneficial results that can be achieved through cryotherapy?

_____

_____

_____

15. What is the process by which thermotherapy promotes healing?

_____

_____

_____

16. What are two types of dry heat therapy?

_____

_____

_____

17. What are two benefits of manual traction?

_____

_____

_____

18. What is the difference between active and passive mobility exercises?

_____

_____

_____

19. To make sure that crutches fit a patient properly, what conditions should you check before the patient leaves the office?

_____

_____

_____

20. What factors determine the type of mobility aid chosen for a patient?

_____

_____

_____

Critical Thinking

Write the answer to each question on the lines provided.

1. Why is it important to check a chemical cold pack for leaks before applying the pack to the patient?

_____

_____

_____

2. How might a reduction in a patient's ROM affect the type of mobility device the patient should be using?

_____

_____

_____

3. Why is it important that a patient not lie on a heating pad?

_____

_____

_____

4. Why is it important to ensure that a patient knows how to perform exercises correctly?

_____

_____

_____

5. Why might a doctor prescribe cryotherapy, thermotherapy, or some other type of therapy in addition to exercise therapy for a patient with a sports injury?

_____

_____

_____

6. What should you do if a patient who uses a walker tells you there are steps in his house?

_____

_____

_____

APPLICATION

Follow the directions for each application.

1. Teaching a Patient How to Use a Walker

Work with two partners to teach a patient how to use a mobility aid. One partner should take the role of the patient, one should take the role of a medical assistant who is teaching the patient how to use a mobility aid, and the third should serve as observer and evaluator.

a. Role-play teaching a patient to use a walker. The medical assistant should assist the patient in stepping into the walker and explain how to grip the sides of the walker. The assistant should then instruct the patient in how to position his feet and to walk securely. The patient should ask questions during the instruction. The observer should refer to the steps outlined in Procedure 11-4 while observing the teaching.

b. The medical assistant should next explain how to maneuver the walker for sitting down in a chair or on a bed.

c. The medical assistant should then teach the patient how to ascend and descend stairs.

d. Following the teaching, the observer should critique the session, pointing out any errors or omissions in the instruction. The three partners should then discuss the session and the evaluator's comments.

e. Team members should exchange roles and review the use of another mobility aid. The new observer should evaluate the session, and all three partners should discuss the session.

f. Team members should exchange roles one more time and go through the use of a third mobility aid. Each student should have the opportunity to play each role.

2. Learning Crutch Walking and Preparing an Educational Brochure

Workings in pairs, teach each other various gaits:

a. Two-point gait

b. Three-point gait

c. Four-point gait

d. Swing-to gait

e. Swing-through gait

Follow these steps:

1. First review text Figures 11-10 and 11-11 and Procedure 11-5.

2. Discuss the steps necessary to perform each type of gait. Write a list of the steps to use for each gait while performing the instruction.

3. Practice teaching and performing the various gaits.

4. Practice getting up and sitting down.

5. Practice ascending and descending stairs.

6. After you have mastered the gaits, create a patient teaching brochure for each of the types of gaits.

CASE STUDIES

Write your response to each case study on the lines provided.

Case 1

The doctor has prescribed use of a chemical ice pack for a 62-year-old patient with a sprained ankle. After the ice pack has been on the ankle for 15 minutes, the patient complains of increased pain in the ankle. What should you do?

_____

_____

_____

Case 2

While applying a moist heat pack, you notice that the patient is shivering. What should you do?

_____

_____

_____

Case 3

After a few minutes, the patient from Case 2 complains of being uncomfortably hot. What should you do?

_____

_____

_____

Case 4

A patient with paraplegia needs crutches. What type of crutches will most likely be prescribed? Why?

_____

_____

_____

Case 5

A patient who is having difficulty recovering from a leg injury sustained in an automobile accident is considering dance therapy. What will you tell her?

_____

_____

_____

CHAPTER 12

Emergency Preparedness and First Aid

REVIEW

Vocabulary Review

Matching

Match the key terms in the right column with the definitions in the left column by placing the letter of each correct answer in the space provided.

_____ 1. A condition resulting from massive, widespread infection that affects the ability of the blood vessels to circulate blood

_____ 2. The vomiting of blood

_____ 3. Low blood sugar

_____ 4. A condition that results from insufficient blood volume in the circulatory system

_____ 5. A jarring injury to the brain

_____ 6. A muscle injury that results from overexertion

_____ 7. A swelling caused by blood under the skin

_____ 8. A brain attack caused by impaired blood supply to the brain

_____ 9. Unusually rapid, strong, or irregular pulsations of the heart

_____ 10. A nosebleed.

a. strain
b. hematemesis
c. palpitations
d. hypoglycemia
e. epistaxis
f. hematoma
g. hypovolemic shock
h. concussion
i. septic shock
j. stroke

True or False

Decide whether each statement is true or false. In the space at the left, write T for true or F for false. On the lines provided, rewrite the false statements to make them true.

_____ 11. A splint is used to bandage a laceration or an incision.

_____

_____ 12. A cast is a rigid, external dressing that is molded to the contours of the body part to which it is applied.

_____

_____ 13. The displacement of a bone end from the joint is a sprain.

_____

_____ 14. Botulism is a life-threatening allergic reaction.

_____

_____ **15.** When caring for a person who has a poisonous snakebite, it is important to apply ice to the bite.

_____

_____ **16.** A contusion is a type of closed wound.

_____

_____ **17.** A person having a seizure should be positioned on the floor with his head turned toward the side.

_____

_____ **18.** Ventricular fibrillation is an unusually rapid, strong, or irregular pulsation of the heart.

_____

_____ **19.** The first priority for medical assistants in an emergency is a victim's airway.

_____

_____ **20.** When assisting in a disaster, you should accept an assignment that is appropriate to your age.

_____

_____ **21.** Hyperglycemia is a lack of adequate water in the body.

_____

_____ **22.** The lower extension of the breastbone is the xiphoid process.

_____

_____ **23.** Establishing a chain of custody is important in cases of rape and when testing for illicit drug use.

_____

_____ **24.** An automated external defibrillator (AED) is used during a cardiac emergency to correct abnormal rhythms such as ventricular fibrillation (VF).

_____

_____ **25.** A person is placed in the recovery position when a fracture, dislocation, sprain, or strain is suspected.

_____

_____ **26.** When treating a bee sting, use tweezers to remove the stinger.

_____

_____ **27.** Bioterrorism is the intentional release of a chemical agent with the intent to harm individuals.

_____

Content Review

Multiple Choice

In the space provided, write the letter of the choice that best completes each statement or answers each question.

_____ **1.** Dry mouth, intense thirst, muscle weakness, and blurred vision are symptoms of
   A. hypoglycemia.
   B. dehydration.
   C. hyperglycemia.
   D. hyperthermia.

_____ **2.** Which of the following is the main symptom of a choking emergency?

    A. A fearful look

    B. The inability to speak

    C. Coughing

    D. Unconsciousness

    E. Pallor

_____ **3.** Which of the following is a type of head injury?

    A. A contusion

    B. A dislocation

    C. Viral encephalitis

    D. Epistaxis

_____ **4.** The most common abnormal rhythm that occurs during cardiac arrest is

    A. tachycardia.

    B. ventricular fibrillation.

    C. palpitations.

    D. CVA.

    E. myocardial infarction.

_____ **5.** Asthma is a common disorder caused by

    A. wheezing and coughing.

    B. electrolyte imbalances.

    C. diabetes.

    D. narrowing of the bronchi.

_____ **6.** An insufficient blood volume in the circulatory system causes

    A. insulin shock.

    B. ventricular fibrillation.

    C. septic shock.

    D. myocardial infarction.

    E. hypovolemic shock.

_____ **7.** A series of violent and involuntary contractions of the muscles is known as

    A. epilepsy.

    B. stroke.

    C. strain.

    D. concussion.

_____ **8.** A symptom specific to toxic shock syndrome is

    A. high fever.

    B. vomiting.

    C. a decreased level of consciousness.

    D. a red rash on the hands and feet.

    E. seizures.

_____ **9.** A life-threatening allergic reaction is known as

    A. asthma.

    B. botulism.

    C. anaphylaxis.

    D. sepsis.

_____ **10.** Which of the following is an electrical device that shocks the heart to restore normal beating?
  A. CVA
  B. MI
  C. AED
  D. PPE
  E. EMT

Sentence Completion

In the space provided, write the word or phrase that best completes each sentence.

11. An important ally in providing emergency care is your local _____ system.

12. A partial thickness burn produces _____.

13. A scalp hematoma can be reduced by applying _____ immediately after the injury.

14. If you suspect bioterrorism, your facility should first contact _____.

15. Acute abdominal pain in the right upper quadrant may signal _____.

16. A _____ is a rolling cart of emergency supplies and equipment.

17. A severe condition that is the end result of severe hyperglycemia is known as _____.

11. _____

12. _____

13. _____

14. _____

15. _____

16. _____

17. _____

Short Answer

Write the answer to each question on the lines provided.

18. What are four ways in which first aid can benefit victims of accidents or sudden illness?

_____

_____

_____

19. How should you position a person who is having a seizure?

_____

_____

_____

20. Name and describe the types of wounds that are depicted in the following illustrations.

A. _____

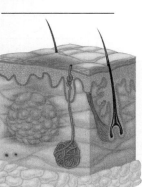

B. _____

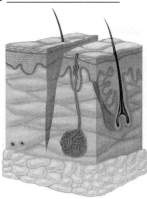

C. _____

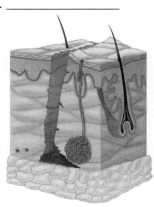

D. _____

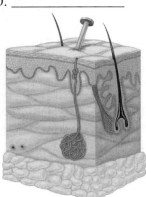

E. _____

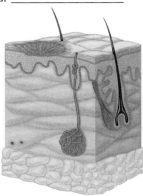

21. Describe four steps to follow when treating a patient who has swallowed poison but who is alert and not having convulsions.

_____

_____

_____

22. What are the five symptoms of dehydration?

_____

_____

_____

23. What are the symptoms of a sprain?

_____

_____

_____

24. What actions are medical personnel required to take when treating a victim of rape?

_____

_____

_____

25. Briefly describe the process of triage during a disaster.

_____

_____

_____

Critical Thinking

Write the answer to each question on the lines provided.

1. Your neighbor has been cutting down trees today. He comes to your door and says that a tree limb slid by his head and amputated his ear. What should you do?

_____

_____

_____

2. Three patients arrive in the office of a general practitioner at about the same time. One is suffering from a second-degree burn on her hand, another has been bitten by a spider, and the third is experiencing chest pain. In what order should these patients be treated? Why?

_____

_____

_____

3. Why should you look for additional symptoms when a patient complains of headache, dizziness, or vomiting?

_____

_____

_____

4. A patient arrives at your office feeling restless and confused. She has a rapid pulse; shallow respirations; hunger; profuse sweating; pale, cool, clammy skin; double vision; and tremors. She states that she took her regular does of insulin this morning but was not able to eat breakfast. What could be wrong with this patient? What should you do?

_____

_____

_____

5. When performing an emergency assessment, why should you check for a medical identification card, necklace, or bracelet?

_____

_____

_____

APPLICATION

Follow the directions for each application.

1. Performing Emergency Procedures

Each of the following descriptions of emergency procedures contains at least one error. On the lines provided, rewrite the procedures to make them correct.

a. When treating a dog bite that has caused a puncture wound, wash the area with antiseptic soap and water and use pressure to stop the bleeding.

_____

_____

b. When treating a spider bite, wash the area thoroughly with soap and water and apply a hot pack to the area to reduce swelling and pain.

_____

_____

c. When treating a first-degree burn, immerse the affected area in cold water. Then pat the area dry and apply petroleum jelly or ointment.

_____

_____

d. When treating a scalp laceration, apply indirect pressure, wash the area with soap and water, and apply a moist, sterile dressing over the area.

_____

_____

2. Choosing Personal Protective Equipment for Emergencies

For each emergency described below, list personal protective equipment that should be worn.

a. Vomiting _____

b. Childbirth _____

c. Heart attack _____

d. Eye injury _____

e. Bleeding _____

CASE STUDIES

Write your response to each case study on the lines provided.

Case 1

While eating dinner in a restaurant, you hear a commotion across the dining room. A man appears to be choking. A woman is slapping him on the back. What, if anything, should you do?

_____

_____

_____

Case 2

While walking at the local park, you see a woman stumble and fall. You notice that she catches herself with her arms extended. As you reach the victim, you notice that her right wrist looks swollen and she is complaining of severe pain in her arm. What should you do?

_____

_____

_____

Case 3

A patient who has been sitting in the waiting room comes to the reception desk and asks you for a glass of water. She seems disoriented and short of breath and her skin appears flushed. When you lean forward to ask the patient whether she is all right, you notice that her breath has a sweet odor. What might be happening, and how should you handle the situation?

_____

_____

_____

Case 4

An infant comes in your office with a high fever. While her mother is talking to you, the infant begins to have a seizure. What should you do?

_____

_____

_____

Case 5

Your neighbor, Jane Chung, has been working in her garage for most of the morning, spray-painting some patio furniture. You notice that she has had the door closed while she was working. You decide to check on her and find her sitting down, holding her chest. She says that she feels dizzy and nauseated and has a headache. What could be wrong with Jane? What should you do?

_____

_____

_____

CHAPTER 13

Complementary and Alternative Medicine

REVIEW

Vocabulary Review

Matching

Match the key terms in the right column with the definitions in the left column by placing the letter of each correct answer in the space provided.

_____ 1. The use of essential oils extracts or essences from flowers, herbs, and trees to promote health and well-being

_____ 2. Vitamins, minerals, herbals, and other substances taken by mouth without a prescription to promote health and well-being

_____ 3. The practice of inserting needles into various areas of the body to restore balance

_____ 4. A state in which the body is consciously relaxed and the mind becomes calm and focused

_____ 5. A series of poses and breathing exercises that provide awareness of the unity of the whole being

_____ 6. A form of medicine, originated in India, that uses herbal preparations, dietary changes, exercises, and meditation to restore health and promote well-being

_____ 7. A therapy in which pressure is applied to zones mapped out on the feet or hands

_____ 8. Adjustments of the spine made to relieve pressure and/or pain

_____ 9. A system of medicine that uses remedies in an attempt to stimulate the body to recover itself

_____ 10. A type of therapy in which an individual learns how to control involuntary body responses to promote health and treat disease

_____ 11. A trance-like state usually induced by another person to access the subconscious mind and promote healing

_____ 12. The use of visualization and touch to balance energy flow and bring healthy energy to affected body parts

a. reflexology
b. acupuncture
c. aroma therapy
d. Ayurveda
e. biofeedback
f. chiropractic medicine
g. dietary supplements
h. homeopathy
i. hypnosis
j. meditation
k. Reiki
l. yoga

True or False

Decide whether each statement is true or false. In the space at the left, write T *for true or* F *for false. On the lines provided, rewrite the false statements to make them true.*

_____ 13. CAM is a set of practices and products that are considered part of conventional medicine.

_____

_____ 14. Integrative medicine is the combination of conventional therapies and CAM therapies.

_____

_____ 15. There are four categories of CAM according to the NCCAM.

_____

_____ 16. Homeopathy is a biologically based therapy.

_____

_____ 17. Homeopathic remedies are regulated by the federal government.

_____

_____ 18. Qi regulates the person's spiritual, emotional, mental, and physical balance.

_____

_____ 19. A chiropractor would examine the tongue of a patient for shape and color before starting treatments.

_____

_____ 20. More than 50% of the population uses prayer as a CAM therapy.

_____

_____ 21. In medication, calming of the conscious mind is induced by another person.

_____

_____ 22. In most cases, it is acceptable for the medical assistant to answer questions about CAM therapy for the patients.

_____

_____ 23. Potentization is a process that ensures the consistency and quality of each batch of medication produced.

_____

_____ 24. Health fraud promoters target people who feel desperate about their conditions and make money off of their desperation.

_____

_____ 25. The FDA does not approve claims made by CAM therapies.

_____

Content Review

Multiple Choice

In the space provided, write the letter of the choice that best completes each statement or answers each question.

_____ 1. Which organization supports CAM research and promotes CAM information to health-care providers and the public?
   A. Federal Trade Commission
   B. Food and Drug Administration
   C. Occupational Safety and Health Administration
   D. Health Insurance Portability and Accountability Act
   E. National Center for Complementary and Alternative Medicine

_____ 2. Which of the following is an approved health claim?
   A. Calcium may reduce the risk of the bone disease osteoporosis.
   B. Diets high in sodium reduce the risk of high blood pressure.
   C. Diets low in saturated fats increase the risk of heart disease.
   D. Diets containing foods that are a good source of potassium may increase the risk of high blood pressure and stroke.

_____ 3. If a patient is taking an anticoagulant like coumadin, which of the following dietary supplements might interact?
   A. Ginseng
   B. Valerian
   C. St. John's Wort
   D. Gingko
   E. Glucosamine chondroitin

_____ 4. Which of the following is a type of biofield therapy?
   A. Magnetic therapy
   B. Therapeutic touch
   C. Reflexology
   D. Aromatherapy

_____ 5. Which of the following supplements was taken off the market after being investigated by the FDA?
   A. Echinacea
   B. Black cohosh
   C. Gingko biloba
   D. Ephedra
   E. Milk thistle

_____ 6. Which of the following substances would have been required to provide scientific evidence of effectiveness before being marketed?
   A. Niacin
   B. Lipitor
   C. Folic acid
   D. St. John's wort

_____ 7. Biofeedback is which type of therapy?
    A. Energy therapy
    B. Mind-body therapy
    C. Biologically based therapy
    D. Alternative medical systems therapy
    E. Herbal therapy

_____ 8. Energetic forces called Tridoshas are part of which type of CAM?
    A. Ayurveda
    B. Reiki
    C. Traditional Chinese medicine
    D. Qi

_____ 9. Which of the following is a biologically based therapy?
    A. Meditation
    B. Reiki
    C. Hypnosis
    D. Yoga
    E. Dietary supplements

_____ 10. Energetic pathways are known as
    A. qi.
    B. placebos.
    C. meridians.
    D. remedies.

Sentence Completion

In the space provided, write the word or phrase that best completes each sentence.

11. Naturopathic medicine is considered _____ health care.

12. A(n) _____ inserts hollow needles under the skin to balance the flow of qi.

13. The difference between acupuncture and moxibustion involves the use of _____.

14. Everything in _____ is validated by observation, inquiry, direct exam, and knowledge derived from ancient texts.

15. Up to 35% of the therapeutic response to a medical treatment could be the result of the _____ effect.

11. _____

12. _____

13. _____

14. _____

15. _____

Short Answer

Write the answer to each question on the lines provided.

16. How are dietary supplements defined by the U.S. Congress?

_____

_____

_____

17. Describe the concept of balanced qi as it relates to traditional Chinese medicine.

_____

_____

_____

18. Name and describe the five categories of CAM as identified by NCCAM.

    1. _____

    2. _____

    3. _____

    4. _____

    5. _____

19. What are the similarities among the various types of CAM?

_____

_____

_____

20. Name at least three recommendations of the WHCCAMP regarding CAM practices and products.

_____

_____

_____

Critical Thinking

Write the answer to each question on the lines provided.

    1. What examples could you give a patient about the differences between complementary and alternative therapy?

_____

_____

_____

    2. A patient asks you a specific question about a type of CAM therapy that you have been using personally for a long time. What should you do?

_____

_____

_____

    3. An ND has been hired to work at your clinic. Is he licensed?

_____

_____

_____

4. When would a dietary supplement be taken off the market?

_____

_____

_____

5. You want to research at least three types of CAM therapies used for back pain. Name and describe the three you would choose.

_____

_____

_____

APPLICATION

Follow the directions for each application.

1. A patient is taking each of the following medications in the table below. Determine which dietary supplement he or she should not take and why by completing the table.

Medication Taken (with Classification)	Dietary Supplement That Interacts	Interaction That Can Occur
a. Coumadin (anticoagulant)		
b. Claritin-D (decongestant)		
c. Paxil (antidepressant)		
d. Valium (benzodiazepine)		

2. What are the steps you can take to determine if CAM therapies are covered by insurance?

_____

_____

_____

CASE STUDIES

Write your response to each case study on the lines provided.

Case 1

Your patient is taking three prescription medications, two megadose vitamins, and two other dietary supplements. What should you do?

_____

_____

_____

Case 2

A patient is using a new type of therapy to help her lose weight. How could you determine if the therapy is fraud?

_____

_____

_____

Case 3

A patient has refused prescription medication as treatment for blood pressure and has decided to take an herbal remedy instead. What should you do?

_____

_____

_____

CHAPTER 14

Laboratory Equipment and Safety

REVIEW

Vocabulary Review

Passage Completion

Study the key terms in the box. Use your textbook to find definitions of terms you do not understand.

biohazard symbol	focus controls	optical microscope	quality assurance program
centrifuge	hazard label	physician's office laboratory (POL)	
Certificate of Waiver tests	Material Safety Data Sheet (MSDS)		reference laboratory

In the space provided, complete the following passage, using some of the terms from the box. You may change the form of a term to fit the meaning of the sentence.

Laboratory analysis plays an important role in any medical practice. Some physicians have all laboratory tests performed by a(n) (1) _____, which is owned and operated by an organization outside the practice. Other physicians do some laboratory work in the office, in the (2) _____. This allows quick turnaround of test results.

One piece of equipment used in the laboratory is a(n) (3) _____, which spins a specimen at high speed until it separates into its component parts. The laboratory equipment that is used most often in the POL, however, is the (4) _____. There are two (5) _____ on the optical microscope, coarse and fine.

Safety is a primary concern in the laboratory. One precaution that is required by law is that all containers used to store hazardous waste products must be clearly marked with the (6) _____. For information about hazardous chemicals used in the laboratory, a medical assistant can consult the (7) _____. The shortened version of the MSDS is called a(n) (8) _____. It is permanently attached to each hazardous substance container. A(n) (9) _____ is designed to monitor the quality of patient care that a medical laboratory provides. A laboratory can gain exemption from meeting certain federal standards if it performs only (10) _____.

1. _____

2. _____

3. _____

4. _____

5. _____

6. _____

7. _____

8. _____

9. _____

10. _____

Matching

Match the key terms in the right column with the definitions in the left column by placing the letter of each correct answer in the space provided.

_____ 11. A foreign object visible through a microscope but unrelated to the specimen

_____ 12. A magnifying lens mounted on the nosepiece of a microscope

_____ 13. Measures the accuracy of test results and adherence to standard operating procedures

_____ 14. A laboratory owned and operated by an organization outside the practice

_____ 15. A device that spins a specimen at high speed until it separates into its component parts

_____ 16. A specimen with a known value that is used every time a patient sample is processed

_____ 17. The eyepiece of a microscope through which an image is viewed

_____ 18. A specimen with a known value that is used during calibration

_____ 19. A document that shows all procedures completed during the workday

_____ 20. Ensures accuracy in test results through careful monitoring of test procedures

a. proficiency testing program
b. centrifuge
c. artifact
d. reference laboratory
e. objective
f. standard
g. daily workload log
h. quality control program
i. control sample
j. ocular

True or False

Decide whether each statement is true or false. In the space at the left, write T for true or F for false. On the lines provided, rewrite the false statements to make them true.

_____ 21. The steam autoclave is used to reduce the risk of fire in a laboratory.

_____

_____ 22. Placing the end of the oil-immersion objective in oil reduces the loss of light and produces a much sharper, brighter image.

_____

_____ 23. The Supreme Court enacted the Clinical Laboratory Improvement Amendments of 1988, which established federal regulations for laboratories.

_____

_____ 24. Hazardous waste products include sharps and gloves.

_____

_____ 25. Generally, positive and negative control samples are used with tests that yield a qualitative test response.

_____

Content Review

Multiple Choice

In the space provided, write the letter of the choice that best completes each statement or answers each question.

_____ 1. Objectives are mounted on a swivel base called the
    A. condenser.
    B. objective.
    C. stage.
    D. lens.
    E. nosepiece.

_____ 2. Chemicals or chemically treated substances used in testing procedures are known as
    A. controls.
    B. standards.
    C. reagents.
    D. pipettes.

_____ 3. Which of the following must an employer make available to employees so as to be in compliance with the OSHA Bloodborne Pathogens Standard?
    A. Polio vaccine
    B. Health insurance
    C. Performance ratings for handling bloodborne pathogens
    D. Hepatitis B vaccine

_____ 4. Which of the following is an instrument that measures light intensity?
    A. Artifact
    B. Hemocytometer
    C. Thermometer
    D. Photometer
    E. Pipette

_____ 5. Blood cell counts and cholesterol screening are examples of
    A. Certificate of Waiver tests.
    B. moderate-complexity tests.
    C. high-complexity tests.
    D. quality control tests.

Sentence Completion

In the space provided, write the word or phrase that best completes each sentence.

6. The iris of a microscope is used to _____ the amount of light illuminating the specimen.

7. When not in use, the microscope should be stored _____.

8. For more information about hazardous chemicals used in the laboratory, a medical assistant can consult the _____.

9. A shortened version of the MSDS found on a chemical label is a _____.

10. Tests that have been approved by the Food and Drug Administration (FDA) for use by patients at home are _____ tests.

6. _____

7. _____

8. _____

9. _____

10. _____

11. The _____ requires that employees receive training regarding workplace hazards.

12. A Materials Safety Data Sheet for a hazardous substance must include _____ for safe handling of the substance.

13. In a microscope, the _____ controls the amount of light on the specimen by opening and closing like a shutter.

14. Graduated flasks are used to measure large amounts of _____.

15. Treating patients with respect is part of the medical assistant's _____ skills.

11. _____

12. _____

13. _____

14. _____

15. _____

Short Answer

Write the answer to each question on the lines provided.

16. Where should you store caustic chemicals?

_____

_____

17. Name three regulations you should be familiar with when working in a physician's office laboratory.

_____

_____

18. As a medical assistant, what might your role be in the POL?

_____

_____

19. Describe a biohazard symbol label.

_____

_____

20. Describe four commonsense safeguards that will ensure your physical safety in the laboratory.

_____

_____

_____

21. What steps would you take to deal with a minor accident in the laboratory?

_____

_____

_____

22. How are Certificate of Waiver tests defined? Give examples.

_____

_____

_____

23. Describe the records that must be kept as part of a quality control program in addition to the quality control log, the reagent control log, and the equipment maintenance log.

_____

_____

_____

24. List six hazardous waste products.

_____

_____

_____

25. The illustration below shows the parts of a microscope. Write the name of each part on the line provided.

A. _____

B. _____

C. _____

L. _____

D. _____

E. _____

F. _____

K. _____

G. _____

J. _____

H. _____

I. _____

Critical Thinking

Write the answer to each question on the lines provided.

1. Why is it important to use a systematic approach when troubleshooting equipment problems?

_____

_____

_____

2. What safeguards can you use to help reduce electrical hazards?

_____

_____

_____

3. Why should you change gloves every time you move from patient to patient when collecting specimens for testing?

_____

_____

_____

4. Why do you think mouth pipetting is prohibited at all times?

_____

_____

_____

5. Explain the meaning of the motto "If it is not written down, it was not done."

_____

_____

_____

APPLICATION

Follow the directions for each application.

1. Equipping a Physician's Office Laboratory (POL)

Work with two partners. You are part of a team that is buying equipment for a new POL. Assume the POL will process routine tests involving blood and urine for a practice with two doctors.

a. You and your partners should make a preliminary list of all the laboratory equipment and supplies you think will be needed. Start with major items, such as a microscope. Then consider all the necessary support materials, such as coverslips, test tubes, dipsticks, and cotton swabs.

b. As you work with your partners, consider these questions: What tests are likely to be performed in the POL? What equipment is needed for each type of test that will be performed? What supplies are needed to run a POL? What supplies will be needed to care for and maintain the equipment in the POL? Make a list of all the possible tests the POL might perform and add the equipment needed for each procedure to your list.

c. Next, use medical supply catalogs to help you choose the laboratory equipment and supplies you would recommend for the POL.

d. Start an equipment inventory log and record your selections. Be specific about the type of equipment. Record model numbers, prices, and amounts. Use medical abbreviations as appropriate. Include illustrations as necessary.

e. Share your inventory log with another team and be prepared to justify your selections. Compare selections, prices, and amounts. Discuss items that are on one team's list but not the other. Check for completeness.

f. Then share your log with a different team.

g. On the basis of classmates' feedback, revise your inventory log to make it as complete as possible.

2. Monitoring Safety in the Laboratory

Work with a partner. You are to play the role of an OSHA representative. Your partner should play the role of a medical assistant who works in a POL. Assume that the OSHA representative is investigating a laboratory accident in which an employee's eyes were damaged when a container of caustic chemical fell from a cupboard in the POL.

a. List the questions you would ask to find out how the accident occurred. Include questions concerning OSHA requirements and office rules and policies.

b. Playing the role of the OSHA representative, ask questions of the medical assistant. Record the medical assistant's responses and ask follow-up questions.

c. Working with your partner, use your questions and answers to create a new set of accident prevention guidelines for physical safety in the laboratory.

d. Share your accident prevention guidelines with another pair of students and critique each other's guidelines. The critiques should include questions such as: Do the guidelines provide enough information? Will the guidelines help prevent accidents from occurring? Is the writing clear and concise? Offer suggestions for revisions.

e. As you and your partner discuss the critique, note the accuracy and completeness of your guidelines as written. Revise your guidelines as needed.

f. Exchange roles. Repeat the activity for this accident scenario: A medical assistant working in the laboratory is overcome by fumes from a chemical and must be rushed to the hospital. Create a new set of accident prevention guidelines for chemical safety in the laboratory.

3. Bring some items from home that you think would be interesting to view under the microscope. (Suggested items: newsprint, a feather, threads, dog or cat hair, sugar crystals) Place each item under the microscope and view them using 10X and 40X objectives. Make drawings of each item under both magnifications. Write your observations about the materials underneath each drawing.

CASE STUDIES

Write your response to each case study on the lines provided.

Case 1

Your office is planning to close the POL and send all tests to a reference laboratory. The doctors say that the complexity and expense of meeting federal regulations is forcing them to take this action. In the past, your office has performed urinalyses, pregnancy tests, and blood glucose tests. Instead of closing the POL, what other option is available?

_____

_____

_____

Case 2

You have been put in charge of the care and maintenance of the microscope in the POL. Describe the procedure you would follow at the end of the workday.

_____

_____

_____

Case 3

You have been asked to train new laboratory personnel in the housekeeping duties essential in your lab. What information should you give new employees?

_____

_____

_____

Case 4

You are a medical assistant in a physician's office laboratory that performs Level II tests. Your employer has asked for your help in designing a quality assurance program. Describe the components the program must include.

_____

_____

_____

Case 5

A patient has arrived in the office for a scheduled blood test. Describe how you will communicate with her before, during, and after the test.

_____

_____

_____

Case 6

The physician in your office suspects that one of the tests you have performed is not accurate. What action should you take?

_____

_____

_____

CHAPTER 15

Introduction to Microbiology

REVIEW

Vocabulary Review

Matching

Match the key terms in the right column with the definitions in the left column by placing the letter of each correct answer in the space provided.

_____ 1. An agent that kills or suppresses the growth of a microorganism

_____ 2. An organism that lives on or in another organism and that uses that other organism for its own nourishment or some other advantage, to the detriment of the host organism

_____ 3. A single-celled eukaryotic organism, generally much larger than bacteria and found in soil and water

_____ 4. A substance that contains all the nutrients a particular type of microorganism needs

_____ 5. A distinct group of organisms

_____ 6. The result of a Gram's stain in which the bacteria lose the purple color and pick up the red color of the safranin

_____ 7. A specimen spread thinly and evenly across a slide

_____ 8. Bacteria that appear blue after the Gram's stain procedure

_____ 9. A procedure that involves culturing a specimen and then testing the isolated bacterium's susceptibility to certain antibiotics

_____ 10. A gelatin-like substance derived from seaweed that gives a medium its consistency

_____ 11. A preparation of a specimen in a liquid that allows organisms to remain alive and mobile while they are examined under a microscope

_____ 12. Fungi that grow mainly as single-celled organisms and reproduce by budding

_____ 13. A eukaryotic organism that has a rigid cell wall at some stage in the life cycle

_____ 14. A comma-shaped bacterium

_____ 15. A staining procedure for identifying bacteria that have a waxy cell wall

_____ 16. A solution of a dye or group of dyes that imparts a color to microorganisms

_____ 17. A spiral-shaped bacterium

_____ 18. A spherical, round, or ovoid bacterium

a. antimicrobial
b. coccus
c. acid-fast stain
d. yeast
e. spirillum
f. parasite
g. agar
h. vibrio
i. fungus
j. culture and sensitivity (C&S)
k. protozoan
l. colony
m. gram-negative
n. smear
o. stain
p. wet mount
q. culture medium
r. gram-positive

True or False

Decide whether each statement is true or false. In the space at the left, write T *for true or* F *for false. On the lines provided, rewrite the false statements to make them true.*

_____ **19.** Viruses are large, prokaryotic organisms.

_____

_____ **20.** Keratin is a tough, hard protein.

_____

_____ **21.** Eukaryotic microorganisms have a simple cell structure with no nucleus and no organelles in the cytoplasm.

_____

_____ **22.** When performing a quantitative analysis of a urine specimen, incubate the plates at 20°C.

_____

_____ **23.** Gram's stain is used to differentiate bacteria according to the chemical composition of their cell walls.

_____

_____ **24.** Aerobes are bacteria that grow best in the presence of oxygen.

_____

_____ **25.** Facultative organisms grow well when oxygen is present or absent.

_____

_____ **26.** A protozoan is a multiple-celled eukaryotic organism that is generally smaller than a bacterium.

_____

_____ **27.** A mordant is a substance that can intensify or deepen the response of a specimen to a stain.

_____

_____ **28.** A parasite is an organism that lives on or in another organism and uses that other organism for its own nourishment.

_____

_____ **29.** Chlamydiae are bacteria that completely lack the rigid cell wall of other bacteria.

_____

_____ **30.** When performing a quantitative analysis of a urine specimen, mix the urine specimen well before taking the sample.

_____

_____ **31.** Trichinosis is an infection caused by *Trichinella spiralis,* a kind of virus.

_____

_____ **32.** An O&P specimen is a urine specimen that is examined for the presence of protozoans or parasites, including their eggs.

_____

_____ **33.** An etiologic agent is a living microorganism or its toxin that can cause human disease.

_____

_____ 34. An ongoing system to evaluate the quality of medical care provided in a medical office is known as qualitative analysis.

_____

_____ 35. A Gram's stain result is referred to as gram-positive when the bacteria appear red.

_____

Content Review

Multiple Choice

In the space provided, write the letter of the choice that best completes each statement or answers each question.

_____ 1. A bacterium that grows best in the absence of oxygen is
   A. a protozoan.
   B. an anaerobe.
   C. an aerobe.
   D. a vibrio.

_____ 2. A procedure to test a bacterium's susceptibility to certain antibiotics is
   A. a culture.
   B. an antimicrobial.
   C. a culture and sensitivity.
   D. a qualitative analysis.
   E. a quantitative analysis.

_____ 3. The label on a collection specimen container should include the patient's name and identification number, source of the specimen, doctor's name, your initials, and the
   A. patient's insurance billing information.
   B. names of medications the patient is currently receiving.
   C. date and time of collection.
   D. doctor's presumptive diagnosis.

_____ 4. A KOH mount is prepared with
   A. a 0.9% solution of sodium chloride.
   B. a 10% solution of potassium hydroxide.
   C. iodine as a mordant.
   D. alcohol as a mordant.

_____ 5. A gelatin-like substance derived from seaweed that is used to give culture medium its consistency is known as
   A. agar.
   B. smear.
   C. safranin.
   D. gentian violet.
   E. inoculum.

Sentence Completion

In the space provided, write the word or phrase that best completes each sentence.

6. Specific microorganisms are named with two words; the first word refers to the microorganism's _____ and the second word refers to its species.

7. Spherical, round, or ovoid bacteria are known as _____.

6. _____

7. _____

8. A doctor makes a(n) _____ clinical diagnosis on the basis of a patient's vital signs, complaints, and exam.

9. To _____ a culture medium, you place a sample of a specimen in or on the medium.

10. Rod-shaped bacteria are known as _____.

11. A(n) _____ is an agent that kills microorganisms or suppresses their growth.

12. A _____ loop is a type of inoculating loop that measures a specific amount of fluid.

13. A fungus that grows mainly as a single-celled organism that reproduces by budding is referred to as a _____.

14. The most common type of culture medium used in the laboratory is _____, a nonselective medium.

15. Antimicrobial sensitivity tests are reported as sensitive (no growth), intermediate (little growth), or _____ (overgrown).

8. _____

9. _____

10. _____

11. _____

12. _____

13. _____

14. _____

15. _____

Short Answer

Write the answer to each question on the lines provided.

16. What are three ways a patient can collect a stool specimen?

_____

_____

_____

17. Compare and contrast prokaryotic and eukaryotic cells, and give examples of each.

_____

_____

18. The four different bacterial shapes are shown here. On the lines provided, write the names of the bacteria that display these shapes.

A. _____   B. _____   C. _____   D. _____

19. What are the six steps in diagnosing and treating an infection?

_____

_____

_____

20. Why is it important to process urine samples within 1 hour?

_____

_____

_____

21. What are the three main objectives for collecting and transporting a microbiologic specimen to an outside laboratory?

_____

_____

_____

22. What is the procedure for preparing a KOH mount?

_____

_____

_____

23. Where should you label a culture plate? Why?

_____

_____

_____

24. Describe how you would prepare a microbiological specimen for transport by the US Postal Service.

_____

_____

_____

25. What are the most common types of culture specimens?

_____

_____

_____

Critical Thinking

Write the answer to each question on the lines provided.

1. Why are cotton swabs no longer used for culture swabs?

_____

_____

_____

2. Why is it more difficult to grow and identify viruses than bacteria?

_____

_____

_____

3. Why is it important to properly collect a stool sample so that it is not contaminated by water from the toilet or urine?

_____

_____

_____

4. Why is it important to develop an up-to-date laboratory procedures manual?

_____

_____

_____

5. Why are cultures usually incubated at 35° to 37°C?

_____

_____

_____

APPLICATION

Follow the directions for the application.

Collecting a Specimen, Preparing a Specimen Smear, and Performing a Gram's Stain

Working with a partner, you are to take a throat culture from your partner, prepare a smear of the specimen for staining, and perform a Gram's stain. Your partner should serve as observer and evaluator.

a. Using a sterile swab, obtain a throat culture from your partner. Follow all safety precautions. Your partner should monitor the procedure while referring to Procedure 15-1 in the textbook and taking notes as needed for later discussion.

b. After you have obtained the specimen, prepare a specimen smear. Your partner should refer to the steps outlined in Procedure 15-3.

c. After you have prepared the smear, your partner should provide a critique of the procedure. Discuss any omissions or errors in the procedure.

d. Using the prepared smear, perform a Gram's stain. Your partner should observe your technique while referring to Procedure 15-4 in the textbook and assess your performance on completion of the stain.

e. Exchange roles and allow your partner to collect a specimen, prepare a smear, and perform a Gram's stain.

CASE STUDIES

Write your response to each case study on the lines provided.

Case 1

The doctor asks you to obtain a urine specimen from a patient. As you explain the procedure to the patient, he tells you that he is currently taking antibiotics that were prescribed by a doctor he visited for the same ailment while out of town on business. Should you have the patient collect the specimen? If not, what should you do?

_____

_____

_____

Case 2

You forgot to break the vial in the CULTURETTE before you sent it out to the lab. The lab rejected the specimen. Why?

_____

_____

_____

Case 3

While you are collecting a throat specimen, the patient gags and accidentally touches the swab with her tongue. What should you do? Why?

_____

_____

_____

Case 4

You have been asked to educate a mother about collecting a stool sample from her 1-year-old child. What tips can you give the mother about collecting the sample?

_____

_____

_____

CHAPTER 16

Collecting, Processing, and Testing Urine Specimens

REVIEW

Vocabulary Review

Matching

Match the key terms in the right column with the definitions in the left column by placing the letter of each correct answer in the space provided.

_____ 1. Excessive nighttime urination

_____ 2. Excess protein in urine

_____ 3. Excess glucose in the urine

_____ 4. A tube used to collect specimens or instill medications

_____ 5. The presence of myoglobin in urine

_____ 6. A tube inserted in the ureter after plastic repair

_____ 7. A bile pigment formed from hemoglobin

_____ 8. An optical instrument that measures the bending of light as it passes through liquid

_____ 9. The functional unit of the kidney

_____ 10. Absence of urine production

_____ 11. A measure of the degree of acidity or alkalinity of urine

_____ 12. Insufficient production (or volume) of urine

_____ 13. Blood in the urine

_____ 14. The presence of bilirubin in urine

_____ 15. A cylinder-shaped element that forms when protein accumulates in the kidney tubules and is washed into the urine

_____ 16. A test using antigens and antibodies conjugated to an enzyme

_____ 17. A naturally produced solid of definite form that is commonly found in urine specimens

_____ 18. The liquid portion of a centrifuged urine sample

_____ 19. A genetically inherited disorder in which the body cannot properly metabolize the nutrient phenylalanine

a. drainage catheter
b. nocturia
c. supernatant
d. anuria
e. enzyme immunoassay (EIA)
f. splinting catheter
g. bilirubin
h. proteinuria
i. crystal
j. cast
k. hematuria
l. bilirubinuria
m. phenylketonuria (PKU)
n. refractometer
o. oliguria
p. glycosuria
q. myoglobinuria
r. urinary pH
s. nephron

True or False

Decide whether each statement is true or false. In the space at the left, write T *for true or* F *for false. On the lines provided, rewrite the false statements to make them true.*

_____ **20.** When a timed urine specimen is obtained, only the first specimen and the last specimen are collected during a 2- to 24-hour period.

_____

_____ **21.** The normal water content of urine is about 50%.

_____

_____ **22.** Hyaline casts form as a result of increased urine flow.

_____

_____ **23.** A clean-catch midstream urine specimen is obtained after special cleansing of the external genitalia.

_____

_____ **24.** Hemoglobinuria is a rare condition in which free hemoglobin is present in urine.

_____

_____ **25.** Glomerular filtration occurs as blood moves through a tight ball of capillaries called the tubule.

_____

_____ **26.** A first morning urine specimen contains lesser concentrations of substances that collect over time than do specimens taken during the day.

_____

_____ **27.** Hemoglobin breaks down into urea in the intestines.

_____

_____ **28.** A random urine specimen is a single urine specimen that can be taken at any time of the day.

_____

_____ **29.** With adequate fluid intake, the average daily output volume of urine is 1250 mL.

_____

_____ **30.** A 24-hour urine specimen is used to complete a quantitative and qualitative analysis of one or more substances.

_____

_____ **31.** Yeast cells are often seen in the urine of patients with diabetes.

_____

Content Review

Multiple Choice

In the space provided, write the letter of the choice that best completes each statement or answers each question.

_____ **1.** The tube that carries urine from the bladder to the outside of the body is the
   A. ureter.
   B. urethra.
   C. glomerulus.
   D. collecting tubule.

_____ **2.** A single urine specimen taken at any time of the day is
  A. a clean-catch.
  B. timed.
  C. random.
  D. 24-hour.

_____ **3.** Fresh urine specimens should be processed within
  A. 1 minute.
  B. 1 hour.
  C. 3 hours.
  D. 1 day.
  E. 1 week.

_____ **4.** The first part of the urinalysis, a visual inspection of color, volume, odor, and specific gravity, is known as what type of test?
  A. Microscopic
  B. Confirmatory
  C. Physical
  D. Chemical
  E. Metabolic

_____ **5.** The normal pH range of freshly voided urine is
  A. 0–2.9.
  B. 2.4–4.8.
  C. 3.8–6.4.
  D. 4.5–8.0.

Sentence Completion

In the space provided, write the word or phrase that best completes each sentence.

6. The presence of _____ in the urine is one of the first signs of liver disease.

7. _____ is a yellow pigment that gives urine its color.

8. A(n) _____ catheter is designed to remain in place within the bladder.

9. Ketone bodies are intermediary products of fat and _____ metabolism.

10. Leukocyte _____ is a chemical seen when leukocytes are present in urine.

11. An increase in urine specific gravity indicates that the kidneys cannot properly _____ the urine.

12. A reagent strip can be used to test for _____, which are intermediary products of fat and protein metabolism in the body.

13. The three types of cells that are found in urine are epithelial cells, white blood cells, and _____.

14. Urine pregnancy tests determine the presence of the hormone _____.

15. A(n) _____ test should be done on a urine specimen before attempting to identify crystals in the specimen.

6. _____

7. _____

8. _____

9. _____

10. _____

11. _____

12. _____

13. _____

14. _____

15. _____

Short Answer

Write the answer to each question on the lines provided.

16. What conditions can cause hematuria?

_____

_____

_____

17. What should be done to refrigerated urine specimens before processing them?

_____

_____

_____

18. Why is it necessary to clean the external genitalia when collecting a clean-catch midstream urine specimen?

_____

_____

_____

19. Why is catheterization not routinely used for collecting urine specimens instead of the clean-catch midstream method?

_____

_____

_____

20. What are the disadvantages of the nucleic acid amplification urine tests for STDs?

_____

_____

_____

21. What do changes in the color of a patient's urine generally indicate about changes in its specific gravity?

_____

_____

_____

22. What are the advantages of using a refractometer to measure urine specific gravity?

_____

_____

_____

23. Why might a doctor order the chemical testing of urine?

_____

_____

_____

24. After centrifugation, where should you pour the supernatant?

_____

_____

_____

25. What is the most common urinary parasite?

_____

_____

_____

Critical Thinking

Write the answer to each question on the lines provided.

1. During a microscopic urine exam, you find a higher than normal count of renal epithelial cells. What might this indicate?

_____

_____

_____

2. What is the purpose of taking the temperature of urine collected for a drug and alcohol analysis?

_____

_____

_____

3. Why should a glucose test be performed on a fresh urine specimen?

_____

_____

_____

4. Why is blood more commonly tested than urine for glucose?

_____

_____

_____

5. Will refrigeration cause a decrease or an increase in urine specific gravity? Explain.

_____

_____

_____

6. What is the purpose of placing a bluing agent in the toilet prior to having a patient collect a urine drug screen specimen?

_____

_____

_____

APPLICATION

Follow the directions for each application.

1. Collecting a Urine Specimen from an Elderly Patient

Working with two partners, conduct an interview with an elderly patient scheduled for a urine test. One person should play the role of the elderly patient, one should take the role of the medical assistant conducting the interview, and the third should act as an observer and evaluator. Assume that the patient is an incontinent male scheduled for a random urine specimen.

a. Take a history of the patient, noting your questions and the patient's responses. On the basis of the responses, ask appropriate follow-up questions.

b. Explain to the patient the procedure he is to follow. Allow the patient to interrupt at any time with questions, which you should answer to the best of your ability. Again, note your statements, the patient's questions, and your responses.

c. Have the observer critique the interview. The critique should include the medical assistant's attitude, or approach, as well as the appropriateness and accuracy of the questions and responses to the elderly patient. The observer also should evaluate the order in which the assistant took the history and its completeness.

d. As a team, discuss the observer's critique, noting the strengths and weaknesses of the interview.

e. Exchange roles and repeat the interview with an elderly patient (perhaps hearing-impaired) scheduled for another type of urine specimen collection. The type of collection should be chosen by the new observer.

f. Exchange roles one more time so that each team member gets to play the medical assistant, the patient, and the observer.

2. Evaluating a Urine Specimen

Indicate whether each of the following results of a urinalysis is normal or abnormal by writing *normal* or *abnormal* in the space provided.

a. Color: Red   _____

b. Turbidity: Clear   _____

c. Odor: Fruity   _____

d. Volume: 2200 mL/24 hours   _____

e. Specific gravity: 1.022   _____

f. Ketones: Negative   _____

g. pH: 5.2   _____

h. Glucose: Positive   _____

i. Red blood cells: 8/high-power field   _____

j. Crystals: Negative   _____

3. Completing a Laboratory Requisition Form

a. Complete the sample reference laboratory requisition form, example found in the documentation section in the back of the book, using appropriate information from the following case.

The physician has seen a young female patient in the office who has been complaining of vague abdominal pain, slight weight gain, fatigue, some nausea, and occasional fever. You have been asked to collect a urine specimen for this patient for a complete urinalysis and a qualitative urine pregnancy test. Your office does not perform any laboratory testing in-house.

The patient's name is Mary Elizabeth Arnold, age 24. The physician's name is Dr. Travis Buffett; his UPIN number is 123456.

The shaded areas must be completed or the reference laboratory will reject the specimen. Remember that you must fill in the date and time of the collection even though those areas are not shaded in; use today's date and time. Do not forget to mark which tests are being requested. In addition, note the patient's unique control number, which the reference laboratory will use to track the specimen.

b. Complete the sample reference laboratory requisition form, example found in the documentation section in the back of the book, using appropriate information from the following case.

An elderly patient by the name of William Overtell has seen the physician in the office today. The physician suspects that this patient may be entering the early phases of kidney failure based on the patient's clinical picture. A key test in diagnosing a condition of this type can be a 24-hour urine specimen.

After measurement of the total volume of the 24-hour specimen, a small sample is prepared to forward to the reference laboratory for analysis. The physician's name is Dr. Felicia Mills and her UPIN number is 98765443. Because the patient has Medicare, the physician cannot bill the patient for the testing. The patient's Medicare number (112-33-5588B) must be provided in the appropriate block on the requisition form so that the laboratory can bill the insurance carrier directly. The total volume of the specimen was 980 mL.

Identify the test number assigned to this test on the requisition form. Also, to ensure proper collection, detail the specific instructions that should be provided to the patient prior to the collection of the specimen.

CASE STUDIES

Write your response to each case study on the lines provided.

Case 1

A patient telephones and tells you she is concerned about not having a means at home of disinfecting a jar for a urine specimen. How would you respond to the patient?

_____

_____

_____

Case 2

You notice that the lid has been left off a urine specimen container that you are supposed to test for ketone bodies. Should you perform the test? Why or why not?

_____

_____

_____

Case 3

You open a fresh container of reagent test strips 5 months before the expiration date marked on the container. You note that the test strips are not discolored. What should your next step be?

_____

_____

_____

Case 4

Elizabeth comes to the office on a very hot day. She says she has been working outside all day and hasn't had much to drink. After you perform her urinalysis, you note that she has an abnormal urine specific gravity. Would you expect the urine specific gravity to be elevated or decreased? Why?

_____

_____

_____

CHAPTER 17

Collecting, Processing, and Testing Blood Specimens

REVIEW

Vocabulary Review

True or False

Decide whether each statement is true or false. In the space at the left, write T *for true or* F *for false. On the lines provided, rewrite the false statements to make them true.*

_____ 1. The main component of erythrocytes is hemoglobin.

_____

_____ 2. The engulfing of invading bacteria is known as lymphocytosis.

_____

_____ 3. Red blood cells, or microphils, are one component of blood.

_____

_____ 4. The function of B lymphocytes is to produce antibodies that combat specific pathogens.

_____

_____ 5. A white blood cell with a solid nucleus and clear cytoplasm is an agranulocyte.

_____

_____ 6. Monocytes, large white blood cells, have oval or horseshoe-shaped nuclei.

_____

_____ 7. A small, calibrated glass tube that holds a small, precise volume of fluid is a hematocrit.

_____

_____ 8. When counting RBCs and WBCs, you use a concentrated blood sample and a hemocytometer.

_____

_____ 9. Hemoglobin is released during hemolysis, the rupturing of red blood cells.

_____

_____ 10. Capillary puncture requires a superficial puncture of the skin with a sharp point.

_____

_____ 11. Neutrophils have a light green nucleus and pale pink cytoplasm, which contains fine pink or lavender granules.

_____

_____ **12.** Through hematocrit determination, you can identify how much of the volume of a sample of blood is made up of red blood cells after the sample has been spun in a centrifuge.

_____

_____ **13.** In a tube of blood that has been spun in a centrifuge, the packed red blood cells are separated from the white blood cells by the buffy coat.

_____

_____ **14.** A complete blood count is a type of serologic test.

_____

_____ **15.** An erythrocyte sedimentation rate (ESR) test measures the rate at which red blood cells settle to the bottom of a blood sample.

_____

_____ **16.** A hematocrit is a test that measures the percentage of white blood cells in a blood sample.

_____

Matching

Match the key terms in the right column with the definitions in the left column by placing the letter of each correct answer in the space provided.

_____ **17.** The liquid part of blood in which other components are suspended

_____ **18.** The process of blood clotting

_____ **19.** The study of the shape or form of objects

_____ **20.** The portion of blood volume that includes red blood cells, white blood cells, and platelets

_____ **21.** The insertion of a needle into a vein for the purpose of withdrawing blood

_____ **22.** Granular leukocytes that capture invading bacteria and antigenantibody complexes

_____ **23.** The rupturing of blood cells

_____ **24.** A white blood cell

_____ **25.** The fever-producing substance released by a neutrophil

_____ **26.** A white blood cell with a solid nucleus and clear cytoplasm

_____ **27.** A winged infusion set

_____ **28.** Clear, yellow liquid that remains after a blood clot forms

_____ **29.** The area of a spun sample of blood that contains the white blood cells and platelets

_____ **30.** A nongranular leukocyte that regulates immunologic response

_____ **31.** The heaviest part of whole blood, which moves to one end of a microhematocrit tube after being spun in a centrifuge

_____ **32.** A blood collection device that includes a double-pointed needle, a plastic needle holder, and collection tubes

a. agranular leukocyte
b. phlebotomy
c. eosinophils
d. serum
e. morphology
f. pyrogen
g. formed elements
h. buffy coat
i. plasma
j. evacuation system
k. venipuncture
l. packed red blood cells
m. coagulation
n. butterfly system
o. leukocyte
p. T lymphocyte
q. tourniquet
r. hemolysis

_____ 33. A flat, broad length of vinyl or rubber used during venipuncture procedures

_____ 34. The puncture of a vein

Content Review

Multiple Choice

In the space provided, write the letter of the choice that best completes each statement or answers each question.

_____ 1. Blood is transported throughout the body by the
  A. circulatory system.
  B. plasma.
  C. hemoglobin.
  D. transrespiratory system.

_____ 2. Which of the following gives red blood cells their color?
  A. Hemoglobin
  B. Hemolysis
  C. Oxygen
  D. B lymphocyte

_____ 3. The study of blood is known as
  A. morphology.
  B. cytology.
  C. histology.
  D. hematology.
  E. cardiology.

_____ 4. Other than assembling the equipment and supplies necessary, the first step in preparing to draw blood is reviewing the
  A. patient's blood type.
  B. procedure with the patient.
  C. written request for the test.
  D. health of the patient.

_____ 5. A small, disposable instrument with a sharp point used to puncture the skin and make a small incision is a
  A. micropipette.
  B. lancet.
  C. syringe.
  D. tourniquet.
  E. butterfly device.

_____ 6. Fragments of megakaryocytes are known as
  A. neutrophils.
  B. basophils.
  C. red blood cells.
  D. monocytes.
  E. thrombocytes.

_____ 7. Which of the following methods of blood collection would be best to use with patients who have small or fragile veins?
   A. Evacuation system
   B. VACUTAINER system
   C. Butterfly system
   D. Venipuncture

_____ 8. Lancets are used
   A. when the amount of blood required for a procedure is not large.
   B. when the amount of blood required for a procedure is large.
   C. for infants only.
   D. for adults only.

_____ 9. A test used to monitor the health of a patient with diabetes is a
   A. complete blood count.
   B. hemoglobin A1c.
   C. creatine kinase.
   D. ESR.
   E. differential count.

Sentence Completion

In the space provided, write the word or phrase that best completes each sentence.

10. When drawing a patient's blood, you should make no more than _____ attempts.

11. Patients often fear that the more tubes of blood you require, _____.

12. Probably the greatest fear of patients undergoing blood tests is contracting _____.

13. The total volume of plasma and formed elements comprises _____.

14. _____ form a gel-like barrier between serum and the clot in a coagulated blood sample.

15. The process of clotting is called _____.

16. The normal range for a total carbon dioxide blood test is _____.

17. _____ are the first line of defense during a phlebotomy procedure.

10. _____

11. _____

12. _____

13. _____

14. _____

15. _____

16. _____

17. _____

Short Answer

Write the answer to each question on the lines provided.

18. Why might you need to wear a mask during a phlebotomy procedure?

_____

_____

_____

19. What two goals are met by wearing personal protective equipment during phlebotomy procedures?

_____

_____

_____

20. Describe three advantages of an evacuation system of blood drawing.

_____

_____

_____

21. How can you prevent infections caused by phlebotomy?

_____

_____

_____

22. Describe the biggest challenge in blood drawing that children present.

_____

_____

_____

23. Describe how you would determine the concentration of hemoglobin in a blood sample.

_____

_____

_____

24. Describe two desired characteristics of engineered safety devices.

_____

_____

_____

25. The illustration below shows several types of blood cells. On the lines provided, write the name and a brief description of each cell's function.

A. 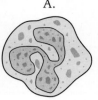 B.  C. 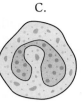 D.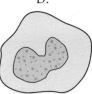

E.   F. 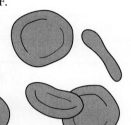 G.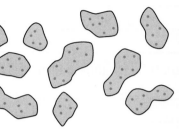

A. _____ B. _____ C. _____

_____ _____ _____

_____ _____ _____

D. _____ E. _____ F. _____

_____ _____ _____

_____ _____ _____

G. _____

_____

_____

Critical Thinking

Write the answer to each question on the lines provided.

1. Why is it important to dispose of sharps promptly using approved sharps containers?

_____

_____

_____

2. What should you do if you suffer a needlestick injury?

_____

_____

_____

3. Why is it important to be absolutely sure of the meaning of any abbreviations used in laboratory work?

_____

_____

_____

4. Why is it important to identify the patient correctly before drawing blood?

_____

_____

_____

5. What are the advantages of pen-like capillary puncture devices?

_____

_____

_____

APPLICATION

Follow the directions for each application.

1. **Identifying Blood Test Collection Tubes**

   For each test listed, name the color and additive of the collection tube used to perform the test.

   a. Creatine kinase _____

   b. Bilirubin _____

   c. Leukocyte count _____

   d. Fasting glucose _____

   e. Phenylalanine _____

   f. Prothrombin _____

   g. Thyroid stimulating hormone _____

   h. Complete blood count _____

2. **Collecting Blood Specimens**

   Practice each technique or role-play each situation below with a partner. Critique each other by using the space provided to note pointers and suggestions that you think will help the other person perform the technique better. For situations in which you draw blood, use a mannequin arm. If a mannequin arm is not available, attach a piece of rubber tubing to a rolled piece of fabric. Then tape over a portion of the tubing to simulate skin.

   a. Venipuncture with a needle and syringe

   _____

   _____

   b. Preparing a smear slide

   _____

   _____

c. Capillary puncture with an automatic puncturing device

_____

_____

d. Preparing patients for blood drawing

_____

_____

e. Handling a patient who faints during blood drawing

_____

_____

3. Completing a Laboratory Requisition Form

a. Complete the sample reference laboratory requisition form, example on page 579, using appropriate information from the following case.

> A female patient was seen in the physician's office today. After examining the patient and reviewing her history, the physician has requested that blood be drawn for the following tests: thyroid profile II, basic chemistry, and total glycohemoglobin.
> The patient's name is Janice Jondahl, age 56. The physician's name is Dr. Rebecca Adamson; her UPIN number is 97644521.

Remember to use today's date and time for the specimen date and time and do not omit any of the shaded areas. After completing the form, name the type of specimen and tube type that are required according to the requisition form. In addition, note the test numbers assigned to each of the tests requested by the physician.

b. Complete the sample reference laboratory requisition form, example on page 579, using appropriate information from the following case.

> Charles Riffe, age 83, has seen Dr. Domingo Krishnan in the office today for a follow-up for high blood cholesterol, which has been an ongoing problem for him. The physician has placed the patient on a cholesterol-reducing medication for six weeks now and has asked that this patient return the next morning without eating to have the following blood tests drawn: lipid profile I to include a lipoprotein analysis, glucose, and a liver profile A (to rule out liver damage from the prescribed medication).
> The patient has Medicare, which means that the physician cannot bill the patient for the service. The patient's Medicare number, 678-35-0022B, must be provided to the reference laboratory in order for the laboratory to bill the insurance carrier directly.

Remember to use today's date and time for the specimen collection date and time. After completing the form, answer the following questions:

1. Why would the physician request that the patient return the next day without having eaten?

2. What are the specimen requirements for the tests requested?

3. Is there any information missing from this scenario that you must have before sending the specimen to the reference laboratory?

CASE STUDIES

Write your response to each case study on the lines provided.

Case 1

While you are preparing a patient for a blood test, she asks whether her symptoms are signs of rheumatoid arthritis. How should you respond?

_____

_____

_____

Case 2

A patient arrived in the office for a blood test. What steps should you follow, from this moment to the time you draw the blood?

_____

_____

_____

Case 3

As you are assembling the equipment for drawing blood from a patient, you notice her eyeing the needle and tubes nervously. She then asks, "Will this hurt?" As you draw the blood, the patient comments, "I guess this test is pretty common, right? I mean, do you usually need so many tubes of blood?" How should you respond to her concerns?

_____

_____

_____

Case 4

While performing a capillary puncture, you notice the patient's hands are very cold. What should you do?

_____

_____

_____

Case 5

You have been asked to prepare a blood sample for transport to an outside lab. How should you do this?

_____

_____

_____

CHAPTER 18

Nutrition and Special Diets

REVIEW

Vocabulary Review

True or False

Decide whether each statement is true or false. In the space at the left, write T for true or F for false. On the lines provided, rewrite the false statements to make them true.

_____ 1. Antigens are chemical agents that fight cell-destroying free radicals.

_____

_____ 2. Amino acids are natural compounds found in plant and animal foods and are used by the body to create protein.

_____

_____ 3. Cholesterol is a fat-related substance that the body produces in the liver and that is also obtained from dietary sources.

_____

_____ 4. Incomplete proteins lack one or more of the essential amino acids.

_____

_____ 5. Starch is the tough, stringy part of vegetables and grains that is not absorbed by the body but aids in a variety of bodily functions.

_____

_____ 6. Proteins that contain all nine essential amino acids are complete proteins.

_____

_____ 7. Complete proteins are also known as polysaccharides.

_____

_____ 8. Lipoproteins are large molecules that are water-soluble on the inside, are fat-soluble on the outside, and carry carbohydrates through the bloodstream.

_____

_____ 9. Saturated fats are derived from animal sources, are clear and liquid at room temperature, and tend to raise blood cholesterol.

_____

_____ 10. Triglycerides are simple lipids that consist of glycerol and three fatty acids.

_____

_____ 11. Minerals are natural, inorganic substances the body needs to help build and maintain body tissues and carry on life functions.

_____

Matching

Match the key terms in the right column with the definitions in the left column by placing the letter of each correct answer in the space provided.

_____ 12. A method of feeding patients who cannot tolerate receiving supplements by way of the digestive tract

_____ 13. The phase of metabolism in which substances are changed into more complex substances and used to build body tissues

_____ 14. An eating disorder in which people starve themselves

_____ 15. The phase of metabolism when complex substances are broken down into simpler substances and converted into energy

_____ 16. A dietary system, used especially with diabetics, in which portions of foods in each of six categories are interchangeable

_____ 17. A large molecule that is fat-soluble on the inside and water-soluble on the outside

_____ 18. A procedure used to measure a person's percentage of body fat

_____ 19. When a person gets too little or loses too much water

_____ 20. Patient with this condition requires a high-fiber diet

_____ 21. A facet of weight loss or weight management that encourages people to change their eating habits

_____ 22. A standard measure for the amount of energy that a food produces in the body

_____ 23. The intolerance of the protein gluten, which causes damage to the intestines

_____ 24. A simple lipid made of glycerol and three fatty acids

_____ 25. An eating disorder in which people binge on food and then try to counter the effects through vomiting, laxatives, and/or excessive exercise

a. anabolism
b. anorexia nervosa
c. behavior modification
d. bulimia
e. calorie
f. catabolism
g. food exchange
h. lipoprotein
i. parenteral nutrition
j. skinfold test
k. triglyceride
l. dehydration
m. diverticulosis
n. celiac disease

Content Review

Multiple Choice

In the space provided, write the letter of the choice that best completes each statement or answers each question.

_____ 1. Which of the following nutrients can help prevent diverticular disease, constipation, and irritable bowel syndrome?

    A. Lipids

    B. Calcium

    C. Fiber

    D. Electrolytes

    E. Complete proteins

_____ 2. An increased risk of heart disease, stroke, and peripheral vascular disease has been linked with high levels of
A. lipoproteins and unsaturated fats.
B. triglycerides and cholesterol.
C. vitamins A and K.
D. iron and fluoride.
E. folate.

_____ 3. Which of the following is *not* a function of water in the human body?
A. Aiding in digestion
B. Promoting the healing of wounds
C. Regulating body temperature
D. Lubricating the body's moving parts

_____ 4. Which of the following statements about diet therapy is false?
A. Diet therapy sometimes involves restricting certain foods.
B. Diet therapy may involve changing the number of meals per day.
C. Physicians and dietitians cooperate to determine which diet therapy is best for a patient.
D. Diet therapy always involves lowering the daily caloric intake.

_____ 5. In terms of general nutrition, elderly patients should
A. decrease their fiber intake.
B. increase their caloric intake.
C. increase their fat intake by 10% to 15%.
D. supplement their diets with massive amounts of iron and vitamin C.
E. decrease their caloric intake but not their protein intake.

_____ 6. Dietary guidelines that aim to lessen the risk of heart attack recommend choosing a diet that is
A. low in saturated fats and cholesterol.
B. low in fiber.
C. moderate in sugars.
D. high in salt.

_____ 7. What is the chief difference between a full-liquid diet and a clear-liquid diet?
A. A full-liquid diet is higher in carbohydrates.
B. A full-liquid diet includes strained cooked cereals and soups.
C. A clear-liquid diet contains large amounts of fiber.
D. A clear-liquid diet is higher in proteins.

_____ 8. The term *reduced cholesterol* on a food label means that the food has
A. less than or equal to 2 mg of cholesterol per serving.
B. less than or equal to 20 mg of cholesterol per serving.
C. at least 25% less cholesterol per serving than the food it replaces.
D. at least 50% less cholesterol per serving than the food it replaces.
E. at least 75% less cholesterol per serving than the food it replaces.

_____ 9. A sign of bulimia is
A. self-starvation.
B. cessation of menstruation.
C. weight gain.
D. the buying and consuming of large quantities of food.

_____ **10.** The 2005 USDA Dietary Guidelines encourage people to do all of the following *except*

  A. get more sleep.

  B. increase physical activity.

  C. eat a well-balanced diet from all food groups.

  D. limit alcohol consumption.

  E. maintain or reduce weight.

Sentence Completion

In the space provided, write the word or phrase that best completes each sentence.

11. A(n) _____ is a health professional who designs ways for people to obtain optimal nourishment on the basis of the science of nutrition.

12. _____ fiber, found in the bran in whole wheat bread and brown rice, promotes regular bowel movements by contributing to stool bulk.

13. The Recommended Daily Allowance of vitamin C for an adult is _____.

14. The _____ on the USDA 2005 Food Guide Pyramid represents physical activity.

15. Iron deficiency can cause _____, a blood disorder that can leave a person fatigued, weak, and mentally impaired.

16. The dietary guidelines developed by the _____ encourage people to be moderate in their consumption of processed and red meats.

17. Wheat, milk, eggs, and chocolate are some of the most common food _____.

18. Patients with diabetes should not miss a meal because skipping meals disturbs the balance of _____.

19. You can learn about a packaged food's caloric, fat, and sodium content per serving by reading the _____.

20. Patient education has become increasingly important because managed care providers want to see documentation of _____ in patients' charts.

11. _____

12. _____

13. _____

14. _____

15. _____

16. _____

17. _____

18. _____

19. _____

20. _____

Short Answer

Write the answer to each question on the lines provided.

21. What are the three major ways in which the human body uses nutrients?

_____

_____

_____

22. What are RDAs? Why do you need to know about them?

_____

_____

_____

23. What is the Food Guide Pyramid? How can you use it to achieve a balanced diet?

_____

_____

_____

24. Under what circumstances might a doctor be likely to prescribe a diet to help a patient gain weight?

_____

_____

_____

25. Describe five guidelines that you can follow when discussing diets with a patient.

_____

_____

_____

26. How is the Diabetes Food Pyramid different from the USDA Food Guide Pyramid?

_____

_____

_____

27. What are the recommendations by the American Cancer Society to prevent cancer?

_____

_____

_____

28. The 2005 Food Guide Pyramid is color-coded. What are the colors and foods represented by them?

_____

_____

_____

29. List the recommended foods for each of the following patients.

    a. 1½-year-old child _____

    _____

    b. 10-month-old infant _____

    _____

    c. 3-month-old infant _____

    _____

Critical Thinking

Write the answer to each question on the lines provided.

  1. Cities that host marathons often provide a spaghetti dinner for participants who want to "carbo-load" the night before the race. Why would marathon runners want to eat a lot of carbohydrates?

_____

_____

_____

2. What is the difference between transfat and saturated fat?

_____

_____

_____

3. Why is behavior modification generally more successful than fad dieting when it comes to long-term weight loss?

_____

_____

_____

4. Why is it important to take factors of culture and religion into account when planning a patient's diet?

_____

_____

_____

5. Explain the key recommendation within the 2005 USDA Dietary Guidelines to "maintain an adequate nutrient intake while monitoring caloric needs."

_____

_____

_____

APPLICATION

Follow the directions for each application.

1. Modifying Diets

Using the Internet, research diabetic diet exchanges and prepare a travel diet for a diabetic patient. Suggestions for research include the American Diabetes Association or American Dietetic Association.

2. Preparing Patient Education Materials

In teams of three or four, choose a disease or condition for each team to research, such as hyperlipidemia, hypertension, food allergies, or another condition. Each team should design a poster or informational booklet describing the disease and diet restrictions. Each team should present their findings to the class for discussion.

3. Educating Patients

Role-play educating a patient about his daily water requirements, food allergies, how to read food labels, and a special diet. Use the sample progress note form on page 591 to document your patient education.

CASE STUDIES

Write your response to each case study on the lines provided.

Case 1

You hear Joe, another medical assistant in your office, talking to a patient about the diet the doctor has prescribed. Joe says, "Well, if you really like red meat, go ahead and eat it. Just try to cut back your fat intake from other foods." What, if anything, has Joe done wrong?

_____

_____

_____

Case 2

"Why is the doctor telling me to cut back on beer?" complains Mr. Kowalski, who is being treated for hypertension. "I've heard that beer can be good for you!" How should you respond?

_____

_____

_____

Case 3

The doctor has just prescribed a low-cholesterol diet for Mrs. Ryan. "But how am I supposed to know how much cholesterol my food has?" she asks you. How could you help Mrs. Ryan?

_____

_____

_____

CHAPTER **19**

Principles of Pharmacology

REVIEW

Vocabulary Review

Matching

Match the key terms in the right column with the definitions in the left column by placing the letter of each correct answer in the space provided.

_____ 1. A drug's official name

_____ 2. The study of what drugs do to the body

_____ 3. A drug or drug product that is categorized as potentially dangerous or addictive

_____ 4. The amount of a drug given at one time

_____ 5. The process of converting a drug from its dose form to a form the body can use

_____ 6. The process of transporting a drug from its administration site to its site of action

_____ 7. A preparation administered to a person to produce reduced sensitivity, or increased immunity, to an infectious disease

_____ 8. Pertaining to medicinal drugs

_____ 9. Produces opium-like effects

_____ 10. Absorption, distribution, metabolism, and excretion

_____ 11. Government term for opioid

_____ 12. The study of drugs

_____ 13. Also called clinical pharmacology

_____ 14. Study of the characteristics of natural drugs and their sources

_____ 15. The study of poisons or poisonous effects of drugs

_____ 16. To give a drug by any route that introduces the drug into a patient's body

_____ 17. A drug's brand or proprietary name

_____ 18. The therapeutic value of a drug

_____ 19. A physician's written order to authorize the dispensing (and, sometimes, administering) of a drug to a patient

_____ 20. The purpose or reason for using a drug

a. toxicology
b. dose
c. pharmacodynamics
d. absorption
e. indication
f. administer
g. vaccine
h. efficacy
i. opioid
j. trade name
k. controlled substance
l. generic name
m. prescription
n. distribution
o. pharmaceutical
p. pharmacokinetics
q. pharmacotherapeutics
r. pharmacognosy
s. prescribe
t. narcotic

True or False

Decide whether each statement is true or false. In the space at the left, write T *for true or* F *for false. On the lines provided, rewrite the false statements to make them true.*

_____ **21.** Pharmacology is the study of the characteristics of natural drugs and their sources.

_____

_____ **22.** The study of what the body does to drugs is known as pharmacokinesis.

_____

_____ **23.** Pharmacotherapeutics is the study of the chemical properties of drugs.

_____

_____ **24.** A doctor prescribes a drug by giving a patient a prescription to be filled by a pharmacy.

_____

_____ **25.** Drugs are eliminated from the body through absorption.

_____

_____ **26.** Labeling for a drug includes the purpose or reason for using the drug and the form of the drug.

_____

_____ **27.** A drug's dosage refers to the size of each dose.

_____

_____ **28.** Prescription drugs are medications that can be used only by order of a physician.

_____

_____ **29.** An opioid is a Schedule I substance.

_____

_____ **30.** Narcotics such as codeine, morphine, and meperidine have a lower abuse potential than Schedule IV drugs.

_____

Content Review

Multiple Choice

In the space provided, write the letter of the choice that best completes each statement or answers each question.

_____ **1.** Bacteria and fungi are simple organisms used to make
 A. antiserums and antitoxins.
 B. antibiotics.
 C. enzymes.
 D. antacids.
 E. ointments.

_____ **2.** Which of the following is the generic name for a medication that lowers cholesterol?
 A. Raloxifene
 B. Toprol XL
 C. Tramadol
 D. Atorvastatin

_____ 3. Administering morphine to reduce the accompanying pain of cancer is an example of
  A. maintenance drug therapy.
  B. curative drug therapy.
  C. supplemental drug therapy.
  D. prophylactic drug therapy.
  E. palliative drug therapy.

_____ 4. The government agency that regulates the manufacture and distribution of all drugs in the United States is known as the
  A. Drug Enforcement Agency.
  B. Federal Drug Administration.
  C. Federal Bureau of Investigation.
  D. Occupational Safety and Health Administration.

_____ 5. The study of adverse reactions or drug interactions is referred to as
  A. toxicology.
  B. pharmacology.
  C. infectious disease.
  D. virology.
  E. pathology.

_____ 6. Which types of drugs cannot be renewed without a written order or prescription?
  A. Schedule I
  B. Schedule II
  C. Schedule III
  D. Schedule IV

_____ 7. A doctor who needs Schedule II drugs for his or her practice must order them using
  A. DEA form 214.
  B. DEA form 41.
  C. DEA form 222.
  D. DEA form 224.
  E. DEA form 41 and DEA form 224.

_____ 8. Which of the following is the generic name for a medication that controls seizures?
  A. Escitalopram oxalate
  B. Zolpidem
  C. Celebrex
  D. Gabapentin

_____ 9. According to the Controlled Substances Act of 1970, physicians are not allowed to prescribe drugs in which of the following schedules?
  A. Schedule IV
  B. Schedule III
  C. Schedule I
  D. Schedule II
  E. Schedule V

_____ **10.** Which of the following generic medications is used for reducing the symptoms and duration of a herpetic infection?
   A. Quinapril
   B. Valacyclovir
   C. Sildenafil citrate
   D. Concerta

_____ **11.** Which of the following is one of the top 50 drugs and is given to treat asthma?
   A. Plavix
   B. Fosamax
   C. Lansoprazole
   D. Zyrtec
   E. Advair Diskus

_____ **12.** What is the most likely reason someone would take the medication Zetia?
   A. to reduce blood pressure
   B. to reduce cholesterol
   C. to reduce depression
   D. to replace a hormone

Sentence Completion

In the space provided, write the word or phrase that best completes each sentence.

13. Antiserums and antitoxins for vaccines are examples of _____ substances used as drugs.

14. Tablets and capsules are absorbed through the stomach or intestines into the _____.

15. Drug metabolism usually takes place in the _____.

16. Distribution can pertain to the length of time between dosing and _____ in the bloodstream.

17. Pharmacotherapeutics is sometimes called _____.

18. A drug's trade name is selected by, is copyrighted by, and is the property of its _____.

19. A nonprescription, or _____, drug is one that the FDA has approved for use without the supervision of a licensed health-care practitioner.

20. A physician's written order that authorizes the dispensing and administering of drugs to a patient is called a(n) _____.

21. The official name of a drug is called the _____.

22. The purpose or reason for using a drug is called the _____.

23. A popular drug reference book used by physician practices is called the _____.

24. A drug that is potentially dangerous and addictive is referred to as a(n) _____.

25. A drug that is used to prevent diseases in children and adults is called _____.

13. _____

14. _____

15. _____

16. _____

17. _____

18. _____

19. _____

20. _____

21. _____

22. _____

23. _____

24. _____

25. _____

Name _____ Class _____ Date _____

Short Answer

Write the answer to each question on the lines provided.

26. What are the regulatory functions of the Food and Drug Administration (FDA) with regard to drugs?

_____

_____

_____

27. What are the four processes of pharmacokinetics?

_____

_____

_____

28. In what ways are drugs excreted?

_____

_____

_____

29. What is out-of-labeling prescribing?

_____

_____

_____

30. What factors determine the safety of a drug?

_____

_____

_____

31. List four main sources of drug information, and describe the contents of each.

a. _____

_____

b. _____

_____

c. _____

_____

d. _____

_____

32. How does regulation of the use of an OTC drug differ from that of a prescription drug?

_____

_____

_____

33. Compare how the five schedules of drugs described in the Controlled Substances Act of 1970 differ according to degree of potential abuse or nontherapeutic effects of the drugs in each schedule.

_____

_____

_____

34. What requirements does the CSA place on doctors who administer, dispense, or prescribe any controlled substance?

_____

_____

_____

35. Explain how controlled substances are identified on their labels.

_____

_____

_____

36. How does the ordering of Schedule II drugs differ from the ordering of drugs from Schedules III, IV, and V?

_____

_____

_____

37. List in order the four parts of a prescription and explain what information is contained in each part.

   a. _____

_____

   b. _____

_____

   c. _____

_____

   d. _____

_____

38. Complete the following chart.

Action of Drug	Drug Category	Example Generic Name	Example Trade Name
a. Counteracts effects of histamine and relieves allergic symptoms	_____	Cetirizine	_____
b. Dilates blood vessels, decreases blood pressure	_____	Nitroglycerin	_____
c. Increases urine output, reduces blood pressure and cardiac output	_____	Furosemide	_____
d. Kills microorganisms or inhibits or prevents their growth	_____	Azithromycin	_____
e. Normalizes heartbeat in cases of certain cardiac arrhythmias	_____	Propafenone Hydrochloride	_____
f. Prevents blood from clotting	_____	Warfarin sodium	_____
g. Prevents or relieves nausea and vomiting	_____	Prochlorperazine	_____
h. Prevents sensation of pain (generally, locally, or topically)	_____	Lidocaine HCl	_____
i. Reduces blood pressure	_____	Quinapril	_____
j. Reduces fever	_____	Acetaminophen	_____
k. Reduces inflammation	_____	Triamcinoline	_____
l. Relieves depression	_____	Escitalopram	_____
m. Relieves diarrhea	_____	Loperamide HCl	_____
n. Relieves mild to severe pain	_____	Oxycodone HCl	_____
o. Relieves or controls convulsions	_____	Divalproex	_____
p. Reduces blood sugar	_____	Metformin	_____

39. Identify the purpose of each part of the package insert pictured here.

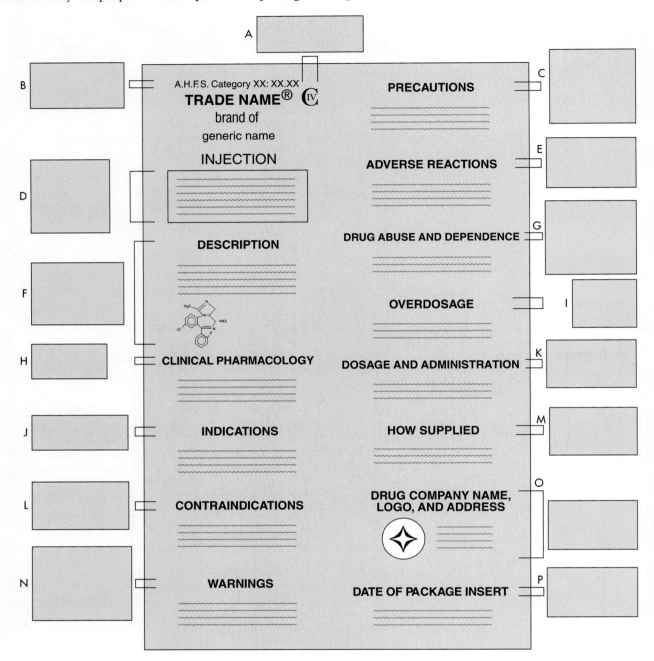

A

B

C — PRECAUTIONS

D

E — ADVERSE REACTIONS

F

G — DRUG ABUSE AND DEPENDENCE

H — CLINICAL PHARMACOLOGY

I — OVERDOSAGE

J — INDICATIONS

K — DOSAGE AND ADMINISTRATION

L — CONTRAINDICATIONS

M — HOW SUPPLIED

N — WARNINGS

O — DRUG COMPANY NAME, LOGO, AND ADDRESS

P — DATE OF PACKAGE INSERT

A.H.F.S. Category XX: XX.XX
TRADE NAME® Ⓒ IV
brand of
generic name
INJECTION

DESCRIPTION

Critical Thinking

Write the answer to each question on the lines provided.

1. Why do clinical studies include both healthy individuals and patients?

_____

_____

_____

2. Why is it important that patients inform their pharmacist of all prescription and OTC drugs they are currently taking when medication is prescribed for them?

_____

_____

_____

3. What are the actions and differences of the following types of antihypertensives? Use the *PDR* or another drug reference.

   a. Calcium channel blockers

   b. ACE inhibitors

   c. Beta blockers

   d. Diuretics

_____

_____

_____

4. Why is it important that the patient chart be consulted before a prescription refill is authorized?

_____

_____

_____

5. What is the first thing a medical assistant does if a patient requests drug samples?

_____

_____

_____

6. A pregnant patient is taking the following medications. Using a drug resource, determine the pregnancy category for each medication and discuss why it should or should not be taken by the patient.

   a. Dilantin

   b. Paracetamol

   c. Amoxicillin

   d. Accutane

   e. Codeine

_____

_____

_____

APPLICATION

Follow the directions for each application.

1. Interpreting Prescriptions

The physician has written the following prescriptions. Interpret each prescription on the lines provided.

a. Proloprim 200 mg 10 caps

Sig l cap po daily. 10 d

_____

b. Nasalide 25 mL nasal sol

Sig ll sprays t.i.d. PRN

_____

c. Furosemide oral sol (10 mg/mL)

Sig 1 tsp po b.i.d.

_____

d. Nitro-Dur 0.3 mg transdermal nitroglycerin infusion system

Sig 1 patch daily

_____

e. Cylert 18.75 mg 14 tabs

Sig ll tabs po qam 7 d

_____

2. Conducting an Inventory of Dispensed Controlled Drugs

On a separate sheet of paper, write an office procedural plan for conducting a controlled drug inventory. The procedure should include the following information:

- How often the inventory is to be conducted
- Information you must have about each drug
- Where this information is obtained for Schedule II drugs
- Where this information is obtained for Schedules III, IV, and V drugs
- How the information for each drug is processed
- What records must be included in the inventory
- How the inventory is retained
- How long the inventory is retained

3. Charting Prescription Refills on a Progress Note

Read each of the cases below and chart the information on the progress note, example provided in the back of the workbook on page 591.

a. A patient calls in a refill for Lexapro 10 mg. She takes one tablet per day. Her pharmacy number is 216-444-0000. She states that she has no known drug allergies. She was authorized 4 refills.

b. The pharmacy calls for a refill for Mr. Smith. He would like his Ativan 1gr refilled. He has not been seen in the office in 6 months and the physician does not authorize the refill.

c. A patient calls to confirm the correct dosage and dosing schedule for her prescription of Zithromax that she received that morning.

d. A patient calls in a refill for Zocor 40 mg, one tablet per day. The physician authorized 3 refills.

CASE STUDIES

Write your response to each case study on the lines provided.

Case 1

You are interviewing a new patient who has arrived with her one-month-old child. The patient tells you that over-the-counter medication she has been taking for allergies does not seem to be working. She thinks she may need a prescription drug for her allergies. What are two important questions you should ask this patient in case the doctor prescribes medication?

_____

_____

_____

Case 2

Your workplace has been burglarized. Schedules III, IV, and V drugs were stolen. (Your workplace does not administer or dispense Schedule II drugs.) What should you do?

_____

_____

_____

Case 3

The physician has written a prescription for Achromycin, 250-mg capsules. After checking a drug reference, you find that Achromycin is a trade name for tetracycline HCl, a generic drug that is available in 250-mg capsules at a lower cost than Achromycin. Returning to the prescription, you note that the physician has failed to check the "Generic Equivalent OK" box on the prescription form. What do you do?

_____

_____

_____

CHAPTER 20

Drug Administration

REVIEW

Vocabulary Review

Matching

Match the key terms in the right column with the definitions in the left column by placing the letter of each correct answer in the space provided.

_____ 1. Liquid used to dissolve and dilute a drug

_____ 2. Beneath the skin

_____ 3. The amount of space a drug occupies

_____ 4. A technique of IM injection that prevents a drug from leaking into the subcutaneous tissue and causing irritation

_____ 5. Between the cheek and gum

_____ 6. Within the upper layers of the skin

_____ 7. The way a drug is introduced into the body

_____ 8. Under the tongue

_____ 9. Slow drip

_____ 10. Salve

_____ 11. Through the skin

_____ 12. Vaginal irrigation

_____ 13. Within a muscle

_____ 14. A homogeneous mixture of a solid, liquid, or gaseous substance in a liquid

_____ 15. Directly into a vein

a. solution
b. intramuscular (IM)
c. Z-track method
d. buccal
e. intravenous (IV)
f. infusion
g. volume
h. intradermal (ID)
i. transdermal
j. douche
k. ointment
l. route
m. diluent
n. sublingual
o. subcutaneous (SC)

Content Review

Multiple Choice

In the space provided, write the letter of the choice that best completes each statement or answers each question.

_____ 1. A volume of 10 cubic centimeters is equal to

    A. 0.01 mL.

    B. 1.0 mL.

    C. 10 mL.

    D. 1000 mL.

    E. 0.001 mL.

_____ **2.** Inhalation therapy can be administered through the nose or
- **A.** ear.
- **B.** eye.
- **C.** mouth.
- **D.** skin.

_____ **3.** Which of the following forms of drugs is administered by a transdermal route?
- **A.** Capsule
- **B.** Pill
- **C.** Spray
- **D.** Patch
- **E.** Suppository

_____ **4.** The office sharps container should be properly disposed of when it is
- **A.** one-third full.
- **B.** two-thirds full.
- **C.** almost full.
- **D.** full.

_____ **5.** What information must you ask a patient every time before administering an injection?
- **A.** Blood pressure results
- **B.** Age
- **C.** Route preference
- **D.** Any known drug allergies
- **E.** Weight

_____ **6.** What is the best site for administering an intramuscular injection for a pediatric patient?
- **A.** Deltoid
- **B.** Dorsogluteal
- **C.** Vastus lateralis
- **D.** Bicep

_____ **7.** You are administering a sublingual medication. Which education statement would be correct?
- **A.** Place the medication between your cheek and gum until it dissolves.
- **B.** Place the medication under you tongue and then take a drink of water.
- **C.** Take a drink of water then swallow this pill with your second drink of water.
- **D.** Inhale the medication, holding your breath for 30 seconds after each inhalation.
- **E.** Place the medication under your tongue until it dissolves.

_____ **8.** Why should you wear gloves during the administration of a transdermal patch?
- **A.** To prevent contamination of the patch
- **B.** To prevent the medication from getting on your skin
- **C.** To keep the patch sterile until it is administered
- **D.** To prevent infection

_____ **9.** When administering eyedrops, how far should the bottle tip or dropper be away from the eye?
- **A.** 1 inch
- **B.** ¾ inch
- **C.** ½ inch
- **D.** ¼ inch
- **E.** It should touch the eye

_____ **10.** How should you hold a 4-year-old's ear when administering eardrops?

    A. Pull the ear upward and outward

    B. Pull the ear outward and downward

    C. Pull the ear down and back

    D. Pull the ear up and back

Sentence Completion

In the space provided, write the word or phrase that best completes each sentence.

11. Topical application is the direct application of a drug on the _____.

12. Drugs that produce systemic effects are administered by routes that allow the drugs to be absorbed and distributed in the _____ throughout the body.

13. Parenteral administration of a drug generally applies to giving drugs by _____.

14. The _____ of a needle is a measure of its inside diameter.

15. The inside diameter of a 23-gauge needle is _____ than the inside diameter of a needle with a lower gauge.

16. Skin tests are usually administered by _____ injection.

17. Physicians usually prescribe vaginal drugs to treat local bacterial or _____ infections.

18. Polypharmacy is common in _____.

11. _____

12. _____

13. _____

14. _____

15. _____

16. _____

17. _____

18. _____

Short Answer

Write the answer to each question on the lines provided.

19. To ensure accuracy, when should you read the label of a drug you are about to administer?

_____

_____

_____

20. Why do drugs that are administered buccally and sublingually produce therapeutic effects more quickly than do orally administered drugs?

_____

_____

_____

21. Why is the tip of an injection needle beveled?

_____

_____

_____

22. Why does parenteral administration of a drug pose more safety risks for patients than administration by other routes?

_____

_____

_____

23. Why do you inject aspirated air from the syringe into the vial of diluent when you are reconstituting a drug for injection?

_____

_____

_____

24. After cleansing the site of an intradermal injection with an alcohol swab, why should you let the skin dry before giving the injection?

_____

_____

_____

25. When administering a subcutaneous injection, why would you avoid an injection site that is hardened or fatty?

_____

_____

_____

26. What is the function of the small amount of air you draw into the syringe when you administer an intramuscular injection?

_____

_____

_____

27. How does a drug-drug interaction differ from the adverse effects of a drug?

_____

_____

_____

28. The illustration below shows a standard syringe. Write the name of each part of the instrument on the lines provided.

C. _____

D. _____

A. _____

B. _____

E. _____

F. _____

29. Why is it important to ask patients about drug allergies every time they come into the office?

_____

_____

_____

30. What is the purpose of a consent form when administering medications?

_____

_____

_____

31. What are some methods to ensure a smooth procedure when administering a pediatric injection?

_____

_____

_____

32. Why is the vastus lateralis the best site for administering an injection to a pediatric patient?

_____

_____

_____

33. What are some important aspects of accurate charting in a medical facility?

_____

_____

_____

34. What information is documented after giving an injection to a patient?

_____

_____

_____

35. On the figure below, label the type of injection that is being given based upon the location of the needle.

A. Intradermal (ID)

Epidermis

Dermis

Subcutaneous

B. Subcutaneous (sub-Q)   **C.** Intravenous (IV)   **D.** Intramuscular (IM)

Critical Thinking

Write the answer to each question on the lines provided.

1. Why do you place a 2 × 2 gauze or cotton ball over the injection site when you withdraw the needle during an intramuscular or subcutaneous injection?

_____

_____

_____

2. The doctor has asked you to administer eye ointment and eyedrops to a patient. In what order should you administer the drugs to the patient? Why?

_____

_____

_____

3. When charting medications in the patient chart, why is it important to refrain from using statements such as "appears" or "seems like"?

_____

_____

_____

4. Why is it important to include the expiration date, lot number, and manufacturer when charting medications?

_____

_____

_____

APPLICATION

Follow the directions for each application.

1. Calculating Conversions

In the spaces provided, perform the necessary calculations for each conversion. Use a table of equivalents, if necessary.

a. 0.51 L = _____ mL   **b.** 75 mg = _____ g

c. 450 mL = _____ L   **d.** 0.205 mg = _____ µg

e. 15 gtt = _____ tsp

f. 500 mg = _____ g

g. 1 tsp = _____ mL

h. 0.125 mg = _____ mcg

2. Calculating Drug Doses

In the spaces provided, use the ratio or fraction method to calculate each of the following drug doses. For the purposes of this application, assume that the medication is being administered at the medical office on written orders from the doctor and is to be administered immediately.

a. For a patient with a urinary tract infection, the doctor orders Cotrim, 800 mg po. The stock container in your office is labeled Cotrim, sulfamethoxazole/trimethoprim, 400-mg tablets. How many tablets should you dispense to the patient?

b. The doctor orders ibuprofen, 600 mg po for a patient with back pain. The stock container of ibuprofen contains 400-mg scored tablets. How many tablets should you dispense to the patient?

c. The doctor orders dimenhydrinate liquid, 50 mg po. The stock container of the drug is labeled 12.5 mg dimenhydrinate/1 mL. What volume of the drug should you dispense to the patient?

d. The doctor orders Valium, 4 mg IM for a patient. The container label reads Valium (diazepam), 5 mg/1 mL. What volume of the drug should you prepare for the patient?

e. A patient is 5 years old and weighs 45 lb. The physician orders 225-mg Augmentin po Q8h. On hand you have Augmentin 125 mg/5 mL. The package insert states for pediatric patients ages 12 weeks and older, but less than 40 kg, the recommended dose is 40 mg/kg/day q8h.

(i) Convert the weight to kilograms.

(ii) Determine if the dosage ordered is within the recommended amount.

(iii) If the dose is within the recommended amount, how much would you administer?

3. Demonstrating the Use of an Epinephrine Autoinjector

Work with two partners to demonstrate the use of the epinephrine autoinjector. One person can play the role of the patient, one should take the role of the medical assistant conducting the demonstration, and the third should act as an observer and evaluator.

a. The medical assistant should explain to the patient that because of his particular allergy, he might inadvertently be exposed to the allergen. Such an exposure could cause a severe allergic reaction, which is called anaphylaxis, or anaphylactic shock. Symptoms of anaphylaxis include flushing, a sharp drop in blood pressure, hives, difficulty breathing, difficulty swallowing, convulsions, vomiting, diarrhea, and abdominal cramps.

b. The medical assistant should explain that autoinjectors, which are prepackaged, deliver 0.3 mg of epinephrine (a single dose for an adult) or 0.15 mg of epinephrine (a single dose for a child).

c. The medical assistant should explain that the injector should be used if exposure to the allergen is confirmed or if exposure is suspected and signs of anaphylaxis appear.

d. The medical assistant should teach the patient to follow these steps when using the autoinjector.
   1. Remove the autoinjector from the packaging.
   2. Pull back the gray cap.
   3. Place the black tip of the injector on the outside of the upper thigh.
   4. Press firmly into the thigh and hold for 10 seconds.
   5. Remove the autoinjector and massage the injection site for a few minutes.
   6. Call the physician or go to the emergency room of a nearby hospital.

e. The patient should identify each part of the autoinjector and explain its use to the medical assistant.

f. The observer should present a critique of the medical assistant's role in the activity. The critique should involve the assistant's attitude, or approach, as well as the appropriateness and accuracy of the assistant's explanation and demonstration.

g. The medical assistant, the patient, and the observer should then discuss the observer's critique, noting the strengths and weaknesses of the assistant's explanations and demonstration.

h. Exchange roles and repeat the activity with another person perhaps acting as the caregiver of an elderly patient or a parent of a pediatric patient.

i. Exchange roles one final time so that each member of the team gets to play medical assistant, patient, and observer once.

4. Demonstrating Proper Medication Administration for Medications Given Orally, Sublingually, and Buccally

Using Procedure Checklists 20.1, Administering Oral Drugs, and 20.2, Administering Buccal or Sublingual Drugs, review and practice administering medications orally, sublingually, and buccally.

Use the following circumstances during your practice.

- Working with a partner, role-play giving the proper instructions for each type of medication.

- Chart the following medications as being administered in the sample progress note or medication flow sheet provided in the back of the workbook on page 587. Make certain your charting is complete, including the date, time, drug name, dosage, expiration date, lot number, manufacturer, route, site, significant patient reactions, and any patient education in the patient's chart. (To make the charting complete, create any information not provided below.)

- 650 mg acetaminophen PO

- Nitroglycerin gr 1/100 SL

- Methyltestosterone 10 mg buccal

5. Demonstrating Proper Medication Preparation for Medications Given by Injection

Using Procedure Checklists 20.3, Drawing a Drug from an Ampule, and 20.4, Reconstituting and Drawing a Drug for Injection, practice preparing medications for administration.

6. Demonstrating Proper Medication Administration for Medications Given by Injection

Using Procedure Checklists 20.5, Giving an Intradermal Injection; 20.6, Giving a Subcutaneous Injection; and 20.7, Giving an Intramuscular Injection, practice administering injections. Use the following circumstances during your practice.

- Working with a partner and a manikin, role-play giving the injections while providing the proper communication to the patient for each type of injection.

- Chart the following injections as being administered in the sample progress note or medication flow sheet provided in the back of the workbook on page 587. Make certain your charting is complete including the date, time, drug name, dosage, expiration date, lot number, manufacturer, route, site, significant patient reactions, and any patient education in the patient's chart. (To make the charting complete, create any information not provided below.)

- Tigan 200 milligram intramuscularly

- Humulin R 20 units subcutaneously

- Mantoux TB test intradermally

7. Demonstrating Proper Medication Administration for Medications Given by Various Routes

Using Procedure Checklists 20.8, Administering Inhalation Therapy; 20.9, Administering and Removing a Transdermal Patch and Providing Instruction; 20.10, Assisting with Administration of Urethral Drug; 20.11, Administering a Vaginal Medication; 20.12, Administering a Rectal Medication; 20.13, Administering Eye Medications; 20.14, Performing Eye Irrigation; 20.15, Administering Eardrops; and 20.16, Performing Ear Irrigation, practice administering medications of various routes. Use the following circumstances for your practice.

- Research names of medications that would be administered by the various routes using Procedures 20.8 through 20.16 or obtain medication names from your instructor.

- Working with a partner and the manikin, when necessary, role-play giving the proper instructions for each procedure performed. Take turns with a partner and review any steps in your instruction you have missed.

- Chart each medication you have researched and/or procedure performed in the sample progress note or medication flow sheet provided in the back of the workbook on page 587. Make certain your charting is complete by creating information based upon your practice session.

CASE STUDIES

Write your response to each case study on the lines provided.

Case 1

A patient received from the pharmacy a prescription for hyoscyamine sulfate tablets for buccal administration. She telephones the office and asks you if it would be all right to take the medication while having her second cup of coffee in the morning. What do you tell her? Why?

_____

_____

_____

Case 2

The physician has given a written order for the application of an ophthalmic drug for a patient. The drug is for local application and systemic absorption should be avoided. How do you prevent the systemic absorption of the drug when administering it?

_____

_____

_____

Case 3

Heparin 1.5 mL SC has been ordered for a patient. What volume syringe and needle (gauge and length) should you prepare?

_____

_____

_____

Case 4

The doctor has written an order for you to administer two 250-g tablets of Trimox (amoxicillin) to a patient who has an infection. The patient reluctantly takes the first tablet but spits out the second. What do you do?

_____

_____

_____

Case 5

You had just administered a drug to a child, and within five minutes the child vomited. Should you readminister the drug?

_____

_____

_____

Case 6

You are explaining the dosage instructions to a mother and the medication is ordered in tablet form. The mother tells you that the child has difficulty swallowing tablets. What should you do?

_____

_____

_____

CHAPTER **21**

Electrocardiography and Pulmonary Function Testing

REVIEW

Vocabulary Review

Matching

Match the key terms in the right column with the definitions in the left column by placing the letter of each correct answer in the space provided.

_____ 1. The condition of having two separate poles, one of which is positive and the other negative

_____ 2. An electrical impulse that initiates a chain reaction, resulting in a contraction of the heart muscle

_____ 3. A period of electrical recovery during which polarity is restored

_____ 4. An instrument that measures and displays the electrical impulses responsible for the cardiac cycle

_____ 5. A wave recorded on an electrocardiogram that is produced by the electrical impulses responsible for the cardiac cycle

_____ 6. An erroneous mark or defect on an ECG tracing

_____ 7. An irregularity in heart rhythm

_____ 8. An instrument that measures the activity of the heart in a 24-hour period

_____ 9. The greatest volume of air that a person can expel when performing rapid, forced expiration

_____ 10. A standardized measuring instrument used to calibrate a spirometer

a. calibration syringe
b. forced vital capacity
c. Holter monitor
d. polarity
e. depolarization
f. arrhythmia
g. repolarization
h. artifact
i. electrocardiogram
j. deflection

True or False

Decide whether each statement is true or false. In the space at the left, write T for true or F for false. On the lines provided, rewrite the false statements to make them true.

_____ 11. Spirometry measures the air taken in by and expelled from the lungs.

_____

_____ 12. A spirometer or peak flow meter is used to measure breathing capacity.

_____

_____ 13. A heart attack is referred to as a myocardial infarction.

_____

_____ **14.** A lead is attached to the patient's skin during electrocardiography.

_____

_____ **15.** A pen-like instrument that records movement on ECG paper is called a stylus.

_____

_____ **16.** An instrument that measures and displays the electrical impulses responsible for the cardiac cycle is referred to as an electrocardiography.

_____

_____ **17.** An electrolyte is a substance that decreases transmission of electrical impulses.

_____

_____ **18.** The atrioventricular node is a mass of specialized conducting cells located at the bottom of the right atrium that delays transmission of electrical impulses so the atria can completely contract.

_____

_____ **19.** The bundle of His is an area of specialized conductive tissue in the heart that sends impulses through a series of bundle branches.

_____

_____ **20.** The sequence of contraction and relaxation is referred to as a pulmonary cycle.

_____

_____ **21.** A procedure that measures and evaluates a patient's lung capacity and volume is referred to as a pulmonary function test.

_____

_____ **22.** The process by which a graphic pattern is created from the electrical impulses generated within the heart as it pumps is called repolarization.

_____

Content Review

Multiple Choice

In the space provided, write the letter of the choice that best completes each statement or answers each question.

_____ **1.** When performing routine electrocardiography, you place electrodes on the
   A. right arm, left arm, right leg, left leg, and six on the chest.
   B. right arm, left arm, right temple, left temple, and six on the chest.
   C. right arm, right leg, and five on the chest.
   D. right arm, left arm, and one on the chest, which is moved to six different positions.

_____ **2.** Augmented leads monitor
   A. bipolar leads.
   B. one electrode and a point within the heart.
   C. one limb electrode and a point midway between two other limb electrodes.
   D. electrical activity between two limb electrodes.

_____ 3. A flat line on the ECG tracing of one of the leads is typically caused by
   A. switching two of the wires.
   B. a loose or disconnected wire.
   C. a loose or disconnected patient cable.
   D. cardiac arrest.
   E. None of the above.

_____ 4. A patient who is to wear a Holter monitor should be instructed
   A. to take baths rather than showers.
   B. to avoid excessive or unusual exercise.
   C. in how to remove the electrodes before going to bed and how to replace them in the morning.
   D. to keep a written record of activities, emotional upsets, physical symptoms, and medications.

_____ 5. When administering spirometry,
   A. emergency resuscitation equipment should always be in the room.
   B. explain the procedure, but once the test begins, avoid coaching patients on their performance.
   C. position the patient with the chin slightly elevated and the neck slightly extended.
   D. position the patient with the chin bent slightly toward the chest and the back straight.

_____ 6. Electrocardiography records the transmission, _____, and duration of the various electrical impulses of the heart.
   A. heart rate
   B. magnitude
   C. amplification
   D. blood pressure
   E. Strength

_____ 7. A single-channel electrocardiograph records the electrical activity of one lead, whereas a(n) _____ electrocardiograph records more than one lead at a time.
   A. deflection
   B. pulse oximeter
   C. multichannel
   D. electronic
   E. rhythm strip

_____ 8. To ensure the conductivity of electrical impulses from the skin, you must apply _____ to each electrode before placing it on the patient's body.
   A. alcohol
   B. soap and water
   C. talcum powder
   D. lotion
   E. an electrolyte

_____ 9. On an electrocardiograph, the _____ is used to adjust the position of the stylus.
   A. sensitivity selector
   B. amplifier
   C. centering control
   D. default switch
   E. interpretative mode

_____ 10. Exercise electrocardiography typically continues until the patient reaches a(n) _____, has chest pain or fatigue, or develops complications.
   A. arrhythmia
   B. target heart rate
   C. personal best peak expiratory flow rate
   D. exhaustion rate

_____ 11. Why is it important for a medical assistant to recognize abnormal heart rhythms?
   A. To effectively triage a medical emergency
   B. To alert the physician or nurse that the patient has an irregular ECG
   C. To take control of the medical emergency
   D. Both A and B
   E. Both A and C

_____ 12. The cardiac arrhythmia that resembles a "saw tooth" is
   A. a bundle branch block.
   B. ventricular fibrillation.
   C. atrial fibrillation.
   D. bradycardia.

_____ 13. The green zone on the peak flow zone chart indicates
   A. good asthma control.
   B. that airways are beginning to narrow.
   C. that airways are constricted.
   D. low oxygen saturation.

_____ 14. Patient symptoms that include wheezing, shortness of breath, and difficulty talking and/or walking indicate patients in the _____ zone.
   A. green
   B. red
   C. yellow
   D. black
   E. safe

_____ 15. The noninvasive procedure that measures oxygen saturation in blood is
   A. peak flow.
   B. arterial blood gasses.
   C. pulse oximetry.
   D. ECG.
   E. forced vital capacity.

Short Answer

Write the answer to each question on the lines provided.

16. Briefly describe the heart's process of conduction.

_____

_____

_____

17. Examine the following ECG tracings. Then follow the directions.

    a. Circle and label the QRS complex on part A.

    b. Label the R wave on part A.

    c. Label the T wave on part A.

    d. Label the P wave on part A.

    e. On part B, draw lines and label the tracing to show when atrial relaxation occurs.

    f. On part B, draw an arrow and label the tracing to show when atrial contraction takes place.

    g. On part B, draw an arrow and label the tracing to show when repolarization takes place.

A.   B.

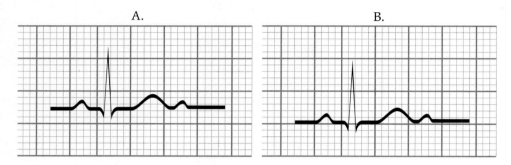

18. Review the abnormal ECG tracings and label each cardiac arrhythmia.

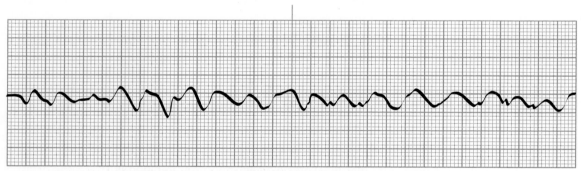

Source: From Shade, B., Wesley, K. Fast and Easy, *ECGs: A Self-Paced Learning Program*, pp. 344, Fig. 11.17.
Copyright 2007 by The McGraw-Hill Companies.

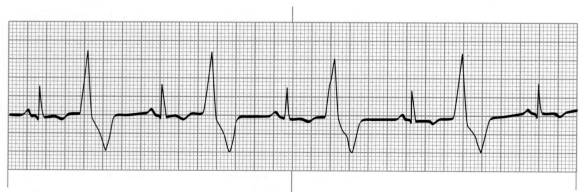

Source: From Shade, B., Wesley, K. Fast and Easy, *ECGs: A Self-Paced Learning Program*, pp. 333, Fig. 11.6a.
Copyright 2007 by The McGraw-Hill Companies.

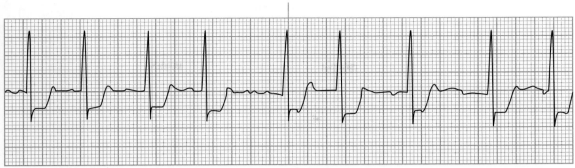

Source: From Shade, B., Wesley, K. Fast and Easy, *ECGs: A Self-Paced Learning Program,* pp. 226, Fig. 7.12.
Copyright 2007 by The McGraw-Hill Companies.

19. What are four possible causes of mechanical problems that can result in a wandering baseline?

_____

_____

_____

20. How do muscles cause somatic interference that shows up as artifacts on ECG tracings?

_____

_____

_____

21. How can the heart rate be determined from an ECG?

_____

_____

_____

22. List three conditions in which a bundle branch block would appear on an ECG.

_____

_____

_____

23. What safety precautions must be taken when administering a stress test?

_____

_____

_____

24. What are four conditions and activities that can affect the outcome of a spirometry test?

_____

_____

_____

25. An acceptable maneuver on a spirometer must have what five features?

_____

_____

_____

26. Describe what occurs during a premature ventricular contraction.

_____

_____

_____

27. Describe one treatment method that can correct ventricular defibrillation.

_____

_____

_____

28. List three causes of atrial fibrillation.

_____

_____

_____

29. What should a patient do if his or her peak expiratory flow is in the red zone?

_____

_____

_____

30. What is the normal range for the peak expiratory flow rate?

_____

_____

_____

Critical Thinking

Write the answer to each question on the lines provided.

1. What may happen if you fail to allow the electrocardiograph to warm up properly?

_____

_____

_____

2. Why might a physician order a series of ECGs for a patient after he has changed her medication?

_____

_____

_____

3. In what situation might it be better to position the electrodes on the upper arms and the thighs rather than lower on the arms and legs?

_____

_____

_____

4. A patient has complained of periodic arrhythmias, but repeated ECGs have not shown any evidence of them. Why might the doctor order a Holter monitor to be used by the patient?

_____

_____

_____

5. What is the purpose of coaching the patient to improve performance during spirometry?

_____

_____

_____

6. Why is averaging the readings of the peak expiratory flow rate not recommended?

_____

_____

_____

7. While observing a pulse oximetry, you notice the reading states 89%. What should you do and why?

_____

_____

_____

APPLICATION

Follow the directions for the application.

Preparing a Patient for Electrocardiography

Working with two partners, prepare a patient for electrocardiography. One partner should play the role of the patient, one should take the role of the medical assistant preparing the patient for the procedure, and the third should act as an observer and evaluator. The patient is elderly and is anxious about the procedure.

a. The medical assistant should introduce herself and explain the procedure to the patient. The patient should ask questions and express concerns about what will happen and what he will experience. The medical assistant should answer all questions to the best of her ability and provide help in allaying the patient's anxieties.

b. The medical assistant should help the patient get into position for the procedure, helping him find the position that is most comfortable.

c. Following the preparation, the observer should critique what the medical assistant did. The critique should include the assistant's skill in communicating with the patient, the accuracy of her descriptions of the procedure, her responses to the patient's questions, how well the medical assistant succeeded in allaying the patient's concerns, and the effectiveness of the assistant's positioning of the patient.

d. As a team, discuss the observer's critique, noting the strengths and weaknesses of preparation of the patient for the procedure.

e. Exchange roles and repeat the preparation for another procedure, such as spirometry, peak flow, or providing a patient with a Holter monitor. The new observer should choose the type of procedure.

f. Exchange roles one final time so that each team member plays all three roles once.

CASE STUDIES

Write your response to each case study on the lines provided.

Case 1

After completing an ECG on a patient, you examine the tracing and find the wave peaks are very low, making it difficult to clearly read the tracing. What should you do?

_____

_____

_____

Case 2

While performing an ECG on a 55-year-old female patient, you note that all of the limb electrodes are coming off. What might cause the electrodes to come off of the patient's arms and legs? What action should you take?

_____

_____

_____

Case 3

Sam Smith is recovering from a heart attack. While you are preparing him for a stress test to determine how his heart is functioning, Mr. Smith expresses his fears. He is afraid the test will cause another heart attack. What do you tell him?

_____

_____

_____

Case 4

You are administering spirometry to a patient. She has been very cooperative but is having difficulty achieving the three acceptable maneuvers that are required. After several attempts, she complains of dizziness. You check her pulse and blood pressure and find that both are significantly elevated. What should you do?

_____

_____

_____

Case 5

You are working in an outpatient surgical clinic in the preoperative holding area. Each patient is monitored with a pulse oximeter. You check Mrs. O'Shaughnessy's fingers and notice that they are cold to the touch and have poor blood return. What should you do?

_____

_____

_____

CHAPTER **22**

X-Rays and Diagnostic Radiology

REVIEW

Vocabulary Review

Matching

Match the key terms in the right column with the definitions in the left column by placing the letter of each correct answer in the space provided.

_____ **1.** A type of x-ray developed with a powder toner, similar to the toner in photocopiers

_____ **2.** A type of radiation therapy that allows deep penetration of tissue to treat deep tumors

_____ **3.** The use of radionuclides or radioisotopes to evaluate the bone, brain, lungs, kidneys, liver, pancreas, thyroid, or spleen

_____ **4.** A nuclear medicine procedure used to locate and determine the extent of brain damage from a stroke

_____ **5.** An x-ray exam of the internal breast tissues

_____ **6.** An x-ray of the abdomen used to assess the urinary organs, evaluate urinary system diseases or disorders, and detect kidney stones

_____ **7.** A series of x-rays taken while a contrast medium travels through the kidneys, ureters, and bladder

_____ **8.** A type of radiation therapy that uses radioactive implants close to or directly into cancerous tissue to treat the tumor

_____ **9.** A test used to detect gallstones and other abnormalities of the gallbladder

_____ **10.** An x-ray procedure in which barium sulfate is instilled through the anus into the rectum and then into the colon to help diagnose abnormalities of the colon or rectum

_____ **11.** An invasive procedure that requires the insertion of a catheter, wire, or other testing device into a patient's blood vessel to obtain an image of the vessel

_____ **12.** The use of x-ray technology for diagnostic purposes

_____ **13.** The use of x-ray technology to identify a disease or a medical condition

a. angiography
b. barium enema
c. brachytherapy
d. cholecystography
e. diagnostic radiology
f. intravenous pyelogram
g. diagnostic radiology
h. KUB radiography
i. mammography
j. nuclear medicine
k. SPECT
l. teletherapy
m. xeroradiography

True or False

Decide whether each statement is true or false. In the space at the left, write T for true or F for false. On the lines provided, rewrite the false statements to make them true.

_____ **14.** A contrast medium makes internal organs denser and blocks the passage of x-rays to the photographic film.

_____

_____ **15.** Standard x-rays and ultrasound, which do not require inserting devices or breaking the skin, are types of invasive procedures.

_____

_____ **16.** A MUGA scan is a type of nuclear medicine test used to evaluate the condition of the heart's myocardium.

_____

_____ **17.** For patients with poor kidney function, doctors often use an IVP to evaluate the function of the ureters, bladder, and urethra.

_____

_____ **18.** Myelography is a type of fluoroscopy of the abdomen.

_____

_____ **19.** A dosimeter is a radiation exposure badge that contains a sensitized piece of film.

_____

_____ **20.** In PET, special isotopes emit positrons, which are processed by computer and viewed to diagnose brain-related conditions.

_____

_____ **21.** In ultrasound, low-frequency sound waves directed through the skin produce echoes that are converted by computer into an image on a screen.

_____

_____ **22.** 4-D ultrasound provides live-action images for observation of fetal movement.

_____

_____ **23.** Radiation therapy is used to treat cancer by promoting cellular reproduction.

_____

_____ **24.** A roentgen ray is another name for an x-ray.

_____

_____ **25.** Hysterosalpingography is a radiological exam of a vagina.

_____

Content Review

Multiple Choice

In the space provided, write the letter of the choice that best completes each statement or answers each question.

_____ 1. An x-ray is a type of electromagnetic wave that has a
   A. low energy level and an extremely long wavelength.
   B. low energy level and an extremely short wavelength.
   C. high energy level and an extremely short wavelength.
   D. high energy level and an extremely long wavelength.

_____ 2. A test that utilizes a contrast medium and fluoroscopy to help diagnose abnormalities or injuries in the cartilage, tendons, or ligaments of the joints is called
   A. arthrography.
   B. cholangiography.
   C. thermography.
   D. xeroradiography.

_____ 3. Which of the following duties in connection with diagnostic radiology are medical assistants most likely to perform?
   A. Operating x-ray equipment
   B. Assisting a radiologist with x-ray procedures
   C. Assisting a radiologic technologist with x-ray procedures
   D. Providing preprocedure and postprocedure patient care

_____ 4. Angiography requires insertion of a catheter into a patient's
   A. knee or shoulder.
   B. pancreatic duct.
   C. urethra.
   D. common bile duct.
   E. blood vessel.

_____ 5. During which of the following procedures does the patient eat a specially prepared fatty meal?
   A. Cholecystography
   B. Cholangiography
   C. A barium swallow
   D. An intravenous pyelogram
   E. MUGA scan

_____ 6. The test that uses nonionizing radiation and a strong magnetic field is known as
   A. SPECT.
   B. CT.
   C. PET.
   D. MRI.

_____ 7. Myelography is a fluoroscopic exam of the
   A. heart.
   B. spinal cord.
   C. bone marrow.
   D. gallbladder.
   E. liver.

_____ **8.** The digital storage area where digital images are sent and stored for diagnostic viewing and electronic image storage and distribution is known as

    A. DICOM.

    B. IHE.

    C. PAC.

    D. EHR.

_____ **9.** Stereotaxis is an example of

    A. magnetic resonance imaging.

    B. nuclear medicine.

    C. stereoscopy.

    D. telemedicine technology.

    E. echocardiography.

Sentence Completion

In the space provided, write the word or phrase that best completes each sentence.

10. _____ is a type of ultrasound test used to study the structure and function of the heart.

11. Before an MRI, it is important to determine whether the patient has any internal _____ materials.

12. In a double-contrast barium enema, _____ is forced into the colon to distend the tissue.

13. During an IVP, a radiologist injects a contrast medium into a patient's _____.

14. A test used to help diagnose and evaluate obstructions, ulcers, polyps, diverticulosis, tumors, or motility problems of the esophagus, stomach, duodenum, and small intestine is a _____ swallow.

15. Tumors or inflammations show up lighter on thermographic photographs because they produce more _____ than healthy tissues.

16. The _____ dense areas of an x-ray are the lightest on the film.

17. Annual mammograms are recommended for women after age _____.

10. _____

11. _____

12. _____

13. _____

14. _____

15. _____

16. _____

17. _____

Short Answer

Write the answer to each question on the lines provided.

18. What are four general duties that medical assistants may perform for patients who will undergo radiologic testing?

_____

_____

_____

19. Why are contrast media used in some diagnostic radiologic tests? List three ways that contrast media can be administered.

_____

_____

_____

20. Describe the mechanics of the diagnostic procedure fluoroscopy.

_____

_____

_____

21. Why do some radiologic diagnostic procedures require patients to be admitted to a hospital or same-day surgical facility? Give one example of such a procedure.

_____

_____

_____

22. How are conventional tomography and computed tomography similar? How are they different?

_____

_____

_____

23. Describe three ways for medical assistants to protect themselves against excessive radiation exposure.

_____

_____

_____

24. What four items of information about a patient's x-rays should be documented in the patient report card or record book?

_____

_____

_____

25. How might a cardiologist use electronic medicine to monitor a patient from afar?

_____

_____

_____

26. For what conditions do radiologists assess when performing a hysterosalpingography?

_____

_____

_____

27. What is the difference between PAC and DICOM?

_____

_____

_____

28. Define DICOM and explain how it applies to digital radiology.

_____

_____

_____

Critical Thinking

Write the answer to each question on the lines provided.

1. Why is it important to take an x-ray only within 10 days of the last menstrual period for women of childbearing age?

_____

_____

_____

2. How might a patient undergoing an invasive radiologic diagnostic procedure be at greater risk than a patient undergoing a noninvasive procedure?

_____

_____

_____

3. Why is preprocedure care especially important for patients who are scheduled to undergo an MRI?

_____

_____

_____

4. Why is it important for the patient to remain still during an x-ray exam?

_____

_____

_____

5. How could a radiologist use electronic medicine to interpret and report on a tomogram produced in another country?

_____

_____

_____

6. Why is it important to ask a patient if they have had a previous mammogram when assisting a patient with setting up an appointment for a mammogram?

_____

_____

_____

APPLICATION

Follow the directions for each application.

1. Preparing a Patient for a Radiologic Diagnostic Test

Work with two partners. One student should take the role of a patient scheduled for a radiologic diagnostic procedure in a few days. The second student should assume the role of medical assistant in a radiology facility or medical office. The third student should act as an observer and evaluator.

a. Choose one of the following procedures: arthrography, barium enema, barium swallow, cholecystography, CT scan with contrast medium, or IVP. Review the description of the chosen procedure and the preprocedure care steps.

b. The medical assistant should schedule a time for the procedure with the patient, taking into account such factors as whether the patient's digestive tract must be empty and whether the patient will want to sleep through the procedure to avoid experiencing hunger.

c. The medical assistant should describe the procedure to the patient according to the guidelines presented in the student textbook. The patient should ask questions about the procedure, which the medical assistant should answer clearly and completely.

d. The medical assistant should explain the preparation instructions. The patient should ask questions about the instructions. The medical assistant may want to have the patient repeat the instructions to ensure understanding of them.

e. After the instructions have been given and the patient's questions have been answered, the observer should provide a critique of the medical assistant's preprocedure care. Comments should include positive feedback and suggestions for improvement.

f. Change roles and repeat the exercise, using a different diagnostic test. Then change roles again so that each student has a turn at each role and all students become familiar with various procedures for different tests.

2. Develop an office policy and procedure plan for the proper storage and handling of x-ray film. Present your plan to the class.

CASE STUDIES

Write your response to each case study on the lines provided.

Case 1

A patient arrives in the office for a diagnostic test that will involve the use of a contrast medium that contains iodine. In your preprocedure interview with the patient a week ago, she reported no known allergies to iodine or shellfish. As you are preparing the patient for the procedure, she informs you that 2 days ago, after eating boiled shrimp at a party, she awoke in the middle of the night with nausea and joint pain. She says these symptoms subsided after 24 hours. You suspect the woman had a mild case of food poisoning from eating the shrimp. What should you do and why?

_____

_____

_____

Case 2

An elderly patient has just been examined by the physician, who has momentarily stepped out of the exam room. You are in the room with the patient and his son. The patient has just learned that he must undergo a barium enema in 2 days. When he asks you to explain this procedure, his son tells him that he is better off not knowing because it will only make him anxious. What, if anything, do you say to the patient?

_____

_____

_____

Case 3

A patient's mammogram indicates a small nodule in one breast. Without further testing, the physician cannot know whether the nodule is benign or malignant. He asks you to call the patient to schedule an ultrasound exam of the breast. When you call the patient to make the appointment, she tells you that she has never had an ultrasound and fears additional exposure to radiation. What can you say to the patient to reassure her?

_____

_____

_____

Case 4

You are interviewing a patient before his cholecystography procedure. When you ask if he was able to take the contrast media tablets the night before, he states that he did take them, but he thinks he might have dropped one of the pills. What should you do?

_____

_____

_____

CHAPTER 23

Medical Assisting Externships and Preparing to Find a Position

REVIEW

Vocabulary Review

Matching

Match the key terms in the right column with the definitions in the left column by placing the letter of each correct answer in the space provided.

_____ 1. A résumé format that is used when an individual does not have relevant job experience

_____ 2. The person who organizes and assigns your externship

_____ 3. A document that outlines the expectations of the academic institution and the medical facility

_____ 4. A résumé that highlights specialty areas of accomplishments and strengths

_____ 5. A résumé for individuals who have a strong work history

_____ 6. Making contacts with relatives, friends, and acquaintances that may have information about how to find a job in your field

_____ 7. A type of critique that is aimed at giving an individual feedback about his or her performance in order to improve

_____ 8. A recommendation for employment from a clinical preceptor or medical facility

_____ 9. A collection of an applicant's résumé, reference letter, and other documents of interest to show to a potential employer

a. affiliation agreement
b. chronological résumé
c. clinical coordinator
d. constructive criticism
e. functional résumé
f. networking
g. portfolio
h. reference
i. targeted résumé

Content Review

Sentence Completion

In the space provided, write the word or phrase that best completes each sentence.

1. A(n) _____ is the opportunity to work within a medical facility to gain the on-the-job training that is essential for beginning your new career.

2. Educational institutions in which externships are mandatory are accredited by _____ and _____.

3. The minimum number of hours required for externship by an accredited institution is _____.

1. _____

2. _____

3. _____

4. _____ should be turned off during working hours.

5. Medical assisting extern students are expected to report to the facility _____ they are assigned.

6. Medical facilities expect the extern student to appear as a _____.

7. Accepting all assignments with enthusiasm and looking for extra work when idle is an example of showing _____.

4. _____

5. _____

6. _____

7. _____

Short Answer

Write the answer to each question on the lines provided.

8. What are three job options you might use to learn about open positions in your field?

_____

_____

_____

9. Describe how to prepare for an interview.

_____

_____

_____

10. What types of questions are you not required to answer at a job interview?

_____

_____

_____

11. What is expected of a medical assisting extern student at a medical facility?

_____

_____

_____

12. How does being an extern differ from being a medical assisting student?

_____

_____

_____

13. Name five reasons an employer would not hire a job candidate.

_____

_____

_____

14. What types of documents should be in a portfolio?

_____

_____

_____

15. What is important to remember when filling out a job application?

_____

_____

_____

Critical Thinking

Write the answer to each question on the lines provided.

1. Should a job candidate send résumés to employers whose ads state qualifications that are higher or different from the candidate's experience or education?

_____

_____

_____

2. What might a site ask of a medical assisting extern student prior to beginning his clinical rotation?

_____

_____

_____

3. How can a medical assisting extern student ensure attendance *every day* in her externship?

_____

_____

_____

4. In choosing a résumé, what style might be the best strategy for you?

_____

_____

_____

APPLICATION

Follow the directions for each application.

1. Preparing a Budget

Salary is an important part of accepting a position. Most people do not have an idea of how much income is needed for everyday living expenses. On the worksheet provided, prepare your budget and calculate a yearly income requirement based on your expenses. See the example in the documentation section on page 559.

2. Interview Practice

Work in groups of three to four students. Assign three or four interview questions each and write responses to the questions. Practice interviewing each other and then compile a list of the best responses. Share your group's responses with the class by holding a mock interview with someone in your group. Type an official copy of the findings and pass it out to the class. Refer to the text chapter for interview questions and research additional questions on the Internet.

3. Employment Interview

Working in teams of three or four, contact local temporary employment agencies to come to your class and conduct mock interviews with your class. To begin this process, use the following steps:

1. Assign each team member a duty or role.

2. Contact local employment agencies and speak with a recruiter.

3. Follow up your call with a letter that recaps what was discussed and an invitation to participate in mock interviews on an established date and time. Mail the letter using campus letterhead.

4. Working in teams, use the information in the text about proper interviewing skills to establish a critique form for the interviewer to use during the interview.

5. The day of the mock interviews, supply a light snack for the interviewers.

6. Wear professional interview apparel.

7. Share critiques with the class.

CASE STUDIES

Write your response to each case study on the lines provided.

Case 1

During a job interview, a prospective employer asks you if you are a single mother. Explain whether the question is appropriate and how you might respond to such a question.

_____

_____

_____

Case 2

You are interviewing with a popular, busy surgeon's office. As the interview is wrapping up, the physician tells you that all applicants will be notified either way regarding the candidate selection. Should you phone the physician to follow up? Do you think it will appear that you are motivated to obtain the position if you call often?

_____

_____

_____

Case 3

You have sent out 25 résumés and have not received a single call. Your classmate has sent out the same amount of résumés and has received invitations to 12 interviews, but your friend has not been offered a position. What could be the possible problem with each job candidate?

_____

_____

_____

Instructions for the Procedure Competency Checklists

General Instructions

Review and practice the correct performance of each procedure prior to attempting the procedure. The rationales for all critical steps are given in the performance guidelines within your textbook. Review these steps and rationales carefully before beginning the procedure. As you become more proficient in the procedure, you should perform the procedure without guidance from the textbook or the reviewer. In any procedure, certain steps are considered to be more "important" than others. These steps are referred to as **critical steps.** If any of these steps are missed or performed incorrectly, you should continue to practice the procedure to perfect the technique. Steps with an * are considered critical steps.

Scoring System

To score each step, use the following scoring system:
1 = poor, 2 = fair, 3 = good, 4 = excellent

A minimum score of at least a 3 must be achieved on **each** step to achieve successful completion of the technique. Calculate the final score by dividing the total number of points achieved by the total possible points listed at the top of the grading table and multiply by 100. For example, if the total possible score is 40 (10 × 4) and a score of 36 was achieved it would be 36/40 × 100 or 90. Remember that steps with an * are considered **critical steps.** If a critical step is not done correctly, you will be considered unsuccessful in completing the procedure during that attempt.

The procedure templates allow for three practice attempts and a final performance. The three practice attempts may be judged by other students or lab assistants. There are areas available for observer comments so that you may improve your technique with each procedure attempt. The final performance should be assessed by the instructor or a designated lab assistant.

PROCEDURE 2-1 ASEPTIC HAND WASHING

Procedure Goal

To remove dirt and microorganisms from under the fingernails and from the surface of the skin, hair follicles, and oil glands of the hands

Scoring System

To score each step, use the following scoring system:
1 = poor, 2 = fair, 3 = good, 4 = excellent

A minimum score of at least a 3 must be achieved on **each** step to achieve successful completion of the technique. Detailed instructions on the scoring system are found on page 179.

Materials

Liquid soap, nailbrush or orange stick, paper towels

Procedure

Procedure Steps Total Possible Points - 28 Time Limit: 10 minutes	Practice #1	Practice #2	Practice #3	Final
1. Remove all jewelry (plain wedding bands may be left on and scrubbed).				
2. Turn on the faucets using a paper towel and adjust the water temperature to moderately warm. (Sinks with knee-operated faucet controls prevent contact of the surface with the hands.)				
3. Wet your hands and apply liquid soap. Use a clean, dry paper towel to activate soap pump. Liquid soap, especially when dispensed with a foot pump, is preferable to bar soap.*				
4. Work the soap into a lather, making sure that all of both hands are lathered. Rub vigorously in a circular motion for 2 minutes. Keep your hands lower than your forearms so that dirty water flows into the sink instead of back onto your arms. Your fingertips should be pointing down. Interlace your fingers to clean between them, and use the palm of one hand to clean the back of the other. It is important that you wash every surface of your hands.*				
5. Use a nailbrush or orange stick to dislodge dirt around your nails and cuticles.*				
6. Rinse your hands well, keeping the hands lower than your forearms and not touching the sink or faucets.				
7. With the water still running, dry your hands thoroughly with clean, dry paper towels and then turn off the faucets using a clean, dry paper towel. Discard the towels.				
Total Number of Points Achieved/Final Score				
Initials of Observer:				

(continued)

Comments and Signatures

Reviewer's comments and signatures:

1. _____

2. _____

3. _____

Instructor's comments:

_____

CAAHEP Competency Achieved

III. P (4) Perform hand washing

ABHES Competency Achieved

4 (c) Apply principles of aseptic techniques and infection control

PROCEDURE 2-2 WRAPPING AND LABELING INSTRUMENTS FOR STERILIZATION IN THE AUTOCLAVE

Procedure Goal

To enclose instruments and equipment to be sterilized in appropriate wrapping materials to ensure sterilization and to protect supplies from contamination after sterilization

Scoring System

To score each step, use the following scoring system:
1 = poor, 2 = fair, 3 = good, 4 = excellent

A minimum score of at least a 3 must be achieved on **each** step to achieve successful completion of the technique. Detailed instructions on the scoring system are found on page 179.

Materials

Dry, sanitized, and disinfected instruments and equipment; wrapping material (paper, muslin, gauze, bags, envelopes); sterilization indicators; autoclave tape; labels (if wrapping does not include space for labeling); pen

Procedure

Procedure Steps Total Possible Points - 48 Time Limit: 10 minutes	Practice #1	Practice #2	Practice #3	Final
For wrapping instruments or equipment in pieces of paper or fabric: 1. Wash your hands and put on gloves before beginning to wrap the items to be sterilized.				
2. Place a square of paper or muslin on the table with one point toward you. With muslin, use a double thickness. The paper or fabric must be large enough to allow all four points to cover the instruments or equipment you will be wrapping. It also must be large enough to provide an overlap, which will be used as a handling flap.				
3. Place each item to be included in the pack in the center area of the paper or fabric "diamond." Items that will be used together should be wrapped together. Take care, however, that surfaces of the items do not touch each other inside the pack. Inspect each item to make sure it is operating correctly. Place hinged instruments in the pack in the open position. Wrap a small piece of paper, muslin, or gauze around delicate edges or points to protect against damage to other instruments or to the pack wrapping.*				
4. Place a sterilization indicator inside the pack with the instruments. Position the indicator correctly, following the manufacturer's guidelines.*				
5. Fold the bottom point of the diamond up and over the instruments in to the center. Fold back a small portion of the point.*				
6. Fold the right point of the diamond in to the center. Again, fold back a small portion of the point to be used as a handle.				

(continued)

Procedure Steps Total Possible Points - 48 Time Limit: 10 minutes	Practice #1	Practice #2	Practice #3	Final
7. Fold the left point of the diamond in to the center, folding back a small portion to form a handle. The pack should now resemble an open envelope.				
8. Grasp the covered instruments (the bottom of the envelope) and fold this portion up, toward the top point. Fold the top point down over the pack, making sure the pack is snug but not too tight.				
9. Secure the pack with autoclave tape. A "quick-opening tab" can be created by folding a small portion of the tape back onto itself. The pack must be snug enough to prevent instruments from slipping out of the wrapping or damaging each other inside the pack but loose enough to allow adequate circulation of steam through the pack.				
10. Label the pack with your initials and the date. List the contents of the pack as well. If the pack contains syringes, be sure to identify the syringe size(s).*				
11. Place the pack aside for loading into the autoclave.				
12. Remove gloves, dispose of them in the appropriate waste container, and wash your hands.				
For wrapping instruments and equipment in bags or envelopes: 1. Wash your hands and put on gloves before beginning to wrap the items to be sterilized.				
2. Insert the items into the bag or envelope as indicated by the manufacturer's directions. Hinged instruments should be opened before insertion into the package.*				
3. Close and seal the pack. Make sure the sterilization indicator is not damaged or already exposed.*				
4. Label the pack with your initials and the date. List the contents of the pack as well. The pens or pencils used to label the pack must be waterproof; otherwise, the contents of the pack and date of sterilization will be obliterated.*				
5. Place the pack aside for loading into the autoclave.				
6. Remove gloves, dispose of them in the appropriate waste container, and wash your hands.				
Total Number of Points Achieved/Final Score				
Initials of Observer:				

(continued)

Comments and Signatures

Reviewer's comments and signatures:

1. _____

2. _____

3. _____

Instructor's comments:

_____

CAAHEP Competencies Achieved

III. P (5) Prepare items for autoclaving

III. P (6) Perform sterilization procedures

ABHES Competencies Achieved

4 (o) Wrap items for autoclaving

4 (p) Perform sterilization techniques

PROCEDURE 2-3 RUNNING A LOAD THROUGH THE AUTOCLAVE

Procedure Goal

To run a load of instruments and equipment through an autoclave, ensuring sterilization of items by properly loading, drying, and unloading them

Scoring System

To score each step, use the following scoring system:
1 = poor, 2 = fair, 3 = good, 4 = excellent

A minimum score of at least a 3 must be achieved on **each** step to achieve successful completion of the technique. Detailed instructions on the scoring system are found on page 179.

Materials

Dry, sanitized, and disinfected instruments and equipment, both individual pieces and wrapped packs; oven mitts; sterile transfer forceps; storage containers for individual items

Procedure

Procedure Steps Total Possible Points - 68 Time Limit: 10 minutes	Practice #1	Practice #2	Practice #3	Final
1. Wash your hands and put on gloves before beginning to load items into the autoclave.				
2. Rest packs on their edges, and place jars and containers on their sides.				
3. Place lids for jars and containers with their sterile sides down.				
4. If the load includes plastic items, make sure no other item leans against them.*				
5. If your load is mixed—containing both wrapped packs and individual instruments—place the tray containing the instruments below the tray containing the wrapped packs.*				
6. Close the door and start the unit. For automatic autoclaves, choose the cycle based on the type of load you are running. Consult the manufacturer's recommendations before choosing the load type.				
7. For manual autoclaves, start the timer when the indicators show the recommended temperature and pressure.				
8. Right after the end of the steam cycle and just before the start of the drying cycle, open the door to the autoclave slightly (between ¼ and ½ inch).* Consult the manufacturer's recommendations regarding opening the door. Some automatic autoclaves do not require opening the door during the drying cycle.				
9. Dry according to the manufacturer's recommendations. Packs and large items may require up to 45 minutes for complete drying.				

(continued)

Procedure Steps Total Possible Points - 68 Time Limit: 10 minutes	Practice #1	Practice #2	Practice #3	Final
10. Unload the autoclave after the drying cycle is finished. Do not unload any packs or instruments with wet wrappings, or the object inside will be considered unsterile and must be processed again.*				
11. Unload each package carefully. Wear oven mitts to protect yourself from burns when removing wrapped packs. Use sterile transfer forceps to unload unwrapped individual objects.				
12. Inspect each package or item, looking for moisture on the wrapping, underexposed sterilization indicators, and tears or breaks in the wrapping. Consider the pack unsterile if any of these conditions is present.				
13. Place sterile packs aside for transfer to storage.				
14. Place individual items that are not required to be sterile in clean containers.				
15. Place items that must remain sterile in sterile containers, being sure to close the container covers tightly.				
16. As you unload items, avoid placing them in an overly cool location because the cool temperature could cause condensation on the instruments or packs.				
17. Remove gloves, dispose of them in the appropriate waste container, and wash your hands.				
Total Number of Points Achieved/Final Score				
Initials of Observer:				

Comments and Signatures

Reviewer's comments and signatures:

1. _____

2. _____

3. _____

Instructor's comments:

_____

CAAHEP Competency Achieved

III. P (5) Prepare items for autoclaving

III. P (6) Perform sterilization procedures

ABHES Competencies Achieved

4 (h) Wrap items for autoclaving

4 n. Assist physician with minor office surgical procedures o. Perform: 4) Sterilization techniques

PROCEDURE 3-1 APPLYING UNIVERSAL PRECAUTIONS

Procedure Goal

To take specific protective measures when performing tasks in which a worker may be exposed to blood, body fluids, or tissues

Scoring System

To score each step, use the following scoring system:
1 = poor, 2 = fair, 3 = good, 4 = excellent

A minimum score of at least a 3 must be achieved on **each** step to achieve successful completion of the technique. Detailed instructions on the scoring system are found on page 179.

Materials

Items needed for the specific treatment or procedure being performed

Procedure

Procedure Steps Total Possible Points - 28 Time Limit: 10 minutes	Practice #1	Practice #2	Practice #3	Final
1. Perform aseptic hand washing.				
2. Put on gloves and a gown or a laboratory coat and, if required, eye protection and a mask or a face shield.				
3. Assist with the treatment or procedure as your office policy dictates.				
4. Follow OSHA procedures to clean and decontaminate the treatment area.				
5. Place reusable instruments in appropriate containers for sanitizing, disinfecting, and sterilizing, as appropriate.				
6. Remove your gloves and all personal protective equipment. Place them in waste containers or laundry receptacles, according to OSHA guidelines.				
7. Wash your hands.				
Total Number of Points Achieved/Final Score				
Initials of Observer:				

(continued)

Comments and Signatures

Reviewer's comments and signatures:

1. _____

2. _____

3. _____

Instructor's comments:

_____

CAAHEP Competency Achieved

III. P (2) Practice Standard Precautions

ABHES Competency Achieved

4 (r) Practice Standard Precautions

PROCEDURE 3-2 NOTIFYING STATE AND COUNTY AGENCIES ABOUT REPORTABLE DISEASES

Procedure Goal

To report cases of infection with reportable disease to the proper state or county health department

Scoring System

To score each step, use the following scoring system:
1 = poor, 2 = fair, 3 = good, 4 = excellent

A minimum score of at least a 3 must be achieved on **each** step to achieve successful completion of the technique. Detailed instructions on the scoring system are found on page 179.

Materials

Communicable disease report form (see pages 425–426 for an example), pen, envelope, stamp

Procedure

Procedure Steps Total Possible Points - 16 Time Limit: 10 minutes	Practice #1	Practice #2	Practice #3	Final
1. Check to be sure you have the correct form. Some states have specific forms for each reportable infectious disease or type of disease, as well as a general form. CDC forms may also be used for reporting specific diseases.				
2. Fill in all blank areas unless they are shaded (generally for local health department use).				
3. Follow office procedures for submitting the report to a supervisor or physician before sending it out.				
4. Sign and date the form. Address the envelope, put a stamp on it, and place it in the mail.				
Total Number of Points Achieved/Final Score				
Initials of Observer:				

Comments and Signatures

Reviewer's comments and signatures:

1. _____

2. _____

3. _____

Instructor's comments:

_____

CAAHEP Competencies Achieved

IV. P (2) Report relevant information to others succinctly and accurately

IX. P (8) Apply local, state, and federal health-care legislation and regulation appropriate to the medical assisting practice setting

PROCEDURE 4-1 GUIDELINES FOR DISINFECTING EXAM ROOM SURFACES

Procedure Goal

To reduce the risk of exposure to potentially infectious microorganisms in the exam room

Scoring System

To score each step, use the following scoring system:
1 = poor, 2 = fair, 3 = good, 4 = excellent

A minimum score of at least a 3 must be achieved on **each** step to achieve successful completion of the technique. Detailed instructions on the scoring system are found on page 179.

Materials

Utility gloves, disinfectant (10% bleach solution or EPA-approved disinfecting product), paper towels, dustpan and brush, tongs, forceps, clean sponge or heavy rag

Procedure

Procedure Steps Total Possible Points - 32 Time Limit: 10 minutes	Practice #1	Practice #2	Practice #3	Final
1. Wash your hands and put on utility gloves.				
2. Remove any visible soil from exam room surfaces with disposable paper towels or a rag.*				
3. Thoroughly wipe all surfaces with the disinfectant.				
4. In the event of an accident involving a broken glass container, use tongs, a dustpan and brush, or forceps to pick up shattered glass, which may be contaminated.*				
5. Remove and replace protective coverings, such as plastic wrap or aluminum foil, on equipment if the equipment or the coverings have become contaminated. After removing the coverings, disinfect the equipment and allow it to air-dry. (Follow office procedures for the routine changing of protective coverings.)				
6. When you finish cleaning, dispose of the paper towels or rags in a biohazardous waste receptacle. (This step is especially important if you are cleaning surfaces contaminated with blood, body fluids, or tissue.)				
7. Remove the gloves and wash your hands.				
8. If you keep a container of 10% bleach solution on hand for disinfection purposes, replace the solution daily to ensure its disinfecting potency.				
Total Number of Points Achieved/Final Score				
Initials of Observer:				

(continued)

Comments and Signatures

Reviewer's comments and signatures:

1. _____

2. _____

3. _____

Instructor's comments:

_____

CAAHEP Competency Achieved

III. P (2) Practice Standard Precautions

ABHES Competencies Achieved

4 (c) Apply principles of aseptic techniques and infection control

4 (g) Prepare and maintain examination and treatment areas

PROCEDURE 4-2 MAKING THE EXAM ROOM SAFE FOR PATIENTS WITH VISUAL IMPAIRMENTS

Procedure Goal

To ensure that patients with visual impairments are safe in the exam room

Scoring System

To score each step, use the following scoring system:
1 = poor, 2 = fair, 3 = good, 4 = excellent

A minimum score of at least a 3 must be achieved on **each** step to achieve successful completion of the technique. Detailed instructions on the scoring system are found on page 179.

Materials

Reflective tape, if needed

Procedure

Procedure Steps Total Possible Points - 36 Time Limit: 10 minutes	Practice #1	Practice #2	Practice #3	Final
1. Make sure the hallway leading to the exam room is clear of obstacles.*				
2. Increase the amount of lighting in the room. Adjust the shades on windows in the room—if there are any windows—to allow for maximum natural light. Turn on all lights, especially those under cabinets, to dispel shadows.*				
3. Clear a path along which the patient can walk through the room. Make sure the chairs are out of the way. If there is a scale in the room, position it out of the path. If there is a step stool for the examining table, place it right up against the table.				
4. Make sure the floor is not slippery.				
5. Remove furniture that might be easily tipped over, such as a visitors' chair that is lightweight. If the physician will use an exam chair, push it out of the way.				
6. Provide a sturdy chair with arms and a straight back to make it easier for the patient to sit down and stand up.				
7. A wide strip of reflective tape will make the examining-table step visible for all patients. Apply it to the step's edge if tape is not there already. If your office uses a step stool instead of a step, make sure the tape on the stool is facing out.				
8. Alert the patient to protruding equipment or furnishings.				

(continued)

Procedure Steps Total Possible Points - 36 Time Limit: 10 minutes	Practice #1	Practice #2	Practice #3	Final
9. Arrange the supplies for the patient, such as gowns or drapes, with the following guideline in mind: It is easier to see light objects against dark objects or dark objects against light objects than light objects against light objects or dark objects against dark objects. If, for example, there is a dressing cubicle, lay the light-colored gown or drape against a dark bench instead of hanging the gown or drape against a light wall.*				
Total Number of Points Achieved/Final Score				
Initials of Observer:				

Comments and Signatures

Reviewer's comments and signatures:

1. _____

2. _____

3. _____

Instructor's comments:

_____

CAAHEP Competency Achieved

XI. C (2) Identify safety techniques that can be used to prevent accidents and maintain a safe work environment

ABHES Competency Achieved

9 (k) Prepare and maintain examination and treatment areas

PROCEDURE 5-1 USING CRITICAL THINKING SKILLS DURING AN INTERVIEW

Procedure Goal

To be able to use verbal and nonverbal clues and critical thinking skills to optimize the process of obtaining data for the patient's chart

Scoring System

To score each step, use the following scoring system:
1 = poor, 2 = fair, 3 = good, 4 = excellent

A minimum score of at least a 3 must be achieved on **each** step to achieve successful completion of the technique. Detailed instructions on the scoring system are found on page 179.

Materials

Patient chart, pen

Procedure

Procedure Steps Total Possible Points - 68 Time Limit: 10 minutes	Practice #1	Practice #2	Practice #3	Final
Example 1: Getting at an Underlying Meaning				
1. You are interviewing a female patient with type 2 diabetes who has recently started insulin injections. She is in the office for a follow-up visit.				
2. Use open-ended questions such as, "How are you managing your diabetes?"*				
3. The patient states that she "just can't get used to the whole idea of injections."				
4. To encourage her to verbalize her concerns more clearly, you can **mirror** her response, or restate her comments in your own words. For example, you might say, "You seem to be having some difficulty giving yourself injections."*				
5. **Verbalize** the implied, which means that you state what you think the patient is suggesting by her response.*				
6. After you determine the specific problem, you will be able to address it in the interview or note it in the patient's chart for the doctor's attention.*				
Example 2: Dealing with a Potentially Violent Patient				
1. You are interviewing a 24-year-old male patient who is new to the office. He appears agitated. You ask his reason for seeing the doctor today.				
2. The patient explains that he does not want to talk to "some assistant" about his problem. He just wants to see the doctor.				
3. You say that you respect his wish not to discuss his symptoms but explain that you need to ask him a few questions so that the doctor can provide the proper medical care.*				
4. The patient begins to yell at you, saying he wants to see the doctor and doesn't "want to answer stupid questions."				

(continued)

Procedure Steps Total Possible Points - 68 Time Limit: 10 minutes	Practice #1	Practice #2	Practice #3	Final
5. The fact that the patient appears agitated and begins to raise his voice in anger should be a warning to you that he may become violent. It would be best not to handle this patient by yourself.				
6. If you are alone with the patient, leave the room and request assistance from another staff member.				
Example 3: Gathering Symptom Information About a Child				
1. A parent brings a 6-year-old boy to the office because the child is complaining about stomach pain.				

2. To gather the pertinent symptom information, ask the child various types of questions.*
  a. Can he tell you about the pain?*
  b. Can he tell you exactly where it hurts?
  c. Is there anything else that hurts?				

3. To confirm the child's answers, ask the parent to answer similar questions.				

4. You should then ask the parent additional questions. Begin with an open-ended question, as above. Follow up with specific questions such as these.
  a. How long has he had the pain?
  b. Is the pain related to any specific event (such as going to school)?				

5. Ask the child to confirm the parent's answers. He may be able to provide additional information at this time.				
Total Number of Points Achieved/Final Score				
Initials of Observer:				

Comments and Signatures

Reviewer's comments and signatures:

1. _____

2. _____

3. _____

Instructor's comments:

_____

CAAHEP Competencies Achieved

I. A (1) Apply critical thinking skills in performing patient assessment and care

IV. C (4) Identify techniques for overcoming communication barriers

ABHES Competencies Achieved

5 b. Identify and respond appropriately when working/caring for patients with special needs

5 e. Advocate on behalf of family/patients, having ability to deal and communicate with family

6 (bb) Are impartial and show empathy when dealing with patients

PROCEDURE 5-2 USING A PROGRESS NOTE

Procedure Goal

To accurately record a chief complaint on a progress note

Scoring System

To score each step, use the following scoring system:
1 = poor, 2 = fair, 3 = good, 4 = excellent

A minimum score of at least a 3 must be achieved on **each** step to achieve successful completion of the technique. Detailed instructions on the scoring system are found on page 179.

Materials

Progress note, patient chart, pen

Procedure

Procedure Steps Total Possible Points - 36 Time Limit: 5 minutes	Practice #1	Practice #2	Practice #3	Final
1. Wash your hands.				
2. Review the patient's chart notes from the patient's previous office visit. Verify that all results for any previously ordered laboratory work or diagnostics are in the chart.*				
3. Greet the patient and escort her to a private exam room.				
4. Introduce yourself and ask the patient her name.				
5. Using open-ended questions, find out why the patient is seeking medical care today.*				
6. Accurately document the chief complaint on the progress note on page 427 or 428. Document vital signs. Initial the chart entry.				
7. File the progress note in chronological order within the patient's chart.*				
8. Thank the patient and offer to answer any questions she may have. Explain that the physician will come in soon to examine her.				
9. Wash your hands.				
Total Number of Points Achieved/Final Score				
Initials of Observer:				

(continued)

Comments and Signatures

Reviewer's comments and signatures:

1. _____

2. _____

3. _____

Instructor's comments:

_____

CAAHEP Competency Achieved

IX. P (7) Document accurately in the patient record

ABHES Competencies Achieved

4 (a) Document accurately

8 (jj) Perform fundamental writing skills including correct grammar, spelling, and formatting techniques when writing prescriptions, documenting medical records, etc.

PROCEDURE 5-3 OBTAINING A MEDICAL HISTORY

Procedure Goal

To obtain a complete medical history with accuracy and professionalism

Scoring System

To score each step, use the following scoring system:
1 = poor, 2 = fair, 3 = good, 4 = excellent

A minimum score of at least a 3 must be achieved on **each** step to achieve successful completion of the technique. Detailed instructions on the scoring system are found on page 179.

Materials

Medical history form, patient chart, pen

Procedure

Procedure Steps Total Possible Points - 10 Time Limit: 10 minutes	Practice #1	Practice #2	Practice #3	Final
1. Wash your hands.				
2. Assemble the necessary materials. Review the medical history form and plan your interview.*				
3. Invite the patient to a private exam room and correctly identify the patient by introducing yourself and asking his or her name and date of birth.				
4. Explain the medical history form while maintaining eye contact. Make the patient feel at ease.				
5. Using language that the patient can understand, ask appropriate questions related to the medical history form. Use open-ended questions. Listen actively to the patient's response.				
6. Accurately document the patient's responses on the form on pages 420–430.				
7. Thank the patient for his or her participation in the interview. Offer to answer any questions.				
8. Sign or initial the medical history form and file it in the patient's chart.				
9. Inform the physician that you are finished with the medical history according to the physician's office policy.				
10. Wash your hands.				
Total Number of Points Achieved/Final Score				
Initials of Observer:				

(continued)

Comments and Signatures

Reviewer's comments and signatures:

1. _____

2. _____

3. _____

Instructor's comments:

_____

CAAHEP Competencies Achieved

I. P (6) Perform patient screening using established protocols

I. A (1) Apply critical thinking skills in performing patient assessment and care

I. A (2) Use language/verbal skills that enable patients' understanding

IV. C (4) Identify techniques for overcoming communication barriers

IV. C (6) Differentiate between subjective and objective information

IV. C (7) Identify resources and adaptations that are required based on individual needs, i.e., culture and environment, developmental life stage, language, and physical threats to communication

IV. P (3) Use medical terminology, pronouncing medical terms correctly, to communicate information, patient history, data, and observations

IV. A (1) Demonstrate empathy in communicating with patients, family, and staff

IV. A (2) Apply active listening skills

IV. A (3) Use appropriate body language and other nonverbal skills in communicating with patients, family, and staff

IV. A (4) Demonstrate awareness of the territorial boundaries of the person with whom communicating

IV. A (7) Demonstrate recognition of the patient's level of understanding in communications

IV. A (8) Analyze communications in providing appropriate responses/feedback

IV. A (9) Recognize and protect personal boundaries in communicating with others

IV. A (10) Demonstrate respect for individual diversity, incorporating awareness of one's own biases in areas including gender, race, religion, age, and economic status

ABHES Competencies Achieved

4 (a) Document accurately

8 (ff) Interview effectively

9 (a) Obtain chief complaint, recording patient history

PROCEDURE 6-1 MEASURING AND RECORDING TEMPERATURE

Procedure Goal

To accurately measure the temperature of patients while preventing the spread of infection

Scoring System

To score each step, use the following scoring system:
1 = poor, 2 = fair, 3 = good, 4 = excellent

A minimum score of at least a 3 must be achieved on **each** step to achieve successful completion of the technique. Detailed instructions on the scoring system are found on page 179.

Materials

Thermometer, probe cover if required by thermometer, lubricant for rectal temperature, gloves, trash receptacle, patient's chart, and recording device

Procedure

Procedure Steps Total Possible Points - 40 Time Limit: 5 minutes	Practice #1	Practice #2	Practice #3	Final
1. Gather the equipment and make sure the thermometer is in working order.				
2. Identify the patient and introduce yourself.				
3. Wash your hands and explain the procedure to the patient.				

4. Prepare the patient for the temperature.
  a. Oral. If the patient has had anything to eat or drink, or has been smoking, wait at least 15 minutes before measuring the temperature orally.*
  b. Rectal. Have the patient remove the appropriate clothing; assist as needed. Have the patient lie on his or her left side and drape for comfort.*
  c. Axillary. Assist the patient to expose the axilla. Provide for privacy and comfort. Pat dry the axilla.*
  d. Temporal or Tympanic. Remove the patient's hat if necessary.				

5. Prepare the equipment.
  a. Prepare an electronic thermometer by inserting the probe into the probe cover if necessary.*
  b. Prepare the disposable thermometer by removing the wrapper to expose the handle end. Avoid touching the part of the thermometer that goes in the mouth or on the skin.*
  c. Prepare the temporal scanner by removing the protective cap and making sure the lens is clean.*				

(continued)

Procedure Steps Total Possible Points - 40 Time Limit: 5 minutes	Practice #1	Practice #2	Practice #3	Final

6. Measure the temperature.
  a. Oral. Place the thermometer under the tongue in the back of the mouth on one side. Have the patient hold it in place with his or her lips and tongue. Wait for the electronic thermometer to beep or indicate completion. For a disposable thermometer, wait the required time, usually 60 seconds.
  b. Rectal. Put on gloves. Lubricate the thermometer tip. Raise the buttock to expose the anus with one hand and insert the thermometer into the anal canal, 1½ inches for adults and ½ to 1 inch for infants and children. Hold the thermometer securely in place until the indicator beeps or blinks.*
  c. Axillary. Place the thermometer into the axilla making sure the tip is in direct contact with the top of the axilla and is touching skin on all sides. Hold the arm firmly against the body until the indicator light blinks or beeps or the proper amount of time has passed.*
  d. Tympanic. Hold the outer edge of the ear (pinna) with your free hand. Gently pull the pinna up for adults and down for children. Insert the probe into the ear canal directed to the eardrum and sealing the ear canal. Press the scan button.*
  e. Temporal. Position the probe flat on the center of the exposed forehead. Press and hold the SCAN button and then slide the thermometer straight across the forehead until it beeps and the red light blinks.				

7. Remove and read the measurement in the display or on the thermometer. Discard the disposable thermometer. Eject and discard the probe cover for an electronic thermometer. Replace the cap and/or place the thermometer into the charging base.*				

8. Record the results. Chart by including the date and location where the temperature was taken.
  • Oral: 98.6
  • Rectal: 99.6 R
  • Axillary: 97.6 Ax
  • Temporal: 97.6
  • Tympanic: 97.6 Tymp.				

9. Help the patient to replace clothing as necessary. Clear the area and provide for safety and comfort for the patient.				
10. Wash your hands.				
Total Number of Points Achieved/Final Score				
Initials of Observer:				

(continued)

Comments and Signatures

Reviewer's comments and signatures:

1. _____

2. _____

3. _____

Instructor's comments:

_____

CAAHEP Competencies Achieved

I. P (1) Obtain vital signs

IV. P (2) Report relevant information to others succinctly and accurately

ABHES Competencies Achieved

9 (c) Take vital signs

9 (i) Use Standard Precautions

PROCEDURE 6-2 MEASURING AND RECORDING PULSE AND RESPIRATIONS

Procedure Goal

To accurately measure the pulse and respirations of a patient while keeping the patient unaware the respirations are being counted

Scoring System

To score each step, use the following scoring system:
1 = poor, 2 = fair, 3 = good, 4 = excellent

A minimum score of at least a 3 must be achieved on **each** step to achieve successful completion of the technique. Detailed instructions on the scoring system are found on page 179.

Materials

Watch with a second hand, patient's charts, and recording device.

Procedure

Procedure Steps Total Possible Points - 44 Time Limit: 5 minutes	Practice #1	Practice #2	Practice #3	Final
1. Gather the equipment and wash your hands.				
2. Introduce yourself and identify the patient.				
3. Explain the procedure saying, "I am going to take your vital signs. We'll start with your pulse first." Do not tell him you are counting the respirations.*				
4. Ask the patient to sit or lie in a comfortable position. Have the patient rest the arm on a table. The palm should be facing downward.				
5. Position yourself so you can observe and/or feel the chest wall movements. You may want to lay the patient's arm over the chest to feel the respiratory chest movements.				
6. Place two to three fingers on the radial pulse site. Find the radial bone on the thumb side of the wrist, then slide your fingers into the groove on the inside of the wrist to locate the pulse.				
7. Count the pulse for 15 to 30 seconds if regular. Note the rhythm and volume. If irregular, count for a full minute. Remember or note the number if necessary.*				
8. Without letting go of the wrist, observe and feel the respirations. Count for one full minute. Observe for rhythm, volume, and effort.				
9. Once you are certain of both numbers, release the wrist and record them. If the pulse was taken for less than one minute, obtain the number of beats per minute. Multiply the number of beats counted in 30 seconds by two or the number of beats counted in 15 seconds by 4.				

(continued)

Procedure Steps Total Possible Points - 44 Time Limit: 5 minutes	Practice #1	Practice #2	Practice #3	Final
10. Document results with the date and time.				
11. Report any findings that are a significant change from a previous result or outside the normal values as shown in Table 6-1 in the text.				
Total Number of Points Achieved/Final Score				
Initials of Observer:				

Comments and Signatures

Reviewer's comments and signatures:

1. _____

2. _____

3. _____

Instructor's comments:

_____

CAAHEP Competencies Achieved

I. P (1) Obtain vital signs

IV. P (2) Report relevant information to others succinctly and accurately

ABHES Competencies Achieved

9 (c) Take vital signs

9 (i) Use Standard Precautions

PROCEDURE 6-3 TAKING THE BLOOD PRESSURE OF ADULTS AND OLDER CHILDREN

Procedure Goal

To accurately measure blood pressure in adults and older children

Scoring System

To score each step, use the following scoring system:
1 = poor, 2 = fair, 3 = good, 4 = excellent

A minimum score of at least a 3 must be achieved on **each** step to achieve successful completion of the technique. Detailed instructions on the scoring system are found on page 179.

Materials

Aneroid or mercury sphygmomanometer, stethoscope, alcohol gauze squares, patient's chart, and black pen

Procedure

Procedure Steps Total Possible Points - 96 Time Limit: 5 minutes	Practice #1	Practice #2	Practice #3	Final
1. Gather the equipment and make sure the sphygmomanometer is in working order and is correctly calibrated.*				
2. Identify the patient and introduce yourself.				
3. Wash your hands and explain the procedure to the patient.				
4. Have the patient sit in a quiet area. If she is wearing long-sleeved clothing, have her loosely roll up one sleeve. If she cannot, have her change into a gown.				
5. Have the patient rest her bared arm on a flat surface so that the midpoint of the upper arm is at the same level as the heart.*				
6. Select a cuff that is the appropriate size for the patient. The bladder inside the cuff should encircle 80% of the arm in adults and 100% of the arm in children younger than the age of 13. If you are not sure about the size, use a larger cuff.*				
7. Locate the brachial artery in the antecubital space.				
8. Position the cuff so that the midline of the bladder is above the arterial pulsation. Then wrap and secure the cuff snugly around the patient's bare upper arm. The lower edge of the cuff should be 1 inch above the antecubital space, where the head of the stethoscope is to be placed.*				
9. Place the manometer so that the center of the aneroid dial or mercury column is at eye level and easily visible and so that the tubing from the cuff is unobstructed.				
10. Close the valve of the pressure bulb until it is finger-tight.				
11. Inflate the cuff rapidly to 70 mm Hg with one hand, and increase this pressure by 10 mm Hg increments while				

(continued)

Procedure Steps Total Possible Points - 96 Time Limit: 5 minutes	Practice #1	Practice #2	Practice #3	Final
palpating the radial pulse with your other hand. Note the level of pressure at which the pulse disappears and subsequently reappears during deflation. This procedure, the **palpatory method,** provides an approximation of the systolic blood pressure to ensure an adequate level of inflation when the actual measurement is made.				
12. Open the valve to release the pressure, deflate the cuff completely, and wait 30 seconds or remove and replace the cuff.*				
13. Place the earpieces of the stethoscope in your ear canals, and adjust them to fit snugly and comfortably. When placed in the ears, they should point up or toward the nose. Switch the stethoscope head to the diaphragm position. Confirm the setting by listening as you tap the stethoscope head gently.				
14. Place the head of the stethoscope over the brachial artery pulsation, just above and medial to the antecubital space but below the lower edge of the cuff. Hold the stethoscope firmly in place between the index and middle fingers, making sure the head is in contact with the skin around its entire circumference.*				
15. Inflate the bladder rapidly and steadily to a pressure 20 to 30 mm Hg above the level previously determined by palpation. Then partially open (unscrew) the valve and deflate the bladder at 2 mm per second while you listen for the appearance of the Korotkoff sounds.				
16. As the pressure in the bladder falls, note the level of pressure on the manometer at the first appearance of repetitive sounds. This reading is the systolic pressure.				
17. Continue to deflate the cuff gradually, noting the point at which the sound changes from strong to muffled.				
18. Continue to deflate the cuff and note when the sound disappears. This reading is the diastolic pressure.				
19. Deflate the cuff completely and remove it from the patient's arm.				
20. Record the numbers, separated by slashes, in the patient's chart. Chart the date and time of the measurement, the arm on which the measurement was made, the subject's position, and the cuff size when a nonstandard size is used.*				
21. Fold the cuff and replace it in the holder.				
22. Inform the patient that you have completed the procedure.				
23. Disinfect the earpieces and diaphragm of the stethoscope with gauze squares moistened with alcohol.				
24. Properly dispose of the used gauze squares and wash your hands.				
Total Number of Points Achieved/Final Score				
Initials of Observer:				

(continued)

Comments and Signatures

Reviewer's comments and signatures:

1. _____

2. _____

3. _____

Instructor's comments:

_____

CAAHEP Competencies Achieved

I. P (1) Obtain vital signs

IV. P (2) Report relevant information to others succinctly and accurately

ABHES Competencies Achieved

9 (c) Take vital signs

9 (i) Use Standard Precautions

PROCEDURE 6-4 MEASURING ADULTS AND CHILDREN

Procedure Goal

To accurately measure weight and height of adults and children

Scoring System

To score each step, use the following scoring system:
1 = poor, 2 = fair, 3 = good, 4 = excellent

A minimum score of at least a 3 must be achieved on **each** step to achieve successful completion of the technique. Detailed instructions on the scoring system are found on page 179.

Materials

For an adult or older child, adult scale with height bar, disposable towel; for toddler, adult scale with height bar or height chart, disposable towel

Procedure

Procedure Steps Total Possible Points - 120 Time Limit: 5 minutes	Practice #1	Practice #2	Practice #3	Final
Adult or Older Child: Weight				
1. Identify the patient and introduce yourself.				
2. Wash your hands and explain the procedure to the patient.				
3. Check to see whether the scale is in balance by moving all the weights to the left side. The indicator should be level with the middle mark. If not, check the manufacturer's directions and adjust it to ensure a zero balance. If you are using a scale equipped to measure either kilograms or pounds, check to see that it is set on the desired units and that the upper and lower weights show the same units.*				
4. Place a disposable towel on the scale or have the patient leave her socks on.*				
5. Ask the patient to remove her shoes, if that is the standard office policy.*				
6. Ask the patient to step on the center of the scale, facing forward. Assist as necessary.				
7. Place the lower weight at the highest number that does not cause the balance indicator to drop to the bottom.*				
8. Move the upper weight slowly to the right until the balance bar is centered at the middle mark, adjusting as necessary.*				
9. Add the two weights together to get the patient's weight.				
10. Record the patient's weight in the chart to the nearest quarter of a pound or tenth of a kilogram.				
11. Return the weights to their starting positions on the left side.				

(continued)

Procedure Steps Total Possible Points - 120 Time Limit: 5 minutes	Practice #1	Practice #2	Practice #3	Final
Adult or Older Child: Height				
12. With the patient off the scale, raise the height bar well above the patient's head and swing out the extension.*				
13. Ask the patient to step on the center of the scale and to stand up straight and look forward.*				
14. Gently lower the height bar until the extension rests on the patient's head.				
15. Have the patient step off the scale before reading the measurement.*				
16. If the patient is fewer than 50 inches tall, read the height on the bottom part of the ruler; if the patient is more than 50 inches tall, read the height on the top movable part of the ruler at the point at which it meets the bottom part of the ruler. Note that the numbers increase on the bottom part of the bar and decrease on the top, moveable part of the bar. Read the height in the right direction.				
17. Record the patient's height.				
18. Have the patient put her shoes back on, if necessary.				
19. Properly dispose of the used towel and wash your hands.				
Toddler: Weight				
1. Identify the patient and obtain permission from the parent to weigh the toddler.				
2. Wash your hands and explain the procedure to the parent.				
3. Check to see whether the scale is in balance and place a disposable towel on the scale or have the patient wear shoes or socks, depending upon the policy of the facility.				
4. Ask the parent to hold the patient and to step on the scale. Follow the procedure for obtaining the weight of an adult.				
5. Have the parent put the child down or hand the child to another staff member.*				
6. Obtain the parent's weight.				
7. Subtract the parent's weight from the combined weight to determine the weight of the child.				
8. Record the patient's weight in the chart to the nearest quarter of a pound or tenth of a kilogram.				
Toddler: Height				
9. Measure the child's height in the same manner as you measure adult height, or have the child stand with his back against the height chart. Measure height at the crown of the head.				
10. Record the height in the patient's chart.				
11. Properly dispose of the towel (if used) and wash your hands.*				
Total Number of Points Achieved/Final Score				
Initials of Observer:				

(continued)

Comments and Signatures

Reviewer's comments and signatures:

1. _____

2. _____

3. _____

Instructor's comments:

_____

CAAHEP Competencies Achieved

II. C (7) Analyze charts, graphs, and/or tables in the interpretation of health-care results

II. P (3) Maintain growth charts

IV. P (2) Report relevant information to others succinctly and accurately

ABHES Competency Achieved

2 (c) Assist the physician with the regimen of diagnostic and treatment modalities as they relate to each body system

PROCEDURE 6-5 MEASURING INFANTS

Procedure Goal

To accurately measure weight and length of infants and infant head circumference

Scoring System

To score each step, use the following scoring system:

1 = poor, 2 = fair, 3 = good, 4 = excellent

A minimum score of at least a 3 must be achieved on **each** step to achieve successful completion of the technique. Detailed instructions on the scoring system are found on page 179.

Materials

Pediatric examining table or infant scale, cardboard, pencil, yardstick, tape measure, disposable towel

Procedure

Procedure Steps Total Possible Points - 80 Time Limit: 5 minutes	Practice #1	Practice #2	Practice #3	Final
Weight				
1. Identify the patient and obtain permission from the parent to weigh the infant.				
2. Wash your hands and explain the procedure to the parent.				
3. Ask the parent to undress the infant.*				
4. Check to see whether the infant scale is in balance and place a disposable towel on it.*				
5. Have the parent place the child face up on the scale (or on the examining table if the scale is built into it). Keep one hand over the infant at all times and hold a diaper over a male patient's penis to catch any urine the infant might void.*				
6. Place the lower weight at the highest number that does not cause the balance indicator to drop to the bottom.*				
7. Move the upper weight slowly to the right until the balance bar is centered at the middle mark, adjusting as necessary.*				
8. Add the two weights together to get the infant's weight.				
9. Record the infant's weight in the chart or on the growth chart in pounds and ounces or to the nearest tenth of a kilogram.				
10. Return the weights to their starting positions on the left side.				
Length: Scale with Length (Height) Bar				
11. If the scale has a height bar, move the infant toward the head of the scale or examining table until her head touches the bar.				
12. Have the parent hold the infant by the shoulders in this position.				

(continued)

Procedure Steps Total Possible Points - 80 Time Limit: 5 minutes	Practice #1	Practice #2	Practice #3	Final
13. Holding the infant's ankles, gently extend the legs and slide the bottom bar to touch the soles of the feet.*				
14. Note the length and release the infant's ankles.				
15. Record the length in the patient's chart or on the growth chart.				
Length: Scale or Examining Table Without Length (Height) Bar				
16. If neither the scale nor the examining table has a height bar, have the parent position the infant close to the head of the examining table and hold the infant by the shoulders in this position.				
17. Place a stiff piece of cardboard against the crown of the infant's head and mark a line on the towel or paper, or hold a yardstick against the cardboard.				
18. Holding the infant's ankles, gently extend the legs and draw a line on the towel or paper to mark the heel, or note the measure on the yardstick.*				
19. Release the infant's ankles and measure the distance between the two markings on the towel or paper using the yardstick or a tape measure.				
20. Record the length in the patient's chart or on the growth chart.				
Head Circumference				
Measurement of head circumference may be performed at the same time as weight and length, or it may be part of the general physical exam.				
21. With the infant in a sitting or supine position, place the tape measure around the infant's head at the forehead.				
22. Adjust the tape so that it surrounds the infant's head at its largest circumference.				
23. Overlap the ends of the tape and read the measure at the point of overlap.				
24. Remove the tape, and record the circumference in the patient's chart or on the growth chart.				
25. Properly dispose of the used towel and wash your hands.				
Total Number of Points Achieved/Final Score				
Initials of Observer:				

(continued)

Comments and Signatures

Reviewer's comments and signatures:

1. _____

2. _____

3. _____

Instructor's comments:

_____

CAAHEP Competencies Achieved

II. C (7) Analyze charts, graphs, and/or tables in the interpretation of health-care results

II. P (3) Maintain growth charts

IV. P (2) Report relevant information to others succinctly and accurately

ABHES Competency Achieved

2 (c) Assist the physician with the regimen of diagnostic and treatment modalities as they relate to each body system

PROCEDURE 7-1 POSITIONING THE PATIENT FOR AN EXAM

Procedure Goal

To effectively assist a patient in assuming the various positions used in a general physical exam

Scoring System

To score each step, use the following scoring system:
1 = poor, 2 = fair, 3 = good, 4 = excellent

A minimum score of at least a 3 must be achieved on **each** step to achieve successful completion of the technique. Detailed instructions on the scoring system are found on page 179.

Materials

Adjustable examining table or gynecologic table, step stool, exam gown, drape

Procedure

Procedure Steps Total Possible Points - 40 Time Limit: 10 minutes	Practice #1	Practice #2	Practice #3	Final
1. Identify the patient and introduce yourself.				
2. Wash your hands.				
3. Explain the procedure to the patient.				
4. Provide a gown or drape if the physician has requested one and instruct the patient in the proper way to wear it after disrobing. Allow the patient privacy while disrobing and assist only if the patient requests help.*				
5. Explain to the patient the necessary exam and the position required.				
6. Ask the patient to step on the stool or the pullout step of the examining table. If necessary, assist the patient onto the examining table.				
7. Assist the patient into the required position: a. Sitting. Do not use this position for patients who cannot sit unsupported. b. Supine (Recumbent). Do not use this position for patients with back injuries, low back pain, or difficulty breathing. Place a pillow or other support under the head and knees for comfort, if needed. c. Dorsal Recumbent. This position may be difficult for someone with leg disabilities. It may be used for patients when lithotomy is difficult. d. Lithotomy. This position is used to examine the female genitalia, with the patient's feet placed in stirrups. Assist as necessary. The patient's buttocks should be near the edge of the table. Drape the client with a large drape to help prevent embarrassment. e. Trendelenburg. This position is a supine position with the patient's head lower than her feet. It is used infrequently in the physician's office but may be necessary for low blood pressure or shock.				

(continued)

Procedure Steps Total Possible Points - 40 Time Limit: 10 minutes	Practice #1	Practice #2	Practice #3	Final
f. Fowler's. Adjust the head of the table to the desired angle. Help the patient move toward the head of the table until the patient's buttocks meet the point at which the head of the table begins to incline upward. g. Prone. This position is when the patient lies face down. It is not used for later stages of pregnancy, obese patients, patients with respiratory difficulty, or certain elderly patients. h. Sims'. In this position, the patient lies on her left side with her left leg slightly bent and her left arm behind her back. Her right knee is bent and raised toward her chest and her right arm is bent toward her head. This position may be difficult for patients with joint deformities. i. Knee-Chest. This position is difficult for patients to assume. The patient is face down, supporting his weight on his knees and chest or an alternative knee-elbow position. This position is used for rectal and perineal exams. Keep the patient in this position for the shortest amount of time possible. j. Proctologic. This position is also used for rectal and perineal exams. In this position, the patient bends over the examining table with his chest resting on the table.				
8. Drape the client to prevent exposure and avoid embarrassment. Place pillows for comfort as needed.*				
9. Adjust the drapes during the exam.				
10. On completion of the exam, assist the client as necessary out of the position and provide privacy as the client dresses.				
Total Number of Points Achieved/Final Score				
Initials of Observer:				

Comments and Signatures

Reviewer's comments and signatures:

1. _____

2. _____

3. _____

Instructor's comments:

_____

CAAHEP Competency Achieved

II. P (6) Prepare a patient for procedures and/or treatments

ABHES Competency Achieved

9 (I) Prepare patient for examinations and treatments

PROCEDURE 7-2 COMMUNICATING EFFECTIVELY WITH PATIENTS FROM OTHER CULTURES AND MEETING THEIR NEEDS FOR PRIVACY

Procedure Goal

To ensure effective communication with patients from other cultures while meeting their needs for privacy

Scoring System

To score each step, use the following scoring system:
1 = poor, 2 = fair, 3 = good, 4 = excellent

A minimum score of at least a 3 must be achieved on **each** step to achieve successful completion of the technique. Detailed instructions on the scoring system are found on page 179.

Materials

Exam gown, drapes

Procedure

Procedure Steps Total Possible Points - 44 Time Limit: 10 minutes	Practice #1	Practice #2	Practice #3	Final
Effective Communication				
1. When it is necessary to use a translator, direct conversation or instruction to the translator.*				
2. Direct demonstrations of what to do, such as putting on an exam gown, to the patient.				
3. Confirm with the translator that the patient has understood the instruction or demonstration.				
4. Allow the translator to be present during the exam if that is the patient's preference.				
5. If the patient understands some English, speak slowly, use simple language, and demonstrate instructions whenever possible.				
Meeting the Need for Privacy				
1. Before the procedure, thoroughly explain to the patient or translator the reason for disrobing. Indicate that you will allow the patient privacy and ample time to undress.				
2. If the patient is reluctant, reassure him that the physician respects the need for privacy and will look at only what is necessary for the exam.*				
3. Provide extra drapes if you think doing so will make the patient feel more comfortable.				
4. If the patient is still reluctant, discuss the problem with the physician; the physician may be able to negotiate a compromise with the patient.				
5. During the procedure, ensure that the patient is undraped only as much as necessary.				

(continued)

Procedure Steps Total Possible Points - 44 Time Limit: 10 minutes	Practice #1	Practice #2	Practice #3	Final
6. Whenever possible, minimize the amount of time the patient remains undraped.				
Total Number of Points Achieved/Final Score				
Initials of Observer:				

Comments and Signatures

Reviewer's comments and signatures:

1. _____

2. _____

3. _____

Instructor's comments:

_____

CAAHEP Competency Achieved

X. A (3) Demonstrate awareness of diversity in providing patient care

ABHES Competencies Achieved

5 (b) Identify and respond appropriately when working/caring for patients with special needs

9 (q) Instruct patients with special needs

PROCEDURE 7-3 TRANSFERRING A PATIENT IN A WHEELCHAIR AND PREPARING FOR AN EXAM

Procedure Goal

To assist a patient in transferring from a wheelchair to the examining table safely and efficiently

Scoring System

To score each step, use the following scoring system:
1 = poor, 2 = fair, 3 = good, 4 = excellent

A minimum score of at least a 3 must be achieved on **each** step to achieve successful completion of the technique. Detailed instructions on the scoring system are found on page 179.

Materials

Adjustable examining table or gynecologic table, step stool (optional), exam gown, drape

Procedure

Procedure Steps Total Possible Points - 68 Time Limit: 10 minutes	Practice #1	Practice #2	Practice #3	Final
Never risk injuring yourself; call for assistance when in doubt. As a rule, you should not attempt to lift more than 35% of your body weight. **Preparation Before Transfer** 1. Identify the patient and introduce yourself.				
2. Wash your hands.				
3. Explain the procedure in detail.				
4. Position the wheelchair at a right angle to the end of the examining table. This position reduces the distance between the wheelchair and the end of the examining table across which the patient must move.				
5. Lock the wheels of the wheelchair.*				
6. Lift the patient's feet and fold back the foot and leg supports of the wheelchair.				
7. Place the patient's feet on the floor. The patient should have shoes or slippers with nonskid soles. Place your feet in front of the patient's feet.*				
8. If needed, place a step stool in front of the table and place the patient's feet flat on the stool.				
Transferring the Patient by Yourself 9. Face the patient, spread your feet apart, align your knees with the patient's knees, and bend your knees slightly.*				
10. Have the patient hold on to your shoulders.				
11. Place your arms around the patient, under the patient's arms.				
12. Tell the patient that you will lift on the count of 3 and ask the patient to support as much of his own weight as possible (if he is able).				
13. At the count of 3, lift the patient.				

(continued)

Procedure Steps Total Possible Points - 68 Time Limit: 10 minutes	Practice #1	Practice #2	Practice #3	Final
14. Pivot the patient to bring the back of the patient's knees against the table.				
15. Gently lower the patient into a sitting position on the table. If the patient cannot sit unassisted, help him move into a supine position.				
16. Move the wheelchair out of the way.				
17. Assist the patient with disrobing as necessary, providing a gown and drape.				
Transferring the Patient with Assistance				
9. Working with your partner, both of you face the patient, spread your feet apart, position yourselves so that one of each of your knees is aligned with the patient's knees, and bend your knees slightly.*				
10. Have the patient place one hand on each of your shoulders and hold on.				
11. Each of you places your outermost arm around the patient, one under each of the patient's arms. Then interlock your wrists.				
12. Tell the patient that you will lift on the count of 3 and ask the patient to support as much of his own weight as possible (if he is able).				
13. At the count of 3, you should lift the patient together.				
14. The stronger of the two of you should pivot the patient to bring the back of the patient's knees against the table.				
15. Working together, gently lower the patient into a sitting position on the table. If the patient cannot sit unassisted, help him move into a supine position.				
16. Move the wheelchair out of the way.				
17. Assist the patient with disrobing as necessary, providing a gown and drape.				
Total Number of Points Achieved/Final Score				
Initials of Observer:				

Comments and Signatures

Reviewer's comments and signatures:

1. _____

2. _____

3. _____

Instructor's comments:

_____

CAAHEP Competency Achieved

IV. P (6) Prepare a patient for procedures and/or treatments

ABHES Competency Achieved

9 (I) Prepare patient for examinations and treatments

PROCEDURE 7-4 ASSISTING WITH A GENERAL PHYSICAL EXAM

Procedure Goal

To effectively assist the physician with a general physical exam

Scoring System

To score each step, use the following scoring system:
1 = poor, 2 = fair, 3 = good, 4 = excellent

A minimum score of at least a 3 must be achieved on **each** step to achieve successful completion of the technique. Detailed instructions on the scoring system are found on page 179.

Materials

Supplies and equipment will vary depending on the type and purpose of the exam and the physician's practice preferences. Supplies may include the following: Gown, drape, adjustable examining table, gloves, laryngeal mirror, lubricant, nasal speculum, otoscope and ophthalmoscope, pillow, reflex hammer, tuning fork, sphygmomanometer, stethoscope, tape measure, tongue depressors, penlight

Procedure

Procedure Steps Total Possible Points - 116 Time Limit: 15 minutes	Practice #1	Practice #2	Practice #3	Final
1. Wash your hands and adhere to Standard Precautions throughout the procedure.*				
2. Gather and assemble the equipment and supplies.				
3. Arrange the instruments and equipment in a logical sequence for the physician's use.				
4. Greet and properly identify the patient using at least two patient identifiers.*				
5. Review the patient's medical history with the patient if office policy requires it.				
6. Obtain vital statistics per the physician's preference.				
7. Obtain the patient's weight and height (with shoes removed).				
8. Obtain a urine specimen before the patient undresses for the exam.				
9. Explain the procedure and exam to the patient.*				
10. Obtain blood specimens or other laboratory tests per the chart or verbal order.				
11. Provide the patient with an appropriate gown and drape and explain where the opening for the gown is placed.				
12. Obtain the ECG if ordered by the physician.				
13. Assist patient to a sitting position at the end of the table with the drape placed across his or her legs.				
14. Inform the physician that the patient is ready and remain in the room to assist the physician.				
15. You may be asked to shut off the light in the exam room to allow the patient's pupils to dilate sufficiently for a retinal exam.				

(continued)

Procedure Steps Total Possible Points - 116 Time Limit: 15 minutes	Practice #1	Practice #2	Practice #3	Final
16. Hand the instruments to the physician as requested.				
17. Assist the patient to a supine position and drape him or her for an exam of the front of the body.				
18. If a gynecological exam is needed, assist and drape the patient in the lithotomy position.				
19. If a rectal exam is needed, assist and drape the patient in the Sims' position.				
20. Assist the patient to a prone position for a posterior body exam.				
21. When the exam is complete, assist the patient to a sitting position and ask the patient to sit for a brief period of time.*				
22. Ask the patient if he or she needs assistance in dressing.				
23. Dispose of contaminated materials in an appropriate container.				
24. Remove the table paper and pillow covering and dispose of them in the proper container.				
25. Disinfect and clean counters and the examining table with a disinfectant.				
26. Sanitize and sterilize the instruments, if needed.				
27. Prepare the room for the next patient by replacing the table paper, pillow case, equipment, and supplies.				
28. Document the procedure.				
Total Number of Points Achieved/Final Score				
Initials of Observer:				

Comments and Signatures

Reviewer's comments and signatures:

1. _____

2. _____

3. _____

Instructor's comments:

_____

CAAHEP Competency Achieved

I. P (10) Assist physician with patient care

ABHES Competency Achieved

9 (I) Prepare patient for examinations and treatments

PROCEDURE 7-5 PERFORMING VISION SCREENING TESTS

Objectives

To screen a patient's ability to see distant or close objects, to determine contrast sensitivity, or to detect color blindness

Scoring System

To score each step, use the following scoring system:
1 = poor, 2 = fair, 3 = good, 4 = excellent

A minimum score of at least a 3 must be achieved on **each** step to achieve successful completion of the technique. Detailed instructions on the scoring system are found on page 179.

Materials

Occluder or card; alcohol; gauze squares; appropriate vision charts to test for distance vision, near vision, and color blindness and Progress Note to record results on page 449

Procedure

Procedure Steps Total Possible Points - 128 Time Limit: 10 minutes	Practice #1	Practice #2	Practice #3	Final
Distance Vision 1. Wash your hands, identify the patient, introduce yourself, and explain the procedure.				
2. Mount one of the following eye charts at eye level: Snellen letter or similar chart (for patients who can read); Snellen E, Landolt C, pictorial, or similar chart (for patients who cannot read). If using the Snellen letter chart, verify that the patient knows the letters of the alphabet. With children or nonreading adults, use demonstration cards to verify that they can identify the pictures or direction of the letters.*				
3. Make a mark on the floor 20 feet away from the chart.				
4. Have the patient stand with the heels at the 20-foot mark or sit with the back of the chair at the mark.				
5. Instruct the patient to keep both eyes open and not to squint or lean forward during the test.*				
6. Test both eyes first, then the right eye, and then the left eye. (Different offices may test in a different order. Follow your office policy.)*				
7. Have the patient read the lines on the chart (or identify the picture/direction), beginning with the 20-foot line. If the patient cannot read this line, begin with the smallest line the patient can read. (Some offices use a pointer to select one symbol at a time in random order to prevent patients from memorizing the order. It is common to start with children at the 40- or 30-foot line, or larger if low vision is suspected, and proceed to the 20-foot line.)				

(continued)

Procedure Steps Total Possible Points - 128 Time Limit: 10 minutes	Practice #1	Practice #2	Practice #3	Final
8. Note the smallest line the patient can read or identify. (When testing children, note the smallest line on which they can identify three out of four or four out of six symbols correctly.)				
9. Record the results as a fraction (for example, O.U. 20/40–1 if the patient misses one letter on a line or O.U. 20/40–2 if the patient misses two letters on a line).				
10. Show the patient how to cover the left eye with the occluder or card. Again, instruct the patient to keep both eyes open and not to squint or lean forward during the test.				
11. Have the patient read the lines on the chart.				
12. Record the results of the right eye (for example, Right Eye 20/30).				
13. Have the patient cover the right eye and read the lines on the chart.				
14. Record the results of the left eye (for example, Left Eye 20/20).				
15. If the patient wears corrective lenses, record the results using $\overline{cc}$ (if your office uses this abbreviation for "with correction") in front of the abbreviation (for example, $\overline{cc}$ both eyes 20/20).*				
16. Note and record any observations of squinting, head tilting, or excessive blinking or tearing.				
17. Ask the patient to keep both eyes open and to identify the two colored bars, and record the results in the patient's chart.				
18. Clean the occluder with a gauze square dampened with alcohol.				
19. Properly dispose of the gauze square and wash your hands.*				
Near Vision				
1. Wash your hands, identify the patient, introduce yourself, and explain the procedure.				
2. Have the patient hold one of the following at normal reading distance (approximately 14 to 16 inches): Jaeger, Richmond pocket, or similar chart or card.				
3. Ask the patient to keep both eyes open and to read or identify the letters, symbols, or paragraphs.*				
4. Record the smallest line read without error.				
5. If the card is laminated, clean it with a gauze square dampened with alcohol.				
6. Properly dispose of the gauze square and wash your hands.*				
Color Vision				
1. Wash your hands, identify the patient, introduce yourself, and explain the procedure.				
2. Hold one of the following color charts or books at the patient's normal reading distance (approximately 14 to 16 inches): Ishihara, Richmond pseudoisochromatic, or similar color-testing system.				

(continued)

Procedure Steps Total Possible Points - 128 Time Limit: 10 minutes	Practice #1	Practice #2	Practice #3	Final
3. Ask the patient to tell you the number or symbol within the colored dots on each chart or page.				
4. Proceed through all the charts or pages.				
5. Record the number correctly identified and failed with a slash between them (for example, 13 passed/1 failed).				
6. If the charts are laminated, clean them with a gauze square dampened with alcohol.				
7. Properly dispose of the gauze square and wash your hands.*				
Total Number of Points Achieved/Final Score				
Initials of Observer:				

Comments and Signatures

Reviewer's comments and signatures:

1. _____

2. _____

3. _____

Instructor's comments:

_____

CAAHEP Competency Achieved

I. P (10) Assist physician with patient care

ABHES Competency Achieved

2 (c) Assist the physician with the regimen of diagnostic and treatment modalities as they relate to each body system

PROCEDURE 7-6 MEASURING AUDITORY ACUITY

Objective

To determine how well a patient hears

Scoring System

To score each step, use the following scoring system:
1 = poor, 2 = fair, 3 = good, 4 = excellent

A minimum score of at least a 3 must be achieved on **each** step to achieve successful completion of the technique. Detailed instructions on the scoring system are found on page 179.

Materials

Audiometer, headset, graph pad (if applicable) or Progress Notes, alcohol, gauze squares

Procedure

Procedure Steps Total Possible Points - 140 Time Limit: 10 minutes	Practice #1	Practice #2	Practice #3	Final
Adults and Children				
1. Wash your hands, identify the patient, introduce yourself, and explain the procedure.				
2. Clean the earpieces of the headset with a gauze square dampened with alcohol.*				
3. Have the patient sit with his back to you.				
4. Assist the patient in putting on the headset and adjust it until it is comfortable.				
5. Tell the patient he will hear tones in the right ear.				
6. Tell the patient to raise his finger or press the indicator button when he hears a tone.				
7. Set the audiometer for the right ear.				
8. Set the audiometer for the lowest range of frequencies and the first degree of loudness (usually 15 decibels). (When using automated audiometers, follow the instructions printed in the user's manual.)				
9. Press the tone button or switch and observe the patient.				
10. If the patient does not hear the first degree of loudness, raise it two or three times to greater degrees, up to 50 or 60 decibels.				
11. If the patient indicates that he has heard the tone, record the setting on the graph.				
12. Change the setting to the next frequency. Repeat steps 9, 10, and 11.				
13. Proceed to the mid-range frequencies. Repeat steps 9, 10, and 11.				
14. Proceed to the high-range frequencies. Repeat steps 9, 10, and 11.				

(continued)

Procedure Steps Total Possible Points - 140 Time Limit: 10 minutes	Practice #1	Practice #2	Practice #3	Final
15. Set the audiometer for the left ear.				
16. Tell the patient that he will hear tones in the left ear and ask him to raise his finger or press the indicator button when he hears a tone.				
17. Repeat steps 8 through 14.				
18. Set the audiometer for both ears.				
19. Ask the patient to listen with both ears and to raise his finger or press the indicator button when he hears a tone.				
20. Repeat steps 8 through 14.				
21. Have the patient remove the headset.				
22. Clean the earpieces with a gauze square dampened with alcohol.				
23. Properly dispose of the used gauze square and wash your hands.*				
Infants and Toddlers				
1. Identify the patient and introduce yourself.				
2. Wash your hands.				
3. Pick a quiet location.				
4. The patient can be sitting, lying down, or held by the parent.				
5. Instruct the parent to be silent during the procedure.				
6. Position yourself so your hands are behind the child's right ear and out of sight.*				
7. Clap your hands loudly. Observe the child's response. (Never clap directly in front of the ear because this can damage the eardrum. As an alternative to clapping, use special devices, such as rattles or clickers, which may be available in the office to generate sounds of varying loudness.)				
8. Record the child's response as positive or negative for loud noise.				
9. Position one hand behind the child's right ear, as before.				
10. Snap your fingers. Observe the child's response.				
11. Record the response as positive or negative for moderate noise.				
12. Repeat steps 6 through 11 for the left ear.				
Total Number of Points Achieved/Final Score				
Initials of Observer:				

(continued)

Comments and Signatures

Reviewer's comments and signatures:

1. _____

2. _____

3. _____

Instructor's comments:

_____

CAAHEP Competency Achieved

I. P (10) Assist physician with patient care

ABHES Competency Achieved

2 (c) Assist the physician with the regimen of diagnostic and treatment modalities as they relate to each body system

PROCEDURE 8-1 ASSISTING WITH A GYNECOLOGICAL EXAM

Procedure Goal

To assist the physician and maintain the client's comfort and privacy during a gynecological exam

Scoring System

To score each step, use the following scoring system:
1 = poor, 2 = fair, 3 = good, 4 = excellent

A minimum score of at least a 3 must be achieved on **each** step to achieve successful completion of the technique. Detailed instructions on the scoring system are found on page 179.

Materials

Gown and drape, vaginal speculum, specimen collection equipment, including cervical brush, cervical broom, and/or scraper, cotton-tipped applicator, potassium hydroxide solution (KOH), exam gloves, tissues, laboratory requisition, water-soluble lubricant, examining table with stirrups, exam light, microscopic slide(s), thin-layer collection vial, tissues, spray fixative, pen and pencil

Procedure

Procedure Steps Total Possible Points - 60 Time Limit: 10 minutes	Practice #1	Practice #2	Practice #3	Final
1. Gather equipment and make sure all items are in working order. Correctly label the slide and/or the collection vials.*				
2. Identify the patient and explain the procedure. The patient should remove all clothing, including underwear, and put the gown on with the opening in the front.				
3. Ask the patient to sit on the edge of the examining table with the drape until the physician arrives.				
4. When the physician is ready, have the patient place her feet into the stirrups and move her buttocks to the edge of the table. This is the lithotomy position.*				
5. Provide the physician with gloves and an exam lamp as she examines the genitalia by inspection and palpation.				
6. Pass the speculum to the physician. To increase patient comfort, you may place it in warm water before handing it to the physician. Water-based lubricant is not recommended prior to the Pap smear because it may interfere with the test results.				
7. For the Pap (Papanicolaou) smear, be prepared to pass a cotton-tipped applicator and cervical brush, broom, or scraper for the collection of the specimens. Have the labeled slide or vial available for the physician to place the specimen on the slide. Depending on the physician, the specimen collected, the method of collection, and the method of preparation, two or more slides or collection vials may be necessary. They may be labeled based on where the specimen was collected: endocervical E, vaginal V, and cervical C.				

(continued)

Procedure Steps Total Possible Points - 60 Time Limit: 10 minutes	Practice #1	Practice #2	Practice #3	Final
8. Once the specimen is on the slide, a cytology fixative must be applied immediately. A spray fixative is common, and it should be held 6 inches from the slide and sprayed lightly with a back and forth motion. Allow the slide to dry completely.* Cells collected for thin-layer preparation should be washed into the collection vial and transported to an outside lab for processing and analysis.				
9. After the physician removes the speculum, a digital exam is performed to check the position of the internal organs. Provide the physician with additional lubricant as needed.				
10. Upon completion of the exam, help the patient switch from the lithotomy position to a supine or sitting position.				
11. Provide tissues or moist wipes for the patient to remove the lubricant and ask the patient to get dressed. Assist as necessary or provide for privacy. Explain the procedure for communicating the laboratory results.				
12. After the patient has left, don gloves and clean the exam room and equipment. Dispose of the disposable speculum, specimen collection devices, and other contaminated waste in a biohazardous waste container.				
13. Store the supplies, straighten the room, and discard the used exam paper on the table.				
14. Prepare the laboratory requisition slip and place it and the specimen in the proper place for transport to an outside laboratory.				
15. Remove your gloves and wash your hands.				
Total Number of Points Achieved/Final Score				
Initials of Observer:				

Comments and Signatures

Reviewer's comments and signatures:

1. _____

2. _____

3. _____

Instructor's comments:

_____

CAAHEP Competencies Achieved

I. P (10) Assist physician with patient care

IV. P (6) Prepare a patient for procedures and/or treatments

ABHES Competencies Achieved

I. Prepare patient for examinations and treatments

m. Assist physician with routine and specialty examinations and treatments

PROCEDURE 8-2 ASSISTING WITH A CERVICAL BIOPSY

Procedure Goal

To assist the physician in obtaining a sample of cervical tissue for analysis

Scoring System

To score each step, use the following scoring system:
1 = poor, 2 = fair, 3 = good, 4 = excellent

A minimum score of at least a 3 must be achieved on **each** step to achieve successful completion of the technique. Detailed instructions on the scoring system are found on page 179.

Materials

Gown and drape, tray or Mayo stand, disposable cervical biopsy kit (disposable forceps, curette, and spatula in a sterile pack), transfer forceps, vaginal speculum, biopsy specimen container, clean basin, sterile cotton balls, sterile gauze squares, sanitary napkin

Procedure

Procedure Steps Total Possible Points - 60 Time Limit: 10 minutes	Practice #1	Practice #2	Practice #3	Final
1. Identify the patient and introduce yourself.				
2. Look at the patient's chart and ask the patient to confirm information or explain any changes. Specific patient information you need to ask about and note in the chart includes the following: • Date of birth and Social Security number (verify that you have the correct chart for the correct patient) • Date of last menstrual period • Method of contraception, if any • Previous gynecologic surgery • Use of hormone replacement therapy or other steroids				
3. Describe the biopsy procedure to the patient, noting that a piece of tissue will be removed to diagnose the cause of her problem. Explain that it may be painful but only for the brief moment during which tissue is taken.				
4. Give the patient a gown, if needed, and a drape. Direct her to undress from the waist down and to wrap the drape around herself. Tell her to sit at the end of the examining table.				
5. Wash your hands and put on exam gloves.				
6. Using sterile method, open the sterile pack to create a sterile field on the tray or Mayo stand and arrange the instruments with transfer forceps. Add the vaginal speculum and sterile supplies to the sterile field.*				
7. When the physician arrives in the exam room, ask the patient to lie back, place her heels in the stirrups of the table, and move her buttocks to the edge of the table.*				
8. Assist the physician by arranging the drape so that only the genitalia are exposed and place the light so that the genitalia are illuminated.				

(continued)

Procedure Steps Total Possible Points - 60 Time Limit: 10 minutes	Practice #1	Practice #2	Practice #3	Final
9. Use transfer forceps to hand instruments and supplies to the physician as he requests them. You may don sterile gloves and hand the physician supplies and instruments directly. When he is ready to obtain the biopsy, tell the patient that it may hurt. If she seems particularly fearful, instruct her to take a deep breath and let it out slowly.				
10. When the physician hands you the instrument with the tissue specimen, place the specimen in the specimen container and discard the instrument in the appropriate container.				
11. Label the specimen container with the patient's name, the date and time, cervical or endocervical (as indicated by the physician), the physician's name, and your initials.				
12. Place the container and the cytology laboratory requisition form in the envelope or bag provided by the laboratory.				
13. When the physician has removed the vaginal speculum, place it in the clean basin for later sanitization, disinfection, and sterilization. Properly dispose of used supplies and disposable instruments.				
14. Remove the gloves and wash your hands.				
15. Tell the patient that she may get dressed. Inform her that she may have some vaginal bleeding for a couple of days and provide her with a sanitary napkin. Instruct her not to take tub baths or have intercourse and not to use tampons for 2 days. Encourage her to call the office if she experiences problems or has questions.				
Total Number of Points Achieved/Final Score				
Initials of Observer:				

Comments and Signatures

Reviewer's comments and signatures:

1. _____

2. _____

3. _____

Instructor's comments:

_____

CAAHEP Competencies Achieved

I. P (10) Assist physician with patient care

IV. P (6) Prepare a patient for procedures and/or treatments

ABHES Competencies Achieved

l. Prepare patient for examinations and treatments

m. Assist physician with routine and specialty examinations and treatments

PROCEDURE 8-3 MEETING THE NEEDS OF THE PREGNANT PATIENT DURING AN EXAM

Procedure Goal

To meet the special needs of the pregnant woman during the general physical exam

Scoring System

To score each step, use the following scoring system:
1 = poor, 2 = fair, 3 = good, 4 = excellent

A minimum score of at least a 3 must be achieved on **each** step to achieve successful completion of the technique. Detailed instructions on the scoring system are found on page 179.

Materials

Patient education materials, examining table, exam gown, drape

Procedure

Procedure Steps Total Possible Points - 68 Time Limit: 10 minutes	Practice #1	Practice #2	Practice #3	Final
Providing Patient Information				
1. Identify the patient and introduce yourself.				
2. Assess the patient's need for education by asking appropriate questions and having the patient describe what she already knows about the information you are providing.				
3. Provide any appropriate instructions or materials.				
4. Ask the patient whether she has any special concerns or questions about her pregnancy that she might want to discuss with the physician.				
5. Communicate the patient's concerns or questions to the physician; include all pertinent background information on the patient.*				
Ensuring Comfort During the Exam				
1. Identify the patient and introduce yourself.				
2. Wash your hands.				
3. Explain the procedure to the patient.				
4. Provide a gown or drape and instruct the patient in the proper way to wear it after disrobing. (Allow the patient privacy while disrobing and assist only if she requests help.)				
5. Ask the patient to step on the stool or the pullout step of the examining table.				
6. Assist the patient onto the examining table.*				
7. Keeping position restrictions in mind, help the patient into the position requested by the physician.				

(continued)

Procedure Steps Total Possible Points - 68 Time Limit: 10 minutes	Practice #1	Practice #2	Practice #3	Final
8. Provide and adjust additional drapes as needed.				
9. Keep in mind any difficulties the patient may have in achieving a certain position; suggest alternative positions whenever possible.				
10. Minimize the time the patient must spend in uncomfortable positions.*				
11. If the patient appears to be uncomfortable during the procedure, ask whether she would like to reposition herself or take a break; assist as necessary.				
12. To prevent pelvic pooling of blood and subsequent dizziness or hyperventilation, allow the patient time to adjust to sitting before standing after she has been lying on the examining table.				
Total Number of Points Achieved/Final Score				
Initials of Observer:				

Comments and Signatures

Reviewer's comments and signatures:

1. _____

2. _____

3. _____

Instructor's comments:

_____

CAAHEP Competencies Achieved

I. P (10) Assist physician with patient care

IV. P (6) Prepare a patient for procedures and/or treatments

ABHES Competencies Achieved

I. Prepare patient for examinations and treatments

m. Assist physician with routine and specialty examinations and treatments

PROCEDURE 9-1 ASSISTING WITH A SCRATCH TEST EXAMINATION

Procedure Goal

To determine substances to which a patient has an allergic reaction

Scoring System

To score each step, use the following scoring system:
1 = poor, 2 = fair, 3 = good, 4 = excellent

A minimum score of at least a 3 must be achieved on **each** step to achieve successful completion of the technique. Detailed instructions on the scoring system are found on page 179.

Materials

Disposable sterile needles or lancets, allergen extracts, control solution, cotton balls, alcohol, timer, adhesive tape, ruler, cold packs or ice bag

Procedure

Procedure Steps Total Possible Points - 68 Time Limit: 10 minutes	Practice #1	Practice #2	Practice #3	Final
1. Wash your hands and assemble the necessary materials.				
2. Identify the patient and introduce yourself.				
3. Show the patient into the treatment area. Explain the procedure and discuss any concerns. Confirm whether the patient followed pretesting procedures (discontinuing antihistamines, etc.).*				
4. Put on exam gloves and assist the patient into a comfortable position.				
5. Swab the test site, usually the upper arm or back, with an alcohol prep pad.				
6. Identify the sites (if more than one) with adhesive-tape labels.*				
7. Apply small drops of the allergen extracts and control solution onto the test site at evenly spaced intervals, about 1½ to 2 inches apart.				
8. Open the package containing the first needle or lancet, making sure you do not contaminate the instrument.				
9. Assist the physician with the scratch procedure or perform the procedure if within your scope of practice. Using a new sterile needle or lancet for each site, scratch the skin beneath each drop of allergen, no more than ⅛-inch deep.				
10. Start the timer for the 20-minute reaction period.				
11. After the reaction time has passed, cleanse each site with an alcohol prep pad. (Do not remove identifying labels until the doctor has checked the patient.)				
12. Assist the physician or examine and measure the sites.				

(continued)

Procedure Steps Total Possible Points - 68 Time Limit: 10 minutes	Practice #1	Practice #2	Practice #3	Final
13. Apply cold packs or an ice bag to sites as needed to relieve itching.				
14. Record the test results in the patient's chart and initial your entries.				
15. Properly dispose of used materials and instruments.				
16. Clean and disinfect the area according to OSHA guidelines.				
17. Remove the gloves and wash your hands.				
Total Number of Points Achieved/Final Score				
Initials of Observer:				

Comments and Signatures

Reviewer's comments and signatures:

1. _____

2. _____

3. _____

Instructor's comments:

_____

CAAHEP Competencies Achieved

    I. P (10) Assist physician with patient care

    IV. P (6) Prepare a patient for procedures and/or treatments

ABHES Competencies Achieved

    I. Prepare patient for examinations and treatments

    m. Assist physician with routine and specialty examinations and treatments

PROCEDURE 9-2 ASSISTING WITH A SIGMOIDOSCOPY

Procedure Goal

To assist the doctor during the exam of the rectum, anus, and sigmoid colon using a sigmoidoscope

Scoring System

To score each step, use the following scoring system:
1 = poor, 2 = fair, 3 = good, 4 = excellent

A minimum score of at least a 3 must be achieved on **each** step to achieve successful completion of the technique. Detailed instructions on the scoring system are found on page 179.

Materials

Sigmoidoscope, suction pump, lubricating jelly, drape, patient gown, tissues

Procedure

Procedure Steps Total Possible Points - 72 Time Limit: 10 minutes	Practice #1	Practice #2	Practice #3	Final
1. Wash your hands and assemble and position materials and equipment according to the preference of the doctor.				
2. Test the suction pump.				
3. Identify the patient and introduce yourself.				
4. Show the patient into the treatment room. Explain the procedure and discuss any concerns the patient may have.				
5. Instruct the patient to empty the bladder, take off all clothing from the waist down, and put on the gown with the opening in the back.				
6. Put on exam gloves and assist the patient into the knee-chest or Sims' position. Immediately cover the patient with a drape.				
7. Use warm water to bring the sigmoidoscope to slightly above body temperature; lubricate the tip.*				
8. Assist as needed, including handing the doctor the necessary instruments and equipment.				
9. Monitor the patient's reactions during the procedure and relay any signs of pain to the doctor.				
10. Clean the anal area with tissues after the exam.				
11. Properly dispose of used materials and disposable instruments.				
12. Remove the gloves and wash your hands.				
13. Help the patient gradually assume a comfortable position.*				
14. Instruct the patient to dress.				
15. Put on clean gloves.				
16. Sanitize reusable instruments and prepare them for disinfection and/or sterilization, as necessary.				

(continued)

Procedure Steps Total Possible Points - 72 Time Limit: 10 minutes	Practice #1	Practice #2	Practice #3	Final
17. Clean and disinfect the equipment and the room according to OSHA guidelines.				
18. Remove the gloves and wash your hands.				
Total Number of Points Achieved/Final Score				
Initials of Observer:				

Comments and Signatures

Reviewer's comments and signatures:

1. _____

2. _____

3. _____

Instructor's comments:

_____

CAAHEP Competencies Achieved

I. P (10) Assist physician with patient care

IV. P (6) Prepare a patient for procedures and/or treatments

ABHES Competencies Achieved

l. Prepare patient for examinations and treatments

m. Assist physician with routine and specialty examinations and treatments

PROCEDURE 9-3 PREPARING THE OPHTHALMOSCOPE FOR USE

Procedure Goal

To ensure that the ophthalmoscope is ready for use during an eye exam

Scoring System

To score each step, use the following scoring system:
1 = poor, 2 = fair, 3 = good, 4 = excellent

A minimum score of at least a 3 must be achieved on **each** step to achieve successful completion of the technique. Detailed instructions on the scoring system are found on page 179.

Materials

Ophthalmoscope, lens, spare bulb, spare battery

Procedure

Procedure Steps Total Possible Points - 20 Time Limit: 10 minutes	Practice #1	Practice #2	Practice #3	Final
1. Wash your hands.				
2. Take the ophthalmoscope out of its battery charger. In a darkened room, turn on the ophthalmoscope light.				
3. Shine the large beam of white light on the back of your hand to check that the instrument's tiny lightbulb is providing strong enough light.				
4. Replace the bulb or battery if necessary. (The battery is located in the ophthalmoscope's handle.)				
5. Make sure the instrument's lens is screwed into the handle. If it is not, attach the lens.				
Total Number of Points Achieved/Final Score				
Initials of Observer:				

(continued)

Comments and Signatures

Reviewer's comments and signatures:

1. _____

2. _____

3. _____

Instructor's comments:

_____

CAAHEP Competency Achieved

I. P (10) Assist physician with patient care

ABHES Competencies Achieved

l. Prepare patient for examinations and treatments

m. Assist physician with routine and specialty examinations and treatments

PROCEDURE 9-4 ASSISTING WITH A NEEDLE BIOPSY

Procedure Goal

To remove tissue from a patient's body so that it can be examined in a laboratory

Scoring System

To score each step, use the following scoring system:
1 = poor, 2 = fair, 3 = good, 4 = excellent

A minimum score of at least a 3 must be achieved on **each** step to achieve successful completion of the technique. Detailed instructions on the scoring system are found on page 179.

Materials

Sterile drapes, tray or Mayo stand, antiseptic solution, cotton balls, local anesthetic, disposable sterile biopsy needle or disposable sterile syringe and needle, sterile sponges, specimen bottle with fixative solution, laboratory packaging, sterile wound-dressing materials

Procedure

Procedure Steps Total Possible Points - 56 Time Limit: 10 minutes	Practice #1	Practice #2	Practice #3	Final
1. Identify the patient and introduce yourself; instruct the patient as needed.				
2. Wash your hands and assemble the necessary materials.				
3. Prepare the sterile field and instruments.				
4. Put on exam gloves.				
5. Cleanse the biopsy site. Prepare the patient's skin.*				
6. Remove the gloves, wash your hands, and put on clean exam gloves.				
7. Assist the doctor as she injects anesthetic.				
8. During the procedure, help drape and position the patient.				
9. If you will be handing the doctor the instruments, remove the gloves, perform a surgical scrub, and put on sterile gloves.				
10. Place the sample in a properly labeled specimen bottle, complete the laboratory requisition form, and package the specimen for immediate transport to the laboratory.*				
11. Dress the patient's wound site.				
12. Properly dispose of used supplies and instruments.				
13. Clean and disinfect the room according to OSHA guidelines.				
14. Remove the gloves and wash your hands.				
Total Number of Points Achieved/Final Score				
Initials of Observer:				

(continued)

Comments and Signatures

Reviewer's comments and signatures:

1. _____

2. _____

3. _____

Instructor's comments:

_____

CAAHEP Competency Achieved

I. P (10) Assist physician with patient care

ABHES Competencies Achieved

l. Prepare patient for examinations and treatments

m. Assist physician with routine and specialty examinations and treatments

PROCEDURE 10-1 CREATING A STERILE FIELD

Procedure Goal

To create a sterile field for a minor surgical procedure

Scoring System

To score each step, use the following scoring system:
1 = poor, 2 = fair, 3 = good, 4 = excellent

A minimum score of at least a 3 must be achieved on **each** step to achieve successful completion of the technique. Detailed instructions on the scoring system are found on page 179.

Materials

Tray or Mayo stand, sterile instrument pack, sterile transfer forceps, cleaning solution, sterile drape, additionally packaged sterile items as required

Procedure

Procedure Steps Total Possible Points - 44 Time Limit: 10 minutes	Practice #1	Practice #2	Practice #3	Final
1. Clean and disinfect the tray or Mayo stand.				
2. Wash your hands and assemble the necessary materials.				
3. Check the label on the instrument pack to make sure it is the correct pack for the procedure.				
4. Check the date and sterilization indicator on the instrument pack to make sure the pack is still sterile.*				
5. Place the sterile pack on the tray or stand and unfold the outermost fold away from yourself.				
6. Unfold the sides of the pack outward, touching only the areas that will become the underside of the sterile field.*				
7. Open the final flap toward yourself, stepping back and away from the sterile field.				
8. Place additional packaged sterile items on the sterile field. • Ensure that you have the correct item or instrument and that the package is still sterile. • Stand away from the sterile field. • Grasp the package flaps and pull apart about halfway. • Bring the corners of the wrapping beneath the package, paying attention not to contaminate the inner package or item. • Hold the package over the sterile field with the opening down; with a quick movement, pull the flap completely open and snap the sterile item onto the field.				
9. Place basins and bowls near the edge of the sterile field so you can pour liquids without reaching over the field.*				

(continued)

Procedure Steps Total Possible Points - 44 Time Limit: 10 minutes	Practice #1	Practice #2	Practice #3	Final
10. Use sterile transfer forceps if necessary to add additional items to the sterile field.				
11. If necessary, don sterile gloves after a sterile scrub to arrange items on the sterile field.				
Total Number of Points Achieved/Final Score				
Initials of Observer:				

Comments and Signatures

Reviewer's comments and signatures:

1. _____

2. _____

3. _____

Instructor's comments:

_____

CAAHEP Competency Achieved

III. P (6) Perform sterilization procedures

ABHES Competency Achieved

4 (p) Perform sterilization techniques

Procedure 10-2 Performing a Surgical Scrub

Procedure Goal

To remove dirt and microorganisms from under the fingernails and from the surface of the skin, hair follicles, and oil glands of the hands and forearms

Scoring System

To score each step, use the following scoring system:
1 = poor, 2 = fair, 3 = good, 4 = excellent

A minimum score of at least a 3 must be achieved on **each** step to achieve successful completion of the technique. Detailed instructions on the scoring system are found on page 179.

Materials

Dispenser with surgical soap, sterile surgical scrub brush or sponge, sterile towels

Procedure

Procedure Steps Total Possible Points - 36 Time Limit: 10 minutes	Practice #1	Practice #2	Practice #3	Final
1. Remove all jewelry and roll up your sleeves to above the elbow.				
2. Assemble the necessary materials.				
3. Turn on the faucet using the foot or knee pedal.				
4. Wet your hands from the fingertips to the elbows. You must keep your hands higher than your elbows.*				
5. Under running water, use a sterile brush to clean under your fingernails.				
6. Apply surgical soap and scrub your hands, fingers, areas between the fingers, wrists, and forearms with the scrub sponge, using a firm circular motion. Follow the manufacturer's recommendations to determine appropriate length of time, usually 2 to 6 minutes.*				
7. Rinse from fingers to elbows, always keeping your hands higher than your elbows.				
8. Thoroughly dry your hands and forearms with sterile towels, working from the hands to the elbows.*				
9. Turn off the faucet with the foot or knee pedal. Use a clean paper towel if a foot or knee pedal is not used.				
Total Number of Points Achieved/Final Score				
Initials of Observer:				

(continued)

Comments and Signatures

Reviewer's comments and signatures:

1. _____

2. _____

3. _____

Instructor's comments:

_____

CAAHEP Competencies Achieved

III. P (4) Perform handwashing

III. P (6) Perform sterilization procedures

ABHES Competencies Achieved

4 (c) Apply principles of aseptic techniques and infection control

4 (p) Perform sterilization techniques

PROCEDURE 10-3 DONNING STERILE GLOVES

Procedure Goal

To don sterile gloves without compromising the sterility of the outer surface of the gloves

Scoring System

To score each step, use the following scoring system:
1 = poor, 2 = fair, 3 = good, 4 = excellent

A minimum score of at least a 3 must be achieved on **each** step to achieve successful completion of the technique. Detailed instructions on the scoring system are found on page 179.

Materials

Correctly sized, prepackaged, double-wrapped sterile gloves

Procedure

Procedure Steps Total Possible Points - 76 Time Limit: 10 minutes	Practice #1	Practice #2	Practice #3	Final
1. Obtain the correct size gloves.				
2. Check the package for tears and ensure that the expiration date has not passed.*				
3. Perform a surgical scrub.				
4. Peel the outer wrap from gloves and place the inner wrapper on a clean surface above waist level.				
5. Position gloves so the cuff end is closest to your body.				
6. Touch only the flaps as you open the package.*				
7. Use instructions provided on the inner package, if available.				
8. Do not reach over the sterile inside of the inner package.				

9. Follow these steps if there are no instructions:
   a. Open the package so the first flap is opened away from you.
   b. Pinch the corner and pull to one side.
   c. Put your fingertips under the side flaps and gently pull until the package is completely open.				

10. Use your nondominant hand to grasp the inside cuff of the opposite glove (the folded edge). Do not touch the outside of the glove. If you are right-handed, use your left hand to put on the right glove first, and vice versa.*				
11. Holding the glove at arm's length and waist level, insert the dominant hand into the glove with the palm facing up. Don't let the outside of the glove touch any other surface.				
12. With your sterile gloved hand, slip the gloved fingers into the cuff of the other glove.				
13. Pick up the other glove, touching only the outside. Don't touch any other surfaces.				

(continued)

Procedure Steps Total Possible Points - 76 Time Limit: 10 minutes	Practice #1	Practice #2	Practice #3	Final
14. Pull the glove up and onto your hand. Ensure that the sterile gloved hand does not touch skin.				
15. Adjust your fingers as necessary, touching only glove to glove.				
16. Do not adjust the cuffs because your forearms may contaminate the gloves.				
17. Keep your hands in front of you, between your shoulders and waist. If you move your hands out of this area, they are considered contaminated.				
18. If contamination or the possibility of contamination occurs, change gloves.				
19. Remove gloves the same way you remove clean gloves, by touching only the inside.*				
Total Number of Points Achieved/Final Score				
Initials of Observer:				

Comments and Signatures

Reviewer's comments and signatures:

1. _____

2. _____

3. _____

Instructor's comments:

_____

CAAHEP Competency Achieved

III. P (3) Select appropriate barrier/personal protective equipment (PPE) for potentially infectious situations

ABHES Competency Achieved

None

PROCEDURE 10-4 ASSISTING AS A FLOATER (UNSTERILE ASSISTANT) DURING MINOR SURGICAL PROCEDURES

Procedure Goal

To provide assistance to the doctor during minor surgery while maintaining clean or sterile technique as appropriate

Scoring System

To score each step, use the following scoring system:
1 = poor, 2 = fair, 3 = good, 4 = excellent

A minimum score of at least a 3 must be achieved on **each** step to achieve successful completion of the technique. Detailed instructions on the scoring system are found on page 179.

Materials

Sterile towel, tray or Mayo stand, appropriate instrument pack(s), needles and syringes, anesthetic, antiseptic, sterile water or normal saline, small sterile bowl, sterile gauze squares or cotton balls, specimen containers half-filled with preservative, suture materials, sterile dressings and tape

Procedure

Procedure Steps Total Possible Points - 28 Time Limit: 10 minutes	Practice #1	Practice #2	Practice #3	Final
1. Perform routine hand washing and put on exam gloves.				
2. Monitor the patient during the procedure; record the results in the patient's chart.				
3. During the surgery, assist as needed.				
4. Add sterile items to the tray as necessary.				
5. Pour sterile solution into a sterile bowl as needed.				

6. Assist in administering additional anesthetic.
  a. Check the medication vial two times.
  b. Clean the rubber stopper with an alcohol pad (write the date opened when using a new bottle); leave pad on top.
  c. Present the needle and syringe to the doctor.
  d. Remove the alcohol pad from the vial and show the label to the doctor.
  e. Hold the vial upside down and grasp the lower edge firmly; brace your wrist with your free hand.*
  f. Allow the doctor to fill the syringe.
  g. Check the medication vial a final time.				

7. Receive specimens for laboratory exam.
  a. Uncap the specimen container; present it to the doctor for the introduction of the specimen.
  b. Replace the cap and label the container.
  c. Treat all specimens as infectious.				

(continued)

Procedure Steps Total Possible Points - 28 Time Limit: 10 minutes	Practice #1	Practice #2	Practice #3	Final
d. Place the specimen container in a transport bag or other container. e. Complete the requisition form found on page 455 to send the specimen to the laboratory.				
Total Number of Points Achieved/Final Score				
Initials of Observer:				

Comments and Signatures

Reviewer's comments and signatures:

1. _____

2. _____

3. _____

Instructor's comments:

_____

CAAHEP Competencies Achieved

I. P (10) Assist physician with patient care

III. P (3) Select appropriate barrier/personal protective equipment (PPE) for potentially infectious situations

ABHES Competencies Achieved

4 (b) Prepare patients for procedures

4 (c) Apply principles of aseptic techniques and infection control

4 (h) Prepare patient for and assist physician with routine and specialty examinations and treatments and minor office surgeries

PROCEDURE 10-5 ASSISTING AS A STERILE SCRUB ASSISTANT DURING MINOR SURGICAL PROCEDURES

Procedure Goal

To provide assistance to the doctor during minor surgery while maintaining clean or sterile technique as appropriate

Scoring System

To score each step, use the following scoring system:

1 = poor, 2 = fair, 3 = good, 4 = excellent

A minimum score of at least a 3 must be achieved on **each** step to achieve successful completion of the technique. Detailed instructions on the scoring system are found on page 179.

Materials

Sterile towel, tray or Mayo stand, appropriate instrument pack(s), needles and syringes, anesthetic, antiseptic, sterile water or normal saline, small sterile bowl, sterile gauze squares or cotton balls, specimen containers half-filled with preservative, suture materials, sterile dressings and tape

Procedure

Procedure Steps Total Possible Points - 28 Time Limit: 10 minutes	Practice #1	Practice #2	Practice #3	Final
1. Perform a surgical scrub and put on sterile gloves. (Remember to remove the sterile towel covering the sterile field and instruments before gloving.)*				
2. Close and arrange the surgical instruments on the tray.*				
3. Prepare for swabbing by inserting gauze squares into the sterile dressing forceps.				
4. Pass the instruments as necessary.				
5. Swab the wound as requested.				
6. Retract the wound as requested.				
7. Cut the sutures as requested.				
Total Number of Points Achieved/Final Score				
Initials of Observer:				

Comments and Signatures

Reviewer's comments and signatures:

1. _____

2. _____

3. _____

Instructor's comments:

_____

(continued)

CAAHEP Competencies Achieved

I. P (10) Assist physician with patient care

III. P (3) Select appropriate barrier/personal protective equipment (PPE) for potentially infectious situations

ABHES Competencies Achieved

4 (b) Prepare patients for procedures

4 (c) Apply principles of aseptic techniques and infection control

4 (h) Prepare patient for and assist physician with routine and specialty examinations and treatments and minor office surgeries

PROCEDURE 10-6 ASSISTING AFTER MINOR SURGICAL PROCEDURES

Procedure Goal

To provide assistance to the doctor during minor surgery while maintaining clean or sterile technique as appropriate

Scoring System

To score each step, use the following scoring system:
1 = poor, 2 = fair, 3 = good, 4 = excellent

A minimum score of at least a 3 must be achieved on **each** step to achieve successful completion of the technique. Detailed instructions on the scoring system are found on page 179.

Materials

Examination gloves, antiseptic, tray or Mayo stand, sterile dressings and tape

Procedure

Procedure Steps Total Possible Points - 44 Time Limit: 10 minutes	Practice #1	Practice #2	Practice #3	Final
1. Monitor the patient.				
2. Put on clean exam gloves and clean the wound with antiseptic.				
3. Dress the wound.*				
4. Remove the gloves and wash your hands.				
5. Give the patient oral postoperative instructions in addition to the release packet.*				
6. Discharge the patient.				
7. Put on clean exam gloves.				
8. Properly dispose of used materials and disposable instruments.				
9. Sanitize reusable instruments and prepare them for disinfection and/or sterilization as needed.				
10. Clean equipment and the exam room according to OSHA guidelines.				
11. Remove the gloves and wash your hands.				
Total Number of Points Achieved/Final Score				
Initials of Observer:				

(continued)

Comments and Signatures

Reviewer's comments and signatures:

1. _____

2. _____

3. _____

Instructor's comments:

_____

CAAHEP Competencies Achieved

I. P (10) Assist physician with patient care

III. P (3) Select appropriate barrier/personal protective equipment (PPE) for potentially infectious situations

ABHES Competencies Achieved

4 (b) Prepare patients for procedures

4 (c) Apply principles of aseptic techniques and infection control

4 (h) Prepare patient for and assist physician with routine and specialty examinations and treatments and minor office surgeries

PROCEDURE 10-7 SUTURE REMOVAL

Procedure Goal

To remove sutures from a healing wound while maintaining sterile technique and protecting the integrity of the closed wound

Scoring System

To score each step, use the following scoring system:
1 = poor, 2 = fair, 3 = good, 4 = excellent

A minimum score of at least a 3 must be achieved on **each** step to achieve successful completion of the technique. Detailed instructions on the scoring system are found on page 179.

Materials:

Tray or Mayo stand, suture removal pack (suture scissors and thumb forceps), sterile towel, antiseptic solution, hydrogen peroxide (3%), two small sterile bowls, sterile gauze squares, sterile strips or butterfly closures, sterile dressings and tape

Procedure

Procedure Steps Total Possible Points - 140 Time Limit: 10 minutes	Practice #1	Practice #2	Practice #3	Final
1. Clean and disinfect the tray or Mayo stand.				
2. Wash your hands and assemble the necessary materials.				
3. Check the date and sterilization indicator on the suture removal pack.*				
4. Unwrap the suture removal pack and place it on the tray or stand to create a sterile field.*				
5. Unwrap the sterile bowls and add them to the sterile field.				
6. Pour a small amount of antiseptic solution into one bowl and pour a small amount of hydrogen peroxide into the other bowl.				
7. Cover the tray with a sterile towel to protect the sterile field while you are out of the room.				
8. Escort the patient to the exam room and explain the procedure.				
9. Perform a routine hand wash, remove the towel from the tray, and put on exam gloves.				

10. Remove the old dressing.
  a. Lift the tape toward the middle of the dressing to avoid pulling on the wound.
  b. If the dressing adheres to the wound, cover the dressing with gauze squares soaked in hydrogen peroxide. Leave the wet gauze in place for several seconds to loosen the dressing.
  c. Save the old dressing for the doctor to inspect.				

11. Inspect the wound for signs of infection.				

(continued)

Procedure Steps Total Possible Points - 140 Time Limit: 10 minutes	Practice #1	Practice #2	Practice #3	Final
12. Clean the wound with gauze pads soaked in antiseptic and pat it dry with clean gauze pads.				
13. Remove the gloves and wash your hands.				
14. Notify the doctor that the wound is ready for examination.*				
15. Once the doctor indicates that the wound is sufficiently healed to proceed, put on clean exam gloves.				
16. Place a square of gauze next to the wound for collecting the sutures as they are removed.				
17. Grasp the first suture knot with forceps.				
18. Gently lift the knot away from the skin to allow room for the suture scissors.				
19. Slide the suture scissors under the suture material and cut the suture where it enters the skin.*				
20. Gently lift the knot up and toward the wound to remove the suture without opening the wound.				
21. Place the suture on the gauze pad and inspect to ensure that the entire suture is present.*				
22. Repeat the removal process until all sutures have been removed.				
23. Count the sutures and compare the number with the number indicated in the patient's record.				
24. Clean the wound with antiseptic and allow the wound to air-dry.				
25. Dress the wound as ordered or notify the doctor if the sterile strips or butterfly closures are to be applied.				
26. Observe the patient for signs of distress, such as wincing or grimacing.				
27. Properly dispose of used materials and disposable instruments.				
28. Remove the gloves and wash your hands.				
29. Instruct the patient on wound care.				
30. In the patient's chart, record pertinent information, such as the condition of the wound and the type of closures used, if any. Use Progress Note on page 457.				
31. Escort the patient to the checkout area.				
32. Put on clean gloves.				
33. Sanitize reusable instruments and prepare them for disinfection and/or sterilization as needed.				
34. Clean the equipment and exam room according to OSHA guidelines.				
35. Remove the gloves and wash your hands.				
Total Number of Points Achieved/Final Score				
Initials of Observer:				

Comments and Signatures

Reviewer's comments and signatures:

1. _____

2. _____

3. _____

Instructor's comments:

_____

CAAHEP Competencies Achieved

I. P (10) Assist physician with patient care

III. P (3) Select appropriate barrier/personal protective equipment (PPE) for potentially infectious situations

ABHES Competencies Achieved

4 (b) Prepare patients for procedures

4 (c) Apply principles of aseptic techniques and infection control

4 (h) Prepare patient for and assist physician with routine and specialty examinations and treatments and minor office surgeries

PROCEDURE 11-1 ADMINISTERING CRYOTHERAPY

Procedure Goal

To reduce pain and swelling by safely and effectively administering cryotherapy

Scoring System

To score each step, use the following scoring system:
1 = poor, 2 = fair, 3 = good, 4 = excellent

A minimum score of at least a 3 must be achieved on **each** step to achieve successful completion of the technique. Detailed instructions on the scoring system are found on page 179.

Materials

Gloves, cold application materials required as ordered: ice bag, ice collar, chemical cold pack, washcloth or gauze squares, or ice

Procedure

Procedure Steps Total Possible Points - 60 Time Limit: 10 minutes	Practice #1	Practice #2	Practice #3	Final
1. Double-check the physician's order. Be sure you know where to apply therapy and how long it should remain in place.				
2. Identify the patient and explain the procedure and its purpose. Ask if the patient has any questions.				
3. Have the patient undress and put on a gown, if required; provide privacy or assistance as needed.				
4. Wash your hands and put on gloves.				
5. Position the patient comfortably and drape appropriately.*				

6. Prepare the therapy as ordered.
• Ice bag or collar
  a. Prior to use, check the ice bag or collar for leaks.
  b. Fill the ice bag or collar two-thirds full with ice chips or small ice cubes. Compress the container to expel any air and then close it.*
  c. Dry the bag or collar completely and cover it with a towel. This will absorb moisture and provide comfort.
• Chemical ice pack
  a. Check the pack for leaks.*
  b. Shake or squeeze the pack to activate the chemicals or use a cold chemical pack taken from a refrigerator or freezer.*
  c. Cover the pack with a towel.*
• Cold compress
  a. Place the washcloth or gauze squares under a stream of running water.
  b. Wring them out.
  c. Rewet at frequent intervals.				

7. Place the device on the patient's affected body part. If you are using a compress, place an ice bag on it, if desired, to keep it colder longer.				

(continued)

Procedure Steps Total Possible Points - 60 Time Limit: 10 minutes	Practice #1	Practice #2	Practice #3	Final
8. Ask the patient how the device feels.*				
9. Explain that the cold is of great benefit, although it may be somewhat uncomfortable.				
10. Leave the device in place for the length of time ordered by the physician. Periodically check the skin for color, feeling, and pain. If the area becomes excessively pale or blue, numb, or painful, remove the device and have the physician examine the area. For cold application using ice, limit application time to 20 minutes.*				
11. Remove the application and observe the area for reduced swelling, redness, and pain. If the patient has a dressing, replace it at this time.				
12. Help the patient dress, if needed.				
13. Remove equipment and supplies, properly discarding used disposable materials; sanitize, disinfect, and/or sterilize reusable equipment and materials as needed.				
14. Remove the gloves and wash your hands.				
15. Document the treatment and your observation in the patient's chart. If you teach the patient or the patient's family how to use the device, document your instructions.				
Total Number of Points Achieved/Final Score				
Initials of Observer:				

Comments and Signatures

Reviewer's comments and signatures:

1. _____

2. _____

3. _____

Instructor's comments:

_____

CAAHEP Competencies Achieved

IV. P. (6) Prepare a patient for procedures and/or treatments

IV. P. (8) Document patient care

IV. P. (9) Document patient education

ABHES Competency Achieved

2. c. Assist the physician with the regimen of diagnostic and treatment modalities as they relate to each body system

PROCEDURE 11-2 ADMINISTERING THERMOTHERAPY

Procedure Goal

To administer thermotherapy safely and effectively

Scoring System

To score each step, use the following scoring system:
1 = poor, 2 = fair, 3 = good, 4 = excellent

A minimum score of at least a 3 must be achieved on **each** step to achieve successful completion of the technique. Detailed instructions on the scoring system are found on page 179.

Materials

Gloves, towels, blanket, heat application materials required for order: chemical hot pack, heating pad, hot-water bottle, heat lamp, container and medication for hot soak, container and gauze for hot compress

Procedure

Procedure Steps Total Possible Points - 68 Time Limit: 10 minutes	Practice #1	Practice #2	Practice #3	Final
1. Double-check the physician's order. Be sure you know where to apply therapy, the proper temperature for the application, and how long it should remain in place.				
2. Identify the patient and explain the procedure and its purpose. Ask if the patient has any questions.				
3. Have the patient undress and put on a gown, if required; provide privacy or assistance as needed.				
4. Wash your hands and put on gloves.				
5. Position the patient comfortably and drape appropriately.*				
6. If the patient has a dressing, check the dressing for blood and change as necessary. Alert the physician and ask if treatment should continue.*				
7. Check the temperature by touch and look for the presence of adverse skin conditions (excessive redness, blistering, or irritation) on all applications before and during the treatment.*				
8. As necessary, reheat devices or solutions to provide therapeutic temperatures and then reapply them.				

9. Prepare the therapy as ordered.
 • Chemical hot pack
   a. Check the pack for leaks.*
   b. Activate the pack. (Check manufacturer's directions.)*
   c. Cover the pack with a towel.
 • Heating pad
   a. Turn the heating pad on, selecting the appropriate temperature setting.
   b. Cover the pad with a towel or pillowcase.
   c. Make sure the patient's skin is dry and do not allow the patient to lie on top of the heating pad.*				

(continued)

Procedure Steps Total Possible Points - 68 Time Limit: 10 minutes	Practice #1	Practice #2	Practice #3	Final

• Hot-water bottle
  a. Fill the bottle one-half full with hot water of the correct temperature—usually 110°F to 115°F. Use a thermometer. The physician can provide information on the ideal water temperature that should be used, which will depend on the area being treated.
  b. Expel the air and close the bottle.*
  c. Cover the bottle with a towel or pillowcase.*
• Heat lamp
  a. Place the lamp 2 feet to 4 feet away from the treatment area. (Check manufacturer's directions.)
  b. Follow the treatment time as ordered.
• Hot soak
  a. Select a container of the appropriate size for the area to be treated.
  b. Fill the container with hot water that is no more than 110°F. Use a thermometer. Add medication to the container if ordered.
• Hot compress
  a. Soak a washcloth or gauze in hot water. Wring it out.
  b. Frequently rewarm the compress to maintain the temperature.				

10. Place the device on the patient's affected body part or place the affected body part in the container. If you are using a compress, place a hot-water bottle on top, if desired, to keep it warm longer.				
11. Ask the patient how the device feels. During any heat therapy, remember that dilated blood vessels cause heat loss from the skin and that this heat loss may make the patient feel chilled. Be prepared to cover the patient with sheets or blankets.				
12. Leave the device in place for the length of time ordered by the physician. Periodically check the skin for redness, blistering, or irritation. If the area becomes excessively red or develops blisters, remove the patient from the heat source and have the physician examine the area.				
13. Remove the application and observe the area for inflammation and swelling. Replace the patient's dressing if necessary.				
14. Help the patient dress, if needed.				
15. Remove equipment and supplies, properly discarding used disposable materials, and sanitize, disinfect, and/or sterilize reusable equipment and materials as needed.				
16. Remove the gloves and wash your hands.				
17. Document the treatment and your observation in the patient's chart. If you teach the patient or the patient's family how to use the device, document your instructions.				
Total Number of Points Achieved/Final Score				
Initials of Observer:				

(continued)

Comments and Signatures

Reviewer's comments and signatures:

1. _____

2. _____

3. _____

Instructor's comments:

_____

CAAHEP Competencies Achieved

IV. P. (6) Prepare a patient for procedures and/or treatments

IV. P. (8) Document patient care

IV. P. (9) Document patient education

ABHES Competency Achieved

2. c. Assist the physician with the regimen of diagnostic and treatment modalities as they relate to each body system

PROCEDURE 11-3 TEACHING A PATIENT HOW TO USE A CANE

Procedure Goal

To teach a patient how to use a cane safely

Scoring System

To score each step, use the following scoring system:
1 = poor, 2 = fair, 3 = good, 4 = excellent

A minimum score of at least a 3 must be achieved on **each** step to achieve successful completion of the technique. Detailed instructions on the scoring system are found on page 179.

Materials

Cane suited to the patient's needs

Procedure

Procedure Steps Total Possible Points - 64 Time Limit: 15 minutes	Practice #1	Practice #2	Practice #3	Final
Standing from a Sitting Position				
1. Instruct the patient to slide his buttocks to the edge of the chair.				
2. Tell the patient to place his right foot slightly behind and inside the right front leg of the chair and his left foot slightly behind and inside the left front leg of the chair. (This provides him with a wide, stable stance.)				
3. Instruct the patient to lean forward and use the armrests or seat of the chair to push upward. Caution the patient not to lean on the cane.				
4. Have the patient position the cane for support on the uninjured or strong side of his body as indicated.				
Walking				
1. Teach the patient to hold the cane on the uninjured or strong side of her body with the tip(s) of the cane 4 to 6 inches from the side and in front of her strong foot. Remind the patient to make sure the tip is flat on the ground.*				
2. Have the patient move the cane forward approximately 8 inches and then move her affected foot forward, parallel to the cane.				
3. Next have the patient move her strong leg forward past the cane and her weak leg.				
4. Observe as the patient repeats this process.				
Ascending Stairs				
1. Instruct the patient to always start with his uninjured or strong leg when going up stairs.				

(continued)

Procedure Steps Total Possible Points - 64 Time Limit: 15 minutes	Practice #1	Practice #2	Practice #3	Final
2. Advise the patient to keep the cane on the uninjured or strong side of his body and to use the wall or rail, if available, for support on the weak side. If a rail is not available, the patient may need assistance for safety.				
3. After the patient steps on the strong leg, instruct him to bring up his weak leg and then the cane.				
4. Remind the patient not to rush.				
Descending Stairs				
1. Instruct the patient to always start with her weak leg when going down stairs.				
2. Advise the patient to keep the cane on the uninjured or strong side of her body and to use the wall or rail, if available, for support on the weak side. If a rail is not available, the patient may need assistance for safety.				
3. Have the patient use the uninjured or strong leg and wall or rail to support her body, put the cane on the next step, and bend the strong leg as she lowers the weak leg to the next step.				
4. Instruct the patient to step down with the strong leg.				
Walking on Snow or Ice				
Suggest that the patient try a metal ice-gripping cane or a ski pole. These can be dug into the snow or ice to prevent slipping. Instruct the patient to avoid walking on ice unless absolutely necessary.				
Total Number of Points Achieved/Final Score				
Initials of Observer:				

Comments and Signatures

Reviewer's comments and signatures:

1. _____

2. _____

3. _____

Instructor's comments:

_____

CAAHEP Competencies Achieved

IV. P. (**6**) Prepare a patient for procedures and/or treatments

IV. P. (**8**) Document patient care

IV. P (**9**) Document patient education

ABHES Competencies Achieved

5. b. Identify and respond appropriately when working/caring for patients with special needs

9. q. Instruct patients with special needs

PROCEDURE 11-4 TEACHING A PATIENT HOW TO USE A WALKER

Procedure Goal

To teach a patient how to use a walker safely

Scoring System

To score each step, use the following scoring system:
1 = poor, 2 = fair, 3 = good, 4 = excellent

A minimum score of at least a 3 must be achieved on **each** step to achieve successful completion of the technique. Detailed instructions on the scoring system are found on page 179.

Materials

Walker suited to the patient's needs

Procedure

Procedure Steps Total Possible Points - 44 Time Limit: 10 minutes	Practice #1	Practice #2	Practice #3	Final
Walking				
1. Instruct the patient to step into the walker.				
2. Tell the patient to place her hands on the handgrips on the sides of the walker.				
3. Make sure the patient's feet are far enough apart so that she feels balanced.*				
4. Instruct the patient to pick up the walker and move it forward about 6 inches.				
5. Have the patient move one foot forward and then the other foot.				
6. Instruct the patient to pick up the walker again and move it forward. If the patient is strong enough, explain that she may advance the walker after moving each leg rather than waiting until she has moved both legs.				
Sitting				
1. Teach the patient to turn his back to the chair or bed.				
2. Instruct the patient to take small, careful steps and to back up until he feels the chair or bed at the back of his legs.				
3. Instruct the patient to keep the walker in front of himself, let go of the walker, and place both his hands on the arms or seat of the chair or on the bed.				
4. Teach the patient to balance himself on his arms while lowering himself slowly to the chair or bed.				
5. If the patient has an injured or affected leg, he should keep it forward while bending his unaffected leg and lowering his body to the chair or bed.				

(continued)

Procedure Steps Total Possible Points - 44 Time Limit: 10 minutes	Practice #1	Practice #2	Practice #3	Final
Ascending and Descending Stairs If a patient needs to use a walker on stairs, refer him to a physical therapist for additional training.				
Total Number of Points Achieved/Final Score				
Initials of Observer:				

Comments and Signatures

Reviewer's comments and signatures:

1. _____

2. _____

3. _____

Instructor's comments:

_____

CAAHEP Competencies Achieved

IV. P. **(6)** Prepare a patient for procedures and/or treatments

IV. P. **(8)** Document patient care

IV. P. **(9)** Document patient education

ABHES Competencies Achieved

5. b. Identify and respond appropriately when working/caring for patients with special needs

9. q. Instruct patients with special needs

PROCEDURE 11-5 TEACHING A PATIENT HOW TO USE CRUTCHES

Procedure Goal

To teach a patient how to use crutches safely

Scoring System

To score each step, use the following scoring system:
1 = poor, 2 = fair, 3 = good, 4 = excellent

A minimum score of at least a 3 must be achieved on **each** step to achieve successful completion of the technique. Detailed instructions on the scoring system are found on page 179.

Materials

Crutches suited to the patient's needs

Procedure

Procedure Steps Total Possible Points - 44 Time Limit: 15 minutes	Practice #1	Practice #2	Practice #3	Final
1. Verify the physician's order for the type of crutches and gait to be used.				
2. Wash your hands, identify the patient, and explain the procedure.				
3. Elderly patients or patients with muscle weakness should be taught muscle strength exercises for their arms.				
4. Have the patient stand erect and look straight ahead.				
5. Tell the patient to place the crutch tips 2 to 4 inches in front of and 4 to 6 inches to the side of each foot.				
6. When instructing a patient to use an axillary crutch, make sure the patient has a 2-inch gap between the axilla and the axillary bar and that each elbow is flexed 25 degrees to 30 degrees.*				
7. Teach the patient how to get up from a chair: a. Instruct the patient to hold both crutches on his affected or weaker side. b. Have the patient slide to the edge of the chair. c. Tell the patient to push down on the arm or seat of the chair on his stronger side and use his strong leg to push up. If indicated, keep the affected leg forward. d. Advise the patient to put the crutches under his arms and press down on the hand grips with his hands.				
8. Teach the patient the required gait. Which gait the patient will use depends on the muscle strength and coordination of the patient. It also depends on the type of crutches, the injury, and the patient's condition. Check the physician's orders, and see Figures 11-10 and 11-11 in the text for examples.				

(continued)

Procedure Steps Total Possible Points - 44 Time Limit: 15 minutes	Practice #1	Practice #2	Practice #3	Final

9. Teach the patient how to ascend stairs:
  a. Start the patient close to the bottom step and tell her to push down with her hands.
  b. Instruct the patient to step up on the first step with her good foot.
  c. Tell the patient to lift the crutches to the same step and then lift her other foot. Advise the patient to keep her crutches with her affected limb.
  d. Remind the patient to check her balance before she proceeds to the next step.				

10. Teach the patient how to descend stairs:
  a. Have the patient start at the edge of the steps.
  b. Instruct the patient to bring his crutches and then the affected foot down first. Advise the patient to bend at the hips and knees to prevent leaning forward, which could cause him to fall.
  c. Tell the patient to bring his unaffected foot to the same step.
  d. Remind the patient to check his balance before he proceeds. In some cases, a handrail may be easier and can be used with both crutches in one hand.				

11. Give the patient the following general information related to the use of crutches:
  a. Do not lean on crutches.
  b. Report to the physician any tingling or numbness in the arms, hands, or shoulders.
  c. Support body weight with the hands.
  d. Always stand erect to prevent muscle strain.
  e. Look straight ahead when walking.
  f. Generally, move the crutches not more than 6 inches at a time to maintain good balance.
  g. Check the crutch tips regularly for wear; replace the tips as needed.
  h. Check the crutch tips for wetness; dry the tips if they are wet.
  i. Check all wing nuts and bolts for tightness.
  j. Wear flat, well-fitting, nonskid shoes.
  k. Remove throw rugs and other unsecured articles from traffic areas.
  l. Report any unusual pain in the affected leg.				

Total Number of Points Achieved/Final Score				
Initials of Observer:				

(continued)

Comments and Signatures

Reviewer's comments and signatures:

1. _____

2. _____

3. _____

Instructor's comments:

_____

CAAHEP Competencies Achieved

IV. P. (**6**) Prepare a patient for procedures and/or treatments

IV. P. (**8**) Document patient care

IV. P. (**9**) Document patient education

ABHES Competencies Achieved

5. b. Identify and respond appropriately when working/caring for patients with special needs

9. q. Instruct patients with special needs

PROCEDURE 12-1 STOCKING THE CRASH CART

Procedure Goal

To ensure that the crash cart includes all appropriate drugs, supplies, and equipment needed for emergencies

Scoring System

To score each step, use the following scoring system:
1 = poor, 2 = fair, 3 = good, 4 = excellent

A minimum score of at least a 3 must be achieved on **each** step to achieve successful completion of the technique. Detailed instructions on the scoring system are found on page 179.

Materials

Protocol for or list of crash cart items, crash cart

Procedure

Procedure Steps Total Possible Points - 20 Time Limit: 10 minutes	Practice #1	Practice #2	Practice #3	Final
1. Review the office protocol for or list of items that should be on the crash cart.				
2. Verify each drug on the crash cart and check the amount against the office protocol or list. Restock those that were used and replace those that have passed their expiration date.* Some typical crash cart drugs are listed here: • Activated charcoal • Atropine • Dextrose 50% • Diazepam (Valium) • Digoxin (Lanoxin) • Diphenhydramine hydrochloride (Benadryl) • Epinephrine, injectable • Furosemide (Lasix) • Glucagon • Glucose paste or tablets • Insulin (regular or a variety) • Intravenous dextrose in saline and intravenous dextrose in water • Isoproterenol hydrochloride (Isuprel), aerosol inhaler and injectable • Lactated Ringer's solution • Lidocaine (Xylocaine), injectable • Methylprednisolone tablets • Nitroglycerin tablets • Phenobarbital, injectable • Phenytoin (Dilantin) • Saline solution, isotonic (0.9%) • Sodium bicarbonate, injectable • Sterile water for injection				

(continued)

Procedure Steps Total Possible Points - 20 Time Limit: 10 minutes	Practice #1	Practice #2	Practice #3	Final
3. Check the supplies on the crash cart against the list. Restock items that were used and make sure the packaging of supplies on the cart has not been opened.* Some typical crash cart supplies are listed here: • Adhesive tape • Constricting band or tourniquet • Dressing supplies (alcohol wipes, rolls of gauze, bandage strips, bandage scissors) • Intravenous tubing, venipuncture devices, and butterfly needles • Personal protective equipment • Syringes and needles in various sizes				
4. Check the equipment on the crash cart against the list and examine it to make sure that it is in working order. Restock equipment that is missing or broken.* Some typical crash cart equipment is listed here: • Airways in assorted sizes • Ambu-bag, a trademark for a breathing bag used to assist respiratory ventilation • **Automated external defibrillator** (electrical device that shocks the heart to restore normal beating) • Endotracheal tubes in various sizes • Oxygen tank with oxygen mask and cannula				
5. Check miscellaneous items on the crash cart against the list and restock as needed. Some typical miscellaneous crash cart items are listed here: • Orange juice • Sugar packets				
Total Number of Points Achieved/Final Score				
Initials of Observer:				

Comments and Signatures

Reviewer's comments and signatures:

1. _____

2. _____

3. _____

Instructor's comments:

_____

CAAHEP Competency Achieved

XI. P. (3) Develop a personal (patient and employee) safety plan.

ABHES Competency Achieved

9. k. Prepare and maintain examination and treatment area

PROCEDURE 12-2 PERFORMING AN EMERGENCY ASSESSMENT

Procedure Goal

To assess a medical emergency quickly and accurately

Scoring System

To score each step, use the following scoring system:
1 = poor, 2 = fair, 3 = good, 4 = excellent

A minimum score of at least a 3 must be achieved on **each** step to achieve successful completion of the technique. Detailed instructions on the scoring system are found on page 179.

Materials

Patient's chart, pen, gloves

Procedure

Procedure Steps Total Possible Points - 52 Time Limit: 5 minutes	Practice #1	Practice #2	Practice #3	Final
1. Put on gloves.				
2. Form a general impression of the patient, including his level of responsiveness, level of distress, facial expressions, age, ability to talk, and skin color.				
3. If the patient can communicate clearly, ask what happened. If not, ask someone who observed the accident or injury.				
4. Assess an unresponsive patient by tapping on his shoulder and asking, "Are you OK?" If there is no response, proceed to the next step.*				
5. Assess the patient's airway. If necessary, open the airway by using the head tilt–chin lift maneuver. Give two breaths of 1 second each.				
6. Assess the patient's breathing. If the patient is not breathing, then perform rescue breathing.				
7. Assess the patient's circulation. Determine if the patient has a pulse. Is there any serious external bleeding? Perform CPR as needed (Procedure 12-8). Control any significant bleeding (Procedure 12-5).				
8. If all life-threatening problems have been identified and treated, perform a focused exam. Start at the head and perform the following steps rapidly, taking about 90 seconds. a. Head: Check for deformities, bruises, open wounds, tenderness, depressions, and swelling. Check the ears, nose, and mouth for fluid, blood, or foreign bodies. b. Eyes: Open the eyes and compare the pupils. They should be the same size. c. Neck: Look and feel for deformities, bruises, depressions, open wounds, tenderness, and swelling. Check for a medical alert bracelet or necklace.				

(continued)

Procedure Steps Total Possible Points - 52 Time Limit: 5 minutes	Practice #1	Practice #2	Practice #3	Final
d. Chest: Look and feel for deformities, bruises, open wounds, tenderness, depressions, and swelling. e. Abdomen: Look and feel for deformities, bruises, open wounds, tenderness, depressions, and swelling. f. Pelvis: Look and feel for deformities, bruises, open wounds, tenderness, depressions, and swelling. g. Arms: Look and feel for deformities, bruises, open wounds, depressions, tenderness, and swelling. Compare the arms for any differences in size, color, or temperature. h. Legs: Look and feel for deformities, bruises, open wounds, depressions, tenderness, and swelling. Compare the legs for any differences in size, color, or temperature. i. Back: Look and feel for deformities, bruises, open wounds, depressions, tenderness, and swelling. Feel under the patient for pools of blood.*				
9. Check vital signs and observe the patient for pallor (paleness) or cyanosis (a bluish tint). If the patient is dark-skinned, observe for pallor or cyanosis on the inside of the lips and mouth.*				
10. Document your findings and report them to the doctor or emergency medical technician (EMT).				
11. Assist the doctor or EMT as requested.				
12. Dispose of biohazardous waste according to OSHA guidelines.				
13. Remove your gloves and wash your hands.				
Total Number of Points Achieved/Final Score				
Initials of Observer:				

Comments and Signatures

Reviewer's comments and signatures:

1. _____

2. _____

3. _____

Instructor's comments:

_____

CAAHEP Competency Achieved

XI. P. (10) Perform first aid procedures

ABHES Competencies Achieved

9. e. Recognize emergencies and treatments and minor office surgical procedures

9. o. 5) First aid and CPR

PROCEDURE 12-3 FOREIGN BODY AIRWAY OBSTRUCTION IN A RESPONSIVE ADULT OR CHILD

Procedure Goal

To correctly relieve a foreign body from the airway of an adult or child

Scoring System

To score each step, use the following scoring system:

1 = poor, 2 = fair, 3 = good, 4 = excellent

A minimum score of at least a 3 must be achieved on **each** step to achieve successful completion of the technique. Detailed instructions on the scoring system are found on page 179.

Materials

Choking adult or child patient

Caution: Never perform this procedure on someone who is not choking.

Procedure

Procedure Steps Total Possible Points - 32 Time Limit: 5 minutes	Practice #1	Practice #2	Practice #3	Final
1. Ask, "Are you choking?" If the answer is "Yes," indicated by a nod of the head or some other sign, ask, "Can you speak?" If the answer is "No," tell the patient that you can help. A choking person cannot speak, cough, or breathe and exhibits the universal sign of choking. If the patient is coughing, observe him closely to see if he clears the object. If he is not coughing or stops coughing, use abdominal thrusts.				
2. Position yourself behind the patient. Place your fist against the abdomen just above the navel and below the xiphoid process.				
3. Grasp your fist with your other hand and provide quick inward and upward thrusts into the patient's abdomen.* Note: If a pregnant or obese person is choking, you will need to place your arms around the chest and perform thrusts over the center of the breastbone.				
4. Continue the thrusts until the object is expelled or the patient becomes unresponsive.				
5. If the patient becomes unresponsive, call EMS and position the patient on his back.*				
6. Use the head tilt–chin lift to open the patient's airway.				
7. Look into the mouth. If you see the foreign body, remove it using your index finger. **Do not perform any blind finger sweeps on a child.**				

(continued)

Procedure Steps Total Possible Points - 32 Time Limit: 5 minutes	Practice #1	Practice #2	Practice #3	Final
8. Open the airway and look, listen, and feel for breathing. If the patient is not breathing, attempt a rescue breath. Observe the chest. If it does not rise with the breath, reposition the airway and administer another rescue breath. If the chest does not rise after the second attempt, assume that the airway is still blocked and begin CPR (Procedure 12-8).				
Total Number of Points Achieved/Final Score				
Initials of Observer:				

Comments and Signatures

Reviewer's comments and signatures:

1. _____

2. _____

3. _____

Instructor's comments:

_____

CAAHEP Competencies Achieved

XI. P. (9) Maintain provider/professional level CPR certification.

XI. P. (10) Perform first aid procedures

ABHES Competencies Achieved

9. e. Recognize emergencies and treatments and minor office surgical procedures

9. o. 5) First aid and CPR

PROCEDURE 12-4 FOREIGN BODY AIRWAY OBSTRUCTION IN A RESPONSIVE INFANT

Procedure Goal

To correctly relieve a foreign body from the airway of an infant

Scoring System

To score each step, use the following scoring system:
1 = poor, 2 = fair, 3 = good, 4 = excellent

A minimum score of at least a 3 must be achieved on **each** step to achieve successful completion of the technique. Detailed instructions on the scoring system are found on page 179.

Materials

Choking infant

Caution: Never perform this procedure on an infant who is not choking.

Procedure

Procedure Steps Total Possible Points - 44 Time Limit: 5 minutes	Practice #1	Practice #2	Practice #3	Final
1. Assess the infant for signs of severe or complete airway obstruction, which include: a. Sudden onset of difficulty in breathing. b. Inability to speak, make sounds, or cry. c. A high-pitched, noisy, wheezing sound, or no sounds while inhaling. d. Weak, ineffective coughs. e. Blue lips or skin.				
2. Hold the infant with his head down, supporting the body with your forearm. His legs should straddle your forearm and you should support his jaw and head with your hand and fingers. This is best done in a sitting or kneeling position.				
3. Give up to five back blows with the heel of your free hand. Strike the infant's back forcefully between the shoulder blades. At any point, if the object is expelled, discontinue the back blows.*				
4. If the obstruction is not cleared, turn the infant over as a unit, supporting the head with your hands and the body between your forearms.				
5. Keep the head lower than the chest and perform five chest thrusts.* Place two fingers over the breastbone (sternum), above the xiphoid. Give five quick chest thrusts about ½ to 1 inch deep. Stop the compressions if the object is expelled.				
6. Alternate five back blows and five chest thrusts until the object is expelled or until the infant becomes unconscious. If the infant becomes unconscious, call EMS or have someone do it for you.				

(continued)

Procedure Steps Total Possible Points - 44 Time Limit: 5 minutes	Practice #1	Practice #2	Practice #3	Final
7. Open the infant's mouth by grasping both the tongue and the lower jaw between the thumb and fingers and pull up the lower jawbone. **If you see the object, remove it using your smallest finger. Do not use blind finger sweeps on an infant.***				
8. Open the airway and attempt to provide rescue breaths. If the chest does not rise, reposition the airway (both head and chin) and try to provide another rescue breath.				
9. If the rescue breaths are unsuccessful, begin CPR. Hold the infant, supporting her body with your forearm and her head with your hand and fingers. Deliver 30 chest compressions about ½ to 1 inch deep.				
10. Open the infant's mouth and look for the foreign object. If you see an object, remove it with your smallest finger.				
11. Open the airway and attempt to provide rescue breaths. If the chest does not rise, continue CPR until the doctor or EMS arrives.				
Total Number of Points Achieved/Final Score				
Initials of Observer:				

Comments and Signatures

Reviewer's comments and signatures:

1. _____

2. _____

3. _____

Instructor's comments:

_____

CAAHEP Competencies Achieved

XI. P. (9) Maintain provider/professional level CPR certification.

XI. P. (10) Perform first aid procedures

ABHES Competencies Achieved

9. e. Recognize emergencies and treatments and minor office surgical procedures

9. o. 5) First aid and CPR

PROCEDURE 12-5 CONTROLLING BLEEDING

Procedure Goal

To control bleeding and minimize blood loss

Scoring System

To score each step, use the following scoring system:
1 = poor, 2 = fair, 3 = good, 4 = excellent

A minimum score of at least a 3 must be achieved on **each** step to achieve successful completion of the technique. Detailed instructions on the scoring system are found on page 179.

Materials

Clean or sterile dressings

Procedure

Procedure Steps Total Possible Points - 36 Time Limit: 10 minutes	Practice #1	Practice #2	Practice #3	Final
1. If you have time, wash your hands and put on exam gloves, face protection, and a gown.*				
2. Using a clean or sterile dressing, apply direct pressure over the wound.				
3. If blood soaks through the dressing, do not remove it. Apply an additional dressing over the original one.*				
4. If possible, elevate the body part that is bleeding.				
5. If direct pressure and elevation do not stop the bleeding, apply pressure over the nearest pressure point between the bleeding and the heart. For example, if the wound is on the lower arm, apply pressure on the brachial artery. For a lower-leg wound, apply pressure on the femoral artery in the groin.				
6. When the doctor or EMT arrives, assist as requested.				
7. After the patient has been transferred to a hospital, properly dispose of contaminated materials.				
8. Remove the gloves and wash your hands.				
9. Document your care in the patient's chart. Progress Notes on page 465.				
Total Number of Points Achieved/Final Score				
Initials of Observer:				

(continued)

Comments and Signatures

Reviewer's comments and signatures:

1. _____

2. _____

3. _____

Instructor's comments:

_____

CAAHEP Competency Achieved

XI. P. (10) Perform first aid procedures

ABHES Competencies Achieved

9. e. Recognize emergencies and treatments and minor office surgical procedures

9. o. 5) First aid and CPR

PROCEDURE 12-6 CLEANING MINOR WOUNDS

Procedure Goal

To clean and dress minor wounds

Scoring System

To score each step, use the following scoring system:
1 = poor, 2 = fair, 3 = good, 4 = excellent

A minimum score of at least a 3 must be achieved on **each** step to achieve successful completion of the technique. Detailed instructions on the scoring system are found on page 179.

Materials

Sterile gauze squares, basin, antiseptic soap, warm water, sterile dressing

Procedure

Procedure Steps Total Possible Points - 44 Time Limit: 10 minutes	Practice #1	Practice #2	Practice #3	Final
1. Wash your hands and put on exam gloves.				
2. Dip several gauze squares in a basin of warm, soapy water.				
3. Wash the wound from the center outward.* Use a new gauze square for each cleansing motion.				
4. As you wash, remove debris that could cause infection.				
5. Rinse the area thoroughly, preferably by placing the wound under warm, running water.*				
6. Pat the wound dry with sterile gauze squares.				
7. Cover the wound with a dry, sterile dressing. Bandage the dressing in place.				
8. Properly dispose of contaminated materials.				
9. Remove the gloves and wash your hands.				
10. Instruct the patient on wound care.				
11. Record the procedure in the patient's chart. Progress Notes on page 467.				
Total Number of Points Achieved/Final Score				
Initials of Observer:				

Comments and Signatures

Reviewer's comments and signatures:

1. _____

2. _____

3. _____

Instructor's comments:

_____

(continued)

CAAHEP Competencies Achieved

III. P. (3) Select appropriate barrier/personal protective equipment (PPE) for potentially infectious situations

IV. P. (6) Prepare a patient for procedures and/or treatments

XI. P. (10) Perform first aid procedures

ABHES Competencies Achieved

9. e. Recognize emergencies and treatments and minor office surgical procedures

9. o. 5) First aid and CPR

PROCEDURE 12-7 CARING FOR A PATIENT WHO IS VOMITING

Procedure Goal

To increase comfort and minimize complications, such as aspiration, for a patient who is vomiting

Scoring System

To score each step, use the following scoring system:
1 = poor, 2 = fair, 3 = good, 4 = excellent

A minimum score of at least a 3 must be achieved on **each** step to achieve successful completion of the technique. Detailed instructions on the scoring system are found on page 179.

Materials

Emesis basin, cool compress, cup of cool water, paper tissues or a towel, and (if ordered) intravenous fluids and electrolytes and an antinausea drug

Procedure

Procedure Steps Total Possible Points - 32 Time Limit: 10 minutes	Practice #1	Practice #2	Practice #3	Final
1. Wash your hands and put on exam gloves and other PPE.				
2. Ask the patient when and how the vomiting started and how frequently it occurs. Find out whether she is nauseated or in pain.				
3. Give the patient an emesis basin to collect vomit. Observe and document its amount, color, odor, and consistency. Particularly note blood, bile, undigested food, or feces in the vomit.				
4. Place a cool compress on the patient's forehead to make her more comfortable. Offer water and paper tissues or a towel to clean her mouth.				
5. Monitor for signs of dehydration, such as confusion, irritability, and flushed, dry skin. Also monitor for signs of electrolyte imbalances, such as leg cramps or an irregular pulse.				
6. If requested, assist by laying out supplies and equipment for the physician to use in administering intravenous fluids and electrolytes. Administer an antinausea drug if prescribed.				
7. Prepare the patient for diagnostic tests if instructed.				
8. Remove the gloves and wash your hands.				
Total Number of Points Achieved/Final Score				
Initials of Observer:				

(continued)

Comments and Signatures

Reviewer's comments and signatures:

1. _____

2. _____

3. _____

Instructor's comments:

_____

CAAHEP Competencies Achieved

III. P. (3) Select appropriate barrier/personal protective equipment (PPE) for potentially infectious situations

IV.P. (6) Prepare a patient for procedures and/or treatments

XI. P. (10) Perform first aid procedures

ABHES Competencies Achieved

9. e. Recognize emergencies and treatments and minor office surgical procedures

9. o. 5) First aid and CPR

9. q. Instruct patients with special needs

PROCEDURE 12-8 PERFORMING CARDIOPULMONARY RESUSCITATION (CPR)

Procedure Goal

To provide ventilation and blood circulation for a patient who shows none

Scoring System

To score each step, use the following scoring system:
1 = poor, 2 = fair, 3 = good, 4 = excellent

A minimum score of at least a 3 must be achieved on **each** step to achieve successful completion of the technique. Detailed instructions on the scoring system are found on page 179.

Materials

Mouth shield, or if not in the office, a piece of plastic with a hole for the mouth

Procedure

Procedure Steps Total Possible Points - 32 Time Limit: 10 minutes	Practice #1	Practice #2	Practice #3	Final
1. Check responsiveness. • Tap shoulder. • Ask, "Are you OK?"				
2. If patient is unresponsive, call 911 or the local emergency number or have someone place the call for you.*				
3. Open the patient's airway. • Tilt the patient's head back, using the head tilt–chin lift maneuver.*				

4. Check for breathing.
• Place your ear next to the patient's mouth, turn your head, and watch the chest.
• Look for the chest to rise and fall, listen for sounds coming out of the mouth or nose, and feel for air movement.
• If the patient is breathing and you do not suspect a spinal injury, place him in the **recovery position:**
  • Kneel beside the patient and place the arm closest to you straight out from the body. Position the far arm with the back of the hand against the patient's near cheek.
  • Grab and bend the patient's far knee.
  • Protecting the patient's head with one hand, gently roll him toward you by pulling the opposite knee over and to the ground.
  • Position the top leg to balance the patient onto his side.
  • Tilt his head up slightly so that the airway is open. Make sure that his hand is under his cheek. Place a blanket or coat over the person and stay close until help arrives.				

(continued)

Procedure Steps Total Possible Points - 32 Time Limit: 10 minutes	Practice #1	Practice #2	Practice #3	Final

• If the patient is not breathing or has inadequate breathing, position the patient on his back and give two rescue breaths, each one second long. Each breath should cause the chest to rise. When giving rescue breaths, use one of three methods:
  a. Mouth-to-mouth or mouth-to-nose rescue breathing:
    • Place your mouth around the patient's mouth and pinch the nose, or close the patient's mouth and place your mouth around the patient's nose.
    • Deliver two slow breaths. Use a face shield.
  b. Mouth-to-mask device.
  c. Bag-mask ventilation. Ensure the adequate rise and fall of the patient's chest. If his chest does not rise, reposition the airway and try again. If on the second attempt the chest does not rise, your patient may have an airway obstruction. See Procedure 12-3.				

5. Place the heel of one hand on the patient's sternum between the nipples. Place your other hand over the first, interlacing your fingers.				
6. Give 30 chest compressions 1½ to 2 inches deep. You should compress the chest hard and fast (100 compressions per minute).* Give two breaths.				
7. Continue cycles of 30:2 until the patient begins to move, an AED is available, qualified help arrives, or you are too exhausted to continue.				
8. If the patient starts moving, check for breathing. If the patient is breathing adequately, put him in the recovery position and monitor him until the doctor or EMS arrives.				
Total Number of Points Achieved/Final Score				
Initials of Observer:				

Comments and Signatures

Reviewer's comments and signatures:

1. _____

2. _____

3. _____

Instructor's comments:

_____

(continued)

CAAHEP Competencies Achieved

XI. P. (9) Maintain provider/professional level CPR certification.

XI. P. (10) Perform first aid procedures

ABHES Competencies Achieved

9. e. Recognize emergencies and treatments and minor office surgical procedures

9. o. 5) First aid and CPR

PROCEDURE 12-9 ASSISTING WITH EMERGENCY CHILDBIRTH

Procedure Goal

To assist in performing an emergency childbirth

Scoring System

To score each step, use the following scoring system:
1 = poor, 2 = fair, 3 = good, 4 = excellent

A minimum score of at least a 3 must be achieved on **each** step to achieve successful completion of the technique. Detailed instructions on the scoring system are found on page 179.

Materials

Clean cloths, sterile or clean sheets or towels, two sterile clamps or two pieces of string boiled in water for at least 10 minutes, sterile scissors, plastic bag, soft blankets or towels

Procedure

Procedure Steps Total Possible Points - 84 Time Limit: 10 minutes	Practice #1	Practice #2	Practice #3	Final
1. Ask the woman her name and age, how far apart her contractions are (about two per minute signals that the birth is near), if her water has broken, and if she feels straining or pressure as if the baby is coming. Alert the doctor or call the EMS system.				
2. Help remove the woman's lower clothing.				
3. Explain that you are about to do a visual inspection to see if the baby's head is in position. Ask the woman to lie on her back with her thighs spread, her knees flexed, and her feet flat. Examine her to see if there is crowning (a bulging at the vaginal opening from the baby's head).				
4. If the head is crowning, childbirth is imminent. Place clean cloths under the woman's buttocks and use sterile sheets or towels (if they are available) to cover her legs and stomach.				
5. Wash your hands thoroughly and put on exam gloves. If other PPE is available, put it on now.				
6. At this point the physician would begin to take steps to deliver the baby, and you would position yourself at the woman's head to provide emotional support and help in case she vomited. If no physician is available, position yourself at the woman's side so that you have a constant view of the vaginal opening.				
7. Talk to the woman and encourage her to relax between contractions while allowing the delivery to proceed naturally.				
8. Position your gloved hands at the woman's vaginal opening when the baby's head starts to appear.* Do not touch her skin.				

(continued)

Procedure Steps Total Possible Points - 84 Time Limit: 10 minutes	Practice #1	Practice #2	Practice #3	Final
9. Place one hand below the baby's head as it is delivered. Spread your fingers evenly around the baby's head.* Use your other hand to help cradle the baby's head. Never pull on the baby.				
10. If the umbilical cord is wrapped around the baby's neck, gently loosen the cord and slide it over the baby's head.				
11. If the amniotic sac has not broken by the time the baby's head is delivered, use your finger to puncture the membrane. Then pull the membranes away from the baby's mouth and nose.*				
12. Wipe blood or mucus from the baby's mouth with a clean cloth.				
13. Continue to support the baby's head as the shoulders emerge. The upper shoulder will deliver first, followed quickly by the lower shoulder.				
14. After the feet are delivered, lay the baby on his side with the head slightly lower than the body. Keep the baby at the same level as the mother until you cut the umbilical cord.				
15. If the baby is not breathing, lower the head, raise the lower part of the body, and tap the soles of the feet. If the baby is still not breathing, begin rescue breathing and CPR.				
16. To cut the cord, wait several minutes, until pulsations stop. Use the clamps or pieces of string to tie the cord in two places.				
17. Use sterilized scissors to cut the cord in between the placement of the two clamps or pieces of string.				
18. Within 10 minutes of the baby's birth, the placenta will begin to expel. Save it in a plastic bag for further examination.				
19. Keep the mother and baby warm by wrapping them in towels or blankets. Do not touch the baby any more than necessary.				
20. Massage the mother's abdomen just below the navel every few minutes to control internal bleeding.				
21. Arrange for transport of the mother and baby to the hospital.				
Total Number of Points Achieved/Final Score				
Initials of Observer:				

(continued)

Comments and Signatures

Reviewer's comments and signatures:

1. _____

2. _____

3. _____

Instructor's comments:

_____

CAAHEP Competency Achieved

XI. P. (10) Perform first aid procedures

ABHES Competencies Achieved

9. e. Recognize emergencies and treatments and minor office surgical procedures

9. o. 5) First aid and CPR

9. q. Instruct patients with special needs

PROCEDURE 12-10 PERFORMING TRIAGE IN A DISASTER

Procedure Goal

To prioritize disaster victims

Scoring System

To score each step, use the following scoring system:
1 = poor, 2 = fair, 3 = good, 4 = excellent

A minimum score of at least a 3 must be achieved on **each** step to achieve successful completion of the technique. Detailed instructions on the scoring system are found on page 179.

Materials

Disaster tag and pen

Procedure

Procedure Steps Total Possible Points - 28 Time Limit: 10 minutes	Practice #1	Practice #2	Practice #3	Final
1. Wash your hands and put on exam gloves and other PPE if available.				
2. Quickly assess each victim.				
3. Sort victims by type of injury and need for care, classifying them as emergent, urgent, nonurgent, or dead.*				
4. Label the emergent patients no. 1 and send them to appropriate treatment stations immediately. Emergent patients, such as those who are in shock or who are hemorrhaging, need immediate care.				
5. Label the urgent patients no. 2 and send them to basic first-aid stations. Urgent patients need care within the next several hours. Such patients may have lacerations that can be dressed quickly to stop the bleeding but can wait for suturing.				
6. Label nonurgent patients no. 3 and send them to volunteers who will be empathic and provide refreshments. Nonurgent patients are those for whom timing of treatment is not critical, such as patients who have no physical injuries but who are emotionally upset.				
7. Label patients who are dead no. 4. Ensure that the bodies are moved to an area where they will be safe until they can be identified and proper action can be taken.				
Total Number of Points Achieved/Final Score				
Initials of Observer:				

(continued)

Comments and Signatures

Reviewer's comments and signatures:

1. _____

2. _____

3. _____

Instructor's comments:

_____

CAAHEP Competency Achieved

XI. P. (6) Participate in a mock environmental exposure event with documentation of steps taken.

ABHES Competencies Achieved

2. c. Assist the physician with the regimen of diagnostic and treatment modalities as they relate to each body system

9. e. Recognize emergencies and treatments and minor office surgical procedures

PROCEDURE 14-1 USING A MICROSCOPE

Procedure Goal

To correctly focus the microscope using each of the three objectives for examination of a prepared specimen slide

Scoring System

To score each step, use the following scoring system:
1 = poor, 2 = fair, 3 = good, 4 = excellent

A minimum score of at least a 3 must be achieved on **each** step to achieve successful completion of the technique. Detailed instructions on the scoring system are found on page 179.

Materials

Microscope, lens paper, lens cleaner, prepared specimen slide, immersion oil, tissues

Procedure

Procedure Steps Total Possible Points - 92 Time Limit: 10 minutes	Practice #1	Practice #2	Practice #3	Final
1. Wash your hands and put on exam gloves.				
2. Remove the protective cover from the microscope. Examine the microscope to make sure that it is clean and that all parts are intact.				
3. Plug in the microscope and make sure the light is working. If you need to replace the bulb, refer to the manufacturer's guidelines. (Be sure to note bulb replacements in the maintenance log for the microscope.) Turn the light off before cleaning the lenses.				
4. Clean the lenses and oculars with lens paper. Avoid touching the lenses with anything except lens paper. Pay careful attention to the oculars. They are easily dirtied by dust and eye makeup. If a lens is particularly dirty, use a small amount of lens cleaner. Oil-immersion lenses are prone to oil buildup if not cleaned properly. Too much lens cleaner, however, can loosen the cement that holds the lens in place.*				
5. Place the specimen slide on the stage. Slide the edges of the slide under the slide clips to secure the slide to the stage.				
6. Adjust the distance between the oculars to a position of comfort.				
7. Adjust the objectives so that the low-power (10X) objective points directly at the specimen slide, as shown in Figure 14-4 in the text. Before swiveling the objective assembly, be sure you have sufficient space for the objective. Recheck the distance between the oculars, making sure the field you see through the eyepieces is a merged field, not separate left and right fields. Raise the body tube by using the coarse adjustment control and lower the stage as needed.*				

(continued)

Procedure Steps Total Possible Points - 92 Time Limit: 10 minutes	Practice #1	Practice #2	Practice #3	Final
8. Turn on the light and, using the iris controls, adjust the amount of light illuminating the specimen so that the light fills the field but does not wash out the image. (At this point you are not examining the specimen image for focus but adjusting the overall light level.)				
9. Observe the microscope from one side and slowly lower the body tube to move the objective closer to the stage and specimen slide. This adjustment is shown in Figure 14-5 in the text. If you used the stage controls to lower the stage away from the objectives, you may also need to adjust those controls. Again, take care not to strike the stage with the objective. The objective should almost meet the specimen slide but not touch it.				
10. Look through the oculars and use the coarse focus control to slowly adjust the image. If necessary, adjust the amount of light coming through the iris.				
11. Continue using the fine focus control to adjust the image. When the image is correctly focused, the specimen will be clearly visible and the field illumination will be bright enough to show details but not so bright that it is uncomfortable to view or washed out.				
12. Switch to the high-power (40X) objective. Use the fine focus controls to view the specimen clearly.*				
13. Rotate the objective assembly so that no objective points directly at the stage and specimen slide. You will now have enough room to apply a drop of immersion oil to the slide. (Only dry slides, without coverslips, are used with the oil-immersion objective.)				
14. Apply a small drop of immersion oil to the specimen slide, as shown in Figure 14-6 in the text.				
15. Gently swing the oil-immersion (100X) objective over the stage and specimen slide so that it is surrounded by the immersion oil.				
16. Examine the image and adjust the amount of light and focus as needed. Only use the fine focus adjustment with this objective. To eliminate air bubbles in the immersion oil, gently move the stage left and right.				
17. After you have examined the specimen as required by the testing procedure, lower the stage and raise the objectives.				
18. Remove the slide. Dispose of it or store it as required by the testing procedure. If you must dispose of the slide, be sure to use the appropriate biohazardous waste container. If you must store the slide, remove the immersion oil with a tissue.				
19. Turn off the light. Unplug the microscope if that is your laboratory's standard operating procedure.				

(continued)

Procedure Steps Total Possible Points - 92 Time Limit: 10 minutes	Practice #1	Practice #2	Practice #3	Final
20. Clean the microscope stage, ocular lenses, and objectives. Be careful to remove all traces of immersion oil from the stage and oil-immersion objective.				
21. Rotate the objective assembly so that the low-power objective points toward the stage. Lower the objective so that it comes close to but does not rest on the stage.				
22. Cover the microscope with its protective cover. Check the work area to be sure you have cleaned everything correctly and disposed of all waste material.				
23. Remove the gloves and wash your hands.				
Total Number of Points Achieved/Final Score				
Initials of Observer:				

Comments and Signatures

Reviewer's comments and signatures:

1. _____

2. _____

3. _____

Instructor's comments:

_____

CAAHEP Competency Achieved

III. P. (2) Practice Standard Precautions

ABHES Competencies Achieved

9. b. Apply principles of aseptic techniques and infection control

10. a. Practice quality control

10. c. Dispose of Biohazardous materials

PROCEDURE 14-2 DISPOSING OF BIOHAZARDOUS WASTE

Procedure Goal

To correctly dispose of contaminated waste products, including sharps and contaminated cleaning and paper products

Scoring System

To score each step, use the following scoring system:
1 = poor, 2 = fair, 3 = good, 4 = excellent

A minimum score of at least a 3 must be achieved on **each** step to achieve successful completion of the technique. Detailed instructions on the scoring system are found on page 179.

Materials

Biohazardous waste containers, gloves, waste materials

Procedure

Procedure Steps Total Possible Points - 36 Time Limit: 5 minutes	Practice #1	Practice #2	Practice #3	Final
To dispose of sharps or other materials that pose a danger of cutting, slicing, or puncturing the skin: 1. While wearing gloves, hold the article by the unpointed or blunt end.				
2. Drop the object directly into an approved container. (If you are using an evacuation system, do not unscrew the needle. Drop the entire system with the needle attached and the safety device engaged into the receptacle.) The container should be puncture-proof, with rigid sides and a tight-fitting lid.*				
3. If you are disposing of a needle, do not bend, break, or attempt to recap the needle before disposal. If the needle is equipped with a safety device, activate the device immediately and drop the entire assembly into the sharps container.*				
4. When the container is two-thirds full, replace it with an empty container.*				
5. Depending on your office's procedures, the container and its contents may be sterilized before further disposal, or they may be collected by an authorized waste management agency.				
6. Remove the gloves and wash your hands.				
To dispose of contaminated paper waste: 1. While wearing gloves, deposit the materials in a properly marked biohazardous waste container. A standard biohazardous waste container has an inner plastic liner, either red or orange and marked with the biohazard symbol, and a puncture-proof outer shell, also marked with the biohazard symbol.				

(continued)

Procedure Steps Total Possible Points - 36 Time Limit: 5 minutes	Practice #1	Practice #2	Practice #3	Final
2. If the container is full, secure the inner liner and place it in the appropriate area for biohazardous waste.*				
3. Remove the gloves and wash your hands.				
Total Number of Points Achieved/Final Score				
Initials of Observer:				

Comments and Signatures

Reviewer's comments and signatures:

1. _____

2. _____

3. _____

Instructor's comments:

_____

CAAHEP Competencies Achieved

III. P. (2) Practice Standard Precautions

XI. P. (2) Evaluate the work environment to identify safe vs. unsafe working conditions.

ABHES Competencies Achieved

9. b. Apply principles of aseptic techniques and infection control

10. c. Dispose of Biohazardous materials

PROCEDURE 15-1 OBTAINING A THROAT CULTURE SPECIMEN

Procedure Goal

To isolate a pathogenic microorganism from the throat or to rule out strep throat

Scoring System

To score each step, use the following scoring system:
1 = poor, 2 = fair, 3 = good, 4 = excellent

A minimum score of at least a 3 must be achieved on **each** step to achieve successful completion of the technique. Detailed instructions on the scoring system are found on page 179.

Materials

Tongue depressor, sterile collection system or sterile swab plus blood agar culture plate

Procedure

Procedure Steps Total Possible Points - 64 Time Limit: 10 minutes	Practice #1	Practice #2	Practice #3	Final
1. Identify the patient, introduce yourself, and explain the procedure.				
2. Assemble the necessary supplies; label the culture plate if used.				
3. Wash your hands and put on exam gloves and goggles and a mask or a face shield.*				
4. Have the patient assume a sitting position. (Having a small child lie down rather than sit may make the process easier. If the child refuses to open the mouth, gently squeeze the nostrils shut. The child will eventually open the mouth to breathe. Enlist the help of the parent to restrain the child's hands if necessary.)				
5. Open the collection system or sterile swab package by peeling the wrapper halfway down; remove the swab with your dominant hand.				
6. Ask the patient to tilt back her head and open her mouth as wide as possible.				
7. With your other hand, depress the patient's tongue with the tongue depressor.				
8. Ask the patient to say "Ah."				
9. Insert the swab and quickly swab the back of the throat in the area of the tonsils, twirling the swab over representative areas on both sides of the throat. Avoid touching the uvula, the soft tissue hanging from the roof of the mouth; the cheeks; or the tongue.*				

(continued)

Procedure Steps Total Possible Points - 64 Time Limit: 10 minutes	Practice #1	Practice #2	Practice #3	Final
10. Remove the swab and then the tongue depressor from the patient's mouth.				
11. Discard the tongue depressor in a biohazardous waste container.				
To transport the specimen to a reference laboratory:				
12. Immediately insert the swab back into the plastic sleeve, being careful not to touch the outside of the sleeve with the swab.				
13. Crush the vial of transport medium to moisten the tip of the swab.*				
14. Label the collection system and arrange for transport to the laboratory.				
To prepare the specimen for evaluation in the physician's office laboratory:				
12. Immediately inoculate the culture plate with the swab, using a back-and-forth motion.				
13. Discard the swab in a biohazardous waste container.				
14. Place the culture plate in the incubator.				
To use the specimen for a quick strep screening test:				
12. Collect a throat culture specimen using the swab provided in the quick strep test kit.				
13. Follow manufacturer's instructions in the test kit. Confirm that the controls worked as expected.				
14. Dispose of biohazardous materials according to OSHA guidelines.				
When finished with all specimens:				
15. Remove the gloves and wash your hands.				
16. Document the procedure in the patient's chart. Progress Notes on page 469.				
Total Number of Points Achieved/Final Score				
Initials of Observer:				

Comments and Signatures

Reviewer's comments and signatures:

1. _____

2. _____

3. _____

Instructor's comments:

_____

(continued)

CAAHEP Competencies Achieved

III. P. (7) Obtain specimens for microbiological testing

III. P. (8) Perform CLIA-waived microbiology testing

ABHES Competencies Achieved

9. b. Apply principles of aseptic techniques and infection control

10. b. Perform selected CLIA-waived tests that assist with diagnosis and treatment
     5) Microbiology testing

10. c. Dispose of Biohazardous materials

PROCEDURE 15-2 PREPARING MICROBIOLOGIC SPECIMENS FOR TRANSPORT TO AN OUTSIDE LABORATORY

Procedure Goal

To properly prepare a microbiologic specimen for transport to an outside laboratory

Scoring System

To score each step, use the following scoring system:
1 = poor, 2 = fair, 3 = good, 4 = excellent

A minimum score of at least a 3 must be achieved on **each** step to achieve successful completion of the technique. Detailed instructions on the scoring system are found on page 179.

Materials

Specimen-collection device, requisition form, secondary container or zipper-type plastic bag

Procedure

Procedure Steps Total Possible Points - 44 Time Limit: 10 minutes	Practice #1	Practice #2	Practice #3	Final
1. Wash your hands and put on exam gloves (and goggles and a mask or a face shield if you are collecting a microbiologic throat culture specimen).				
2. Obtain the microbiologic culture specimen. 　a. Use the collection system specified by the outside laboratory for the test requested. 　b. Label the microbiologic specimen-collection device at the time of collection. 　c. Collect the microbiologic specimen according to the guidelines provided by the laboratory and office procedure.*				
3. Remove the gloves and wash your hands.				
4. Complete the test requisition form.				
5. Place the microbiologic specimen container in a secondary container or zipper-type plastic bag.*				
6. Attach the test requisition form to the outside of the secondary container or bag, per laboratory policy. Requisition form on page 471.				
7. Log the microbiologic specimen in the list of outgoing specimens.*				
8. Store the microbiologic specimen according to guidelines provided by the laboratory for that type of specimen (for example, refrigerated, frozen, or 37°C).				
9. Call the laboratory for pickup of the microbiologic specimen, or hold it until the next scheduled pickup.				

(continued)

Procedure Steps Total Possible Points - 44 Time Limit: 10 minutes	Practice #1	Practice #2	Practice #3	Final
10. At the time of pickup ensure that the carrier takes all microbiologic specimens that are logged and scheduled to be picked up.				
11. If you are ever unsure about collection or transportation details, call the laboratory.				
Total Number of Points Achieved/Final Score				
Initials of Observer:				

Comments and Signatures

Reviewer's comments and signatures:

1. _____

2. _____

3. _____

Instructor's comments:

_____

CAAHEP Competency Achieved

III. P. (7) Obtain specimens for microbiological testing

ABHES Competencies Achieved

9. b. Apply principles of aseptic techniques and infection control

10. b. Perform selected CLIA-waived tests that assist with diagnosis and treatment
    5) Microbiology testing

PROCEDURE 15-3 PREPARING A MICROBIOLOGIC SPECIMEN SMEAR

Procedure Goal

To prepare a smear of a microbiologic specimen for staining

Scoring System

To score each step, use the following scoring system:
1 = poor, 2 = fair, 3 = good, 4 = excellent

A minimum score of at least a 3 must be achieved on **each** step to achieve successful completion of the technique. Detailed instructions on the scoring system are found on page 179.

Materials

Glass slide with frosted end, pencil, specimen swab, Bunsen burner, forceps

Procedure

Procedure Steps Total Possible Points - 40 Time Limit: 10 minutes	Practice #1	Practice #2	Practice #3	Final
1. Wash your hands and put on exam gloves.				
2. Assemble all the necessary items.				
3. Use a pencil to label the frosted end of the slide with the patient's name.				
4. Roll the specimen swab evenly over the smooth part of the slide, making sure that all areas of the swab touch the slide.*				
5. Discard the swab in a biohazardous waste container. (Retain the microbiologic specimen for culture as necessary or according to office policy.)				
6. Allow the smear to air-dry. Do not wave the slide to dry it.*				
7. Heat-fix the slide by holding the frosted end with forceps and passing the clear part of the slide, with the smear side up, through the flame of a Bunsen burner three or four times. (Your office may use an alternate procedure for fixing the slide, such as flooding the smear with alcohol, allowing it to sit for a few minutes, and either pouring off the remaining liquid or allowing the smear to air-dry. Chlamydia slides come with their own fixative.)*				
8. Allow the slide to cool before the smear is stained.				
9. Return the materials to their proper location.				
10. Remove the gloves and wash your hands.				
Total Number of Points Achieved/Final Score				
Initials of Observer:				

(continued)

Comments and Signatures

Reviewer's comments and signatures:

1. _____

2. _____

3. _____

Instructor's comments:

_____

CAAHEP Competency Achieved

III. P. (7) Obtain specimens for microbiological testing

ABHES Competencies Achieved

9. b. Apply principles of aseptic techniques and infection control

10. b. Perform selected CLIA-waived tests that assist with diagnosis and treatment
    5) Microbiology testing

10. c. Dispose of Biohazardous materials

PROCEDURE 15-4 PERFORMING A GRAM'S STAIN

Procedure Goal

To make bacteria present in a specimen smear visible for microscopic identification

Scoring System

To score each step, use the following scoring system:
1 = poor, 2 = fair, 3 = good, 4 = excellent

A minimum score of at least a 3 must be achieved on **each** step to achieve successful completion of the technique. Detailed instructions on the scoring system are found on page 179.

Materials

Heat-fixed smear, slide staining rack and tray, crystal violet dye, iodine solution, alcohol or acetone-alcohol decolorizer, safranin dye, wash bottle filled with water, forceps, blotting paper or paper towels (optional)

Procedure

Procedure Steps Total Possible Points - 68 Time Limit: 10 minutes	Practice #1	Practice #2	Practice #3	Final
1. Assemble all the necessary supplies.				
2. Wash your hands and put on examination gloves.				
3. Place the heat-fixed smear on a level staining rack and tray, with the smear side up.				
4. Completely cover the specimen area of the slide with the crystal violet stain. (Many commercially available Gram's stain solutions have flip-up bottle caps that allow you to dispense stain by the drop. If the stain bottle you are using does not have an attached dropper cap, use an eyedropper.)				
5. Allow the stain to sit for 1 minute; wash the slide thoroughly with water from the wash bottle.*				
6. Use the forceps to hold the slide at the frosted end, tilting the slide to remove excess water.				
7. Place the slide flat on the rack again and completely cover the specimen area with iodine solution.				
8. Allow the iodine to remain for 1 minute; wash the slide thoroughly with water.*				
9. Use the forceps to hold and tilt the slide to remove excess water.				
10. While still tilting the slide, apply the alcohol or decolorizer drop by drop until no more purple color washes off. (This step usually takes 10 to 30 seconds.)*				
11. Wash the slide thoroughly with water; use the forceps to hold and tip the slide to remove excess water.				
12. Completely cover the specimen with safranin dye.				

(continued)

Procedure Steps Total Possible Points - 68 Time Limit: 10 minutes	Practice #1	Practice #2	Practice #3	Final
13. Allow the safranin to remain for 1 minute; wash the slide thoroughly with water.*				
14. Use the forceps to hold the stained smear by the frosted end, and carefully wipe the back of the slide to remove excess stain.				
15. Place the smear in a vertical position and allow it to air-dry. (The smear may be blotted lightly between blotting paper or paper towels to hasten drying. Take care not to rub the slide or the specimen may be damaged.)				
16. Sanitize and disinfect the work area.				
17. Remove the gloves and wash your hands.				
Total Number of Points Achieved/Final Score				
Initials of Observer:				

Comments and Signatures

Reviewer's comments and signatures:

1. _____

2. _____

3. _____

Instructor's comments:

_____

CAAHEP Competency Achieved

III. P. (7) Obtain specimens for microbiological testing

ABHES Competencies Achieved

9. b. Apply principles of aseptic techniques and infection control

10. a. Practice quality control

10. b. Perform selected CLIA-waived tests that assist with diagnosis and treatment
    5) Microbiology testing

10. c. Dispose of Biohazardous materials

PROCEDURE 16-1 COLLECTING A CLEAN-CATCH MIDSTREAM URINE SPECIMEN

Procedure Goal

To collect a urine specimen that is free from contamination

Scoring System

To score each step, use the following scoring system:
1 = poor, 2 = fair, 3 = good, 4 = excellent

A minimum score of at least a 3 must be achieved on **each** step to achieve successful completion of the technique. Detailed instructions on the scoring system are found on page 179.

Materials

Dry, sterile urine container with lid; label; written instructions (if the patient is to perform procedure independently); antiseptic towelettes

Procedure

Procedure Steps Total Possible Points - 48 Time Limit: 10 minutes	Practice #1	Practice #2	Practice #3	Final
1. Confirm the patient's identity and be sure all forms are correctly completed.				
2. Label the sterile urine specimen container with the patient's name, ID number, date of birth, the physician's name, the date and time of collection, and the initials of the person collecting the specimen.				
When the patient will be completing the procedure independently: 3. Explain the procedure in detail. Provide the patient with written instructions, antiseptic towelettes, and the labeled sterile specimen container.				
4. Confirm that the patient understands the instructions, especially not to touch the inside of the specimen container and to refrigerate the specimen until bringing it to the physician's office.*				
When you are assisting a patient: 3. Explain the procedure and how you will be assisting in the collection.				
4. Wash your hands and put on exam gloves.				
5. Remove the lid from the specimen container and place the lid upside down on a flat surface.				
6. Use three antiseptic towelettes to clean the perineal area by spreading the labia and wiping from front to back. Wipe with the first towelette on one side and discard it. Wipe with the second towelette on the other side and discard it. Wipe with the third towelette down the middle and discard it. To remove soap residue that could cause a higher pH and affect chemical test results, rinse the area once from front to back with water.*				

(continued)

Procedure Steps Total Possible Points - 48 Time Limit: 10 minutes	Practice #1	Practice #2	Practice #3	Final
7. Keeping the patient's labia spread to avoid contamination, tell her to urinate into the toilet. After she has expressed a small amount of urine, instruct her to stop the flow.*				
8. Position the specimen container close to but not touching the patient.				
9. Tell the patient to start urinating again. Collect the necessary amount of urine in the container. (If the patient cannot stop her urine flow, move the container into the urine flow and collect the specimen anyway.)				
10. Allow the patient to finish urinating. Place the lid back on the collection container.				
11. Remove the gloves and wash your hands.				
12. Complete the test request slip and record the collection in the patient's chart.				
When you are assisting in the collection for male patients: 5. Remove the lid from the specimen container and place the lid upside down on a flat surface.				
6. If the patient is circumcised, use an antiseptic towelette to clean the head of the penis. Wipe with a second towelette directly across the urethral opening. If the patient is uncircumcised, retract the foreskin before cleaning the penis. To remove soap residue that could cause a higher pH and affect chemical test results, rinse the area once from front to back with water.*				
7. Keeping an uncircumcised patient's foreskin retracted, tell the patient to urinate into the toilet. After he has expressed a small amount of urine, instruct him to stop the flow.*				
8. Position the specimen container close to but not touching the patient.				
9. Tell the patient to start urinating again. Collect the necessary amount of urine in the container. (If the patient cannot stop his urine flow, move the container into the urine flow and collect the specimen anyway.)				
10. Allow the patient to finish urinating. Place the lid back on the collection container.				
11. Remove the gloves and wash your hands.				
12. Complete the laboratory request form (page 473) and record the collection in the patient's chart.				
Total Number of Points Achieved/Final Score				
Initials of Observer:				

(continued)

Comments and Signatures

Reviewer's comments and signatures:

1. _____

2. _____

3. _____

Instructor's comments:

_____

CAAHEP Competencies Achieved

I. P. (14) Perform CLIA-waived urinalysis

IV. P. (6) Prepare a patient for procedures and/or treatments

ABHES Competencies Achieved

9. q. Instruct patients with special needs

10. c. Dispose of Biohazardous materials

10. e. Instruct patients in the collection of a clean-catch mid-stream urine specimen

PROCEDURE 16-2 COLLECTING A URINE SPECIMEN FROM A PEDIATRIC PATIENT

Procedure Goal

To collect a urine specimen from an infant or a child who is not toilet-trained

Scoring System

To score each step, use the following scoring system:
1 = poor, 2 = fair, 3 = good, 4 = excellent

A minimum score of at least a 3 must be achieved on **each** step to achieve successful completion of the technique. Detailed instructions on the scoring system are found on page 179.

Materials

Urine specimen bottle or container, label, sterile cotton balls, soapy water, sterile water, plastic disposable urine collection bag

Procedure

Procedure Steps Total Possible Points - 68 Time Limit: 10 minutes	Practice #1	Practice #2	Practice #3	Final
1. Confirm the patient's identity and be sure all forms are correctly completed.				
2. Label the urine specimen container with the patient's name, ID number, and date of birth, the physician's name, the date and time of collection, and your initials.				
3. Explain the procedure to the child (if age-appropriate) and to the parents or guardians.				
4. Wash your hands and put on exam gloves.				
5. Have the parents pull the child's pants down and take off the diaper.				
6. Position the child with the genitalia exposed.				
7. Clean the genitalia. For a male patient, wipe the tip of the penis with a soapy cotton ball and then rinse it with a cotton ball saturated with sterile water. Allow to air-dry. For a female patient, use soapy cotton balls to clean the labia majora from front to back, using one cotton ball for each wipe. Again, use cotton balls saturated in sterile water to rinse the area and allow it to air-dry.*				
8. Remove the paper backing from the plastic urine collection bag and apply the sticky, adhesive surface over the penis and scrotum (in a male patient) or vulva (in a female patient), as shown in Figure 16-3 in the text. Seal tightly to avoid leaks. Do not include the child's rectum within the collection bag or cover it with the adhesive surface.				
9. Diaper the child.				

(continued)

Procedure Steps Total Possible Points - 68 Time Limit: 10 minutes	Practice #1	Practice #2	Practice #3	Final
10. Remove the gloves and wash your hands.				
11. Check the collection bag every half-hour for urine. You must open the diaper to check; do not just feel the diaper.*				
12. If the child has voided, wash your hands and put on exam gloves.				
13. Remove the diaper, take off the urine collection bag very carefully so that you do not irritate the child's skin, wash off the adhesive residue, rinse, and pat dry.				
14. Diaper the child.				
15. Place the specimen in the specimen container and cover it.				
16. Remove the gloves and wash your hands.				
17. Complete the laboratory request form and record the collection in the patient's chart. Progress Notes on page 475.				
Total Number of Points Achieved/Final Score				
Initials of Observer:				

Comments and Signatures

Reviewer's comments and signatures:

1. _____

2. _____

3. _____

Instructor's comments:

_____

CAAHEP Competencies Achieved

I. P. (14) Perform CLIA-waived urinalysis

IV. P. (6) Prepare a patient for procedures and/or treatments

ABHES Competencies Achieved

9. q. Instruct patients with special needs

10. c. Dispose of Biohazardous materials

10. e. Instruct patients in the collection of a clean-catch mid-stream urine specimen

PROCEDURE 16-3 ESTABLISHING CHAIN OF CUSTODY FOR A URINE SPECIMEN

Procedure Goal

To collect a urine specimen for drug testing, maintaining a chain of custody

Scoring System

To score each step, use the following scoring system:
1 = poor, 2 = fair, 3 = good, 4 = excellent

A minimum score of at least a 3 must be achieved on **each** step to achieve successful completion of the technique. Detailed instructions on the scoring system are found on page 179.

Materials

Dry, sterile urine container with lid; chain of custody form (CCF) (pages 477–479); two additional specimen containers

Procedure

Procedure Steps Total Possible Points - 64 Time Limit: 10 minutes	Practice #1	Practice #2	Practice #3	Final
1. Positively identify the patient. (Complete the top part of CCF with the name and address of the drug testing laboratory, the name and address of the requesting company, and the Social Security number of the patient. Make a note on the form if the patient refuses to give her Social Security number.) Ensure that the number on the printed label matches the number at the top of the form.				
2. Ensure that the patient removes any outer clothing and empties her pockets, displaying all items.*				
3. Instruct the patient to wash and dry her hands.				
4. Instruct the patient that no water is to be running while the specimen is being collected. Tape the faucet handles in the *off* position and add bluing agent to the toilet.*				
5. Instruct the patient to provide the specimen as soon as it is collected so that you may record the temperature of the specimen.				
6. Remain by the door of the restroom.				
7. Measure and record the temperature of the urine specimen within 4 minutes of collection. Make a note if its temperature is out of acceptable range.*				
8. Examine the specimen for signs of adulteration (unusual color or odor).				
9. *In the presence of the patient,* check the "single specimen" or "split specimen" box. The patient should witness you transferring the specimen into the transport specimen bottle(s), capping the bottle(s), and affixing the label on the bottle(s).*				

(continued)

Procedure Steps Total Possible Points - 64 Time Limit: 10 minutes	Practice #1	Practice #2	Practice #3	Final
10. The patient should initial the specimen bottle label(s) *after* it is placed on the bottle(s).*				
11. Complete any additional information requested on the form, including the authorization for drug screening. This information will include • Patient's daytime telephone number • Patient's evening telephone number • Test requested • Patient's name • Patient's signature • Date				
12. Sign the CCF; print your full name and note the date and time of the collection and the name of the courier service.				
13. Give the patient a copy of the CCF.				
14. Place the specimen in a leakproof bag with the appropriate copy of the form.				
15. Release the specimen to the courier service.				
16. Distribute additional copies as required.				
Total Number of Points Achieved/Final Score				
Initials of Observer:				

Comments and Signatures

Reviewer's comments and signatures:

1. _____

2. _____

3. _____

Instructor's comments:

_____

CAAHEP Competencies Achieved

IX. P. (7) Document accurately in the patient record

IX. P. (8) Apply local, state, and federal health care legislation and regulation appropriate to the medical assisting practice

ABHES Competencies Achieved

3. d. Recognize and identify acceptable medical abbreviations

9. f. Screen and follow up patient test results

9. q. Instruct patients with special needs

10. e. Instruct patients in the collection of a clean-catch mid-stream urine specimen

PROCEDURE 16-4 MEASURING SPECIFIC GRAVITY WITH A REFRACTOMETER

Procedure Goal

To measure the specific gravity of a urine specimen with a refractometer

Scoring System

To score each step, use the following scoring system:
1 = poor, 2 = fair, 3 = good, 4 = excellent

A minimum score of at least a 3 must be achieved on **each** step to achieve successful completion of the technique. Detailed instructions on the scoring system are found on page 179.

Materials

Urine specimen, refractometer, dropper, laboratory report form

Procedure

Procedure Steps Total Possible Points - 60 Time Limit: 10 minutes	Practice #1	Practice #2	Practice #3	Final
1. Wash your hands and put on exam gloves.				
2. Check the specimen for proper labeling and examine it to make sure that there is no visible contamination and that no more than 1 hour has passed since collection (or since the specimen has been removed from the refrigerator and brought back to room temperature).				
3. Swirl the specimen.*				
4. Confirm that the refractometer has been calibrated that day. If not, you must calibrate it with distilled water. You also must use two standard solutions as controls to check the accuracy of the refractometer. Follow steps 6 through 11, using each of the three samples in place of the specimen. Clean the refractometer and the dropper after each use and record the calibration values in the quality control log.*				
5. Open the hinged lid of the refractometer.				
6. Draw up a small amount of the specimen into the dropper.				
7. Place one drop of the specimen under the cover.				
8. Close the lid.				
9. Turn on the light and look into the eyepiece of the refractometer. As the light passes through the specimen, the refractometer measures the refraction of the light and displays the refractive index on a scale on the right with corresponding specific gravity values on the left.				
10. Read the specific gravity value at the line where light and dark meet.				
11. Record the value on the laboratory report form.				

(continued)

Procedure Steps Total Possible Points - 60 Time Limit: 10 minutes	Practice #1	Practice #2	Practice #3	Final
12. Sanitize and disinfect the refractometer and the dropper. Put them away when they are dry.				
13. Clean and disinfect the work area.				
14. Remove the gloves and wash your hands.				
15. Record the value in the patient's chart. Use form on page 481 of this workbook.				
Total Number of Points Achieved/Final Score				
Initials of Observer:				

Comments and Signatures

Reviewer's comments and signatures:

1. _____

2. _____

3. _____

Instructor's comments:

_____

CAAHEP Competencies Achieved

I. P. (14) Perform CLIA-waived urinalysis

I. P. (16) Screen test results

ABHES Competencies Achieved

9. f. Screen and follow up patient test results

10. a. Practice quality control

10. b. Perform selected CLIA-waived tests that assist with diagnosis and treatment
    1) Urinalysis

Procedure 16-5 Performing a Reagent Strip Test

Procedure Goal

To perform chemical testing on urine specimens (This test is used to screen for the presence of leukocytes, nitrite, urobilinogen, protein, pH, blood, specific gravity, ketones, bilirubin, and glucose.)

Scoring System

To score each step, use the following scoring system:
1 = poor, 2 = fair, 3 = good, 4 = excellent

A minimum score of at least a 3 must be achieved on **each** step to achieve successful completion of the technique. Detailed instructions on the scoring system are found on page 179.

Materials

Urine specimen, laboratory report form, reagent strips, paper towel, timer

Procedure

Procedure Steps Total Possible Points - 44 Time Limit: 10 minutes	Practice #1	Practice #2	Practice #3	Final
1. Wash your hands and put on personal protective equipment.				
2. Check the specimen for proper labeling and examine it to make sure that there is no visible contamination. Perform the test as soon as possible after collection. Refrigerate the specimen if testing will take place more than 1 hour later. Bring the refrigerated specimen back to room temperature prior to testing.				
3. Check the expiration date on the reagent strip container and check the strip for damaged or discolored pads.*				
4. Swirl the specimen.*				
5. Dip a urine strip into the specimen, making sure each pad is completely covered. Briefly tap the strip sideways on a paper towel. *Do not blot* the test pads.*				
6. Read each test pad against the chart on the bottle at the designated time. Note: It is important to read each pad at the appropriate time. Most reagent strip results are invalid after 2 minutes.*				
7. Record the values on the laboratory report form.				
8. Discard the used disposable supplies.				
9. Clean and disinfect the work area.				
10. Remove your gloves and wash your hands.				
11. Record the result in the patient's chart. Use form on page 483 of this workbook.				
Total Number of Points Achieved/Final Score				
Initials of Observer:				

(continued)

Comments and Signatures

Reviewer's comments and signatures:

1. _____

2. _____

3. _____

Instructor's comments:

_____

CAAHEP Competencies Achieved

I. P. (14) Perform CLIA-waived urinalysis

I. P. (16) Screen test results

ABHES Competencies Achieved

3. d. Recognize and identify acceptable medical abbreviations

9. f. Screen and follow up patient test results

10. a. Practice quality control

10. b. Perform selected CLIA-waived tests that assist with diagnosis and treatment
    1) Urinalysis
    6) Kit testing
       c) Dip sticks

10. c. Dispose of Biohazardous materials

PROCEDURE 16-6 PREGNANCY TESTING USING THE EIA METHOD

Procedure Goal

To perform the enzyme immunoassay in order to detect HCG in the urine (or serum) and to interpret results as positive or negative

Scoring System

To score each step, use the following scoring system:
1 = poor, 2 = fair, 3 = good, 4 = excellent

A minimum score of at least a 3 must be achieved on **each** step to achieve successful completion of the technique. Detailed instructions on the scoring system are found on page 179.

Materials

Gloves, urine specimen, timing device, surface disinfectant, pregnancy control solutions, pregnancy test kits

Procedure

Procedure Steps Total Possible Points - 40 Time Limit: 10 minutes	Practice #1	Practice #2	Practice #3	Final
1. Wash your hands and put on exam gloves.				
2. Gather the necessary supplies and equipment.				
3. If materials have been refrigerated, allow all materials to reach room temperature prior to conducting the testing.				
4. Label the test chamber with the patient's name or identification number; label one test chamber for a negative and positive control.				
5. Apply the urine (or serum) to the test chamber per the manufacturer's instructions.*				
6. At the appropriate time, read and interpret the results.*				
7. Document the patient's results in the chart; document the quality control results in the appropriate log book. Use forms on pages 485–486 of this workbook.				
8. Dispose of used reagents in a biohazard container.				
9. Clean the work area with a disinfectant solution.				
10. Wash your hands.				
Total Number of Points Achieved/Final Score				
Initials of Observer:				

(continued)

Comments and Signatures

Reviewer's comments and signatures:

1. _____

2. _____

3. _____

Instructor's comments:

_____

CAAHEP Competencies Achieved

I. P. (6) Perform patient screening using established protocols

I. P. (13) Perform chemistry testing

ABHES Competencies Achieved

9. f. Screen and follow up patient test results

10. a. Practice quality control

10. b. Perform selected CLIA-waived tests that assist with diagnosis and treatment
    6) Kit testing
      a) Pregnancy

10. c. Dispose of Biohazardous materials

Procedure 16-7 Processing a Urine Specimen for Microscopic Examination of Sediment

Objective

To prepare a slide for microscopic examination of urine sediment

Scoring System

To score each step, use the following scoring system:
1 = poor, 2 = fair, 3 = good, 4 = excellent

A minimum score of at least a 3 must be achieved on **each** step to achieve successful completion of the technique. Detailed instructions on the scoring system are found on page 179.

Materials

Fresh urine specimen, two glass or plastic test tubes, water, centrifuge, tapered pipette, glass slide with coverslip, microscope with light source, laboratory report form

Procedure

Procedure Steps Total Possible Points - 80 Time Limit: 15 minutes	Practice #1	Practice #2	Practice #3	Final
1. Wash your hands and put on exam gloves.				
2. Check the specimen for proper labeling and examine it to make sure that there is no visible contamination and that no more than 1 hour has passed since collection (or since the specimen has been removed from the refrigerator and brought back to room temperature).				
3. Swirl the urine specimen.*				
4. Pour approximately 10 mL of urine into one test tube and 10 mL of plain water into the balance tube.				
5. Balance the centrifuge by placing the test tubes on either side.*				
6. Make sure the lid is secure and set the centrifuge timer for 5 to 10 minutes.*				
7. Set the speed as prescribed by your office's protocol (usually 1500 to 2000 revolutions per minute) and start the centrifuge.				
8. After the centrifuge stops, lift out the tube containing the urine and carefully pour most of the liquid portion—called the **supernatant**—down the drain in the sink.				
9. A few drops of urine should remain in the bottom of the test tube with any sediment. Mix the urine and sediment together by gently tapping the bottom of the tube on the palm of your hand.*				
10. Use the tapered pipette to obtain a drop or two of urine sediment. Place the drops in the center of a clean glass slide.				
11. Place the coverslip over the specimen, allow it to settle, and place it on the stage of the microscope.				
12. Correctly focus the microscope as directed in Procedure 14-1. *Note:* Most medical assistants are trained to perform this procedure only up to this point. After this, the physician usually				

(continued)

Procedure Steps Total Possible Points - 80 Time Limit: 15 minutes	Practice #1	Practice #2	Practice #3	Final
examines the specimen. You may, however, be asked to clean the items after the examination is completed. The remaining steps are provided for your information.				
13. Use a dim light and view the slide under the low-power objective. Observe the slide for casts (found mainly around the edges of the coverslip) and count the casts viewed.				
14. Switch to the high-power objective. Identify the casts. Identify any epithelial cells, mucus, protozoa, yeasts, and crystals. Adjust the slide position so that you can view and count the cells, protozoa, yeasts, and crystals from at least 10 different fields. Turn off the light after the examination is completed.				
15. Record the observations on the laboratory report form.				
16. Properly dispose of used disposable materials.				
17. Sanitize and disinfect nondisposable items; put them away when they are dry.				
18. Clean and disinfect the work area.				
19. Remove the gloves and wash your hands.				
20. Record the observations in the patient's chart (pages 487–488).				
Total Number of Points Achieved/Final Score				
Initials of Observer:				

Comments and Signatures

Reviewer's comments and signatures:

1. _____

2. _____

3. _____

Instructor's comments:

_____

CAAHEP Competencies Achieved

I.P. (14) Perform CLIA-waived urinalysis

I. P. (16) Screen test results

ABHES Competencies Achieved

3. d. Recognize and identify acceptable medical abbreviations

9. f. Screen and follow up patient test results

10. a. Practice quality control

10. b. Perform selected CLIA-waived tests that assist with diagnosis and treatment
    1) Urinalysis

10. c. Dispose of Biohazardous materials

Procedure 17-1 Quality Control Procedures for Blood Specimen Collection

Procedure Goal

To follow proper quality control procedures when taking a blood specimen

Scoring System

To score each step, use the following scoring system:
1 = poor, 2 = fair, 3 = good, 4 = excellent

A minimum score of at least a 3 must be achieved on **each** step to achieve successful completion of the technique. Detailed instructions on the scoring system are found on page 179.

Materials

Necessary sterile equipment, specimen-collection container, paperwork related to the type of blood test the specimen is being drawn for, requisition form, marker, proper packing materials for transport

Procedure

Procedure Steps Total Possible Points - 36 Time Limit: 10 minutes	Practice #1	Practice #2	Practice #3	Final
1. Review the request form for the test ordered, verify the procedure, prepare the necessary equipment and paperwork, and prepare the work area.				
2. Identify the patient and explain the procedure. Confirm the patient's identification. Ask the patient to spell her name. Make sure the patient understands the procedure that is to be performed, even if she has had it done before.				
3. Confirm that the patient has followed any pretest preparation requirements such as fasting, taking any necessary medication, or stopping a medication. For example, if a fasting specimen is being taken, the patient should not have eaten anything after midnight of the day before. Some doctors' offices will let the patient drink water or black coffee, however. It often depends on the type of specimen being taken.*				
4. Collect the specimen properly. Collect it at the right time intervals if that applies. Use sterile equipment and proper technique.				
5. Use the correct specimen-collection containers and the right preservatives, if required. For example, blood collected into a test tube with additives should be mixed immediately.*				
6. Immediately label the specimens. The label should include the patient's name, the date and time of collection, the test's name, and the name of the person collecting the specimen. Do not label the containers before collecting the specimen.*				

(continued)

Procedure Steps Total Possible Points - 36 Time Limit: 10 minutes	Practice #1	Practice #2	Practice #3	Final
7. Follow correct procedures for disposing of hazardous specimen waste and decontaminating the work area. Used needles, for instance, should immediately be placed in a biohazard sharps container.				
8. Thank the patient. Keep the patient in the office if any follow-up observation is necessary.				
9. If the specimen is to be transported to an outside laboratory, prepare it for transport in the proper container for that type of specimen, according to OSHA regulations. Place the container in a clear plastic bag with a zip closure and dual pockets with the international biohazard label imprinted in red or orange. The requisition form should be placed in the outside pocket of the bag (page 489). This ensures protection from contamination if the specimen leaks. Have a courier pick up the specimen and place it in an appropriate carrier (such as an insulated cooler) with the biohazard label. Place specimens to be sent by mail in appropriate plastic containers and then place the containers inside a heavy-duty plastic container with a screw-down, nonleaking lid. Then place this container in either a heavy-duty cardboard box or nylon bag. The words *Human Specimen* or *Body Fluids* should be imprinted on the box or bag. Seal with a strong tape strip.*				
Total Number of Points Achieved/Final Score				
Initials of Observer:				

Comments and Signatures

Reviewer's comments and signatures:

1. _____

2. _____

3. _____

Instructor's comments:

_____

CAAHEP Competency Achieved

I. P. (11) Perform quality control measures

ABHES Competencies Achieved

10. a. Practice quality control

10. c. Dispose of Biohazardous materials

10. d. Collect, label, and process specimens
    1) Perform venipuncture
    2) Perform capillary puncture

Procedure 17-2 Performing Venipuncture Using an Evacuation System

Procedure Goal

To collect a venous blood sample using an evacuation system

Scoring System

To score each step, use the following scoring system:
1 = poor, 2 = fair, 3 = good, 4 = excellent

A minimum score of at least a 3 must be achieved on **each** step to achieve successful completion of the technique. Detailed instructions on the scoring system are found on page 179.

Materials

VACUTAINER components (safety needle, needle holder/adapter, collection tubes), antiseptic and cotton balls or antiseptic wipes, tourniquet, sterile gauze squares, sterile adhesive bandages

Procedure

Procedure Steps Total Possible Points - 88 Time Limit: 10 minutes	Practice #1	Practice #2	Practice #3	Final
1. Review the laboratory request form and make sure you have the necessary supplies.				
2. Greet the patient, confirm the patient's identity, and introduce yourself.				
3. Explain the purpose of the procedure and confirm that the patient has followed the pretest instructions.*				
4. Make sure the patient is sitting in a venipuncture chair or is lying down.				
5. Wash your hands. Put on exam gloves.				
6. Prepare the safety needle holder/adapter assembly by inserting the threaded side of the needle into the adapter and twisting the adapter in a clockwise direction. Push the first collection tube into the other end of the needle holder/adapter until the outer edge of the collection tube stopper meets the guideline.*				
7. Ask the patient whether one arm is better than the other for the venipuncture. The chosen arm should be positioned slightly downward.				
8. Apply the tourniquet to the patient's upper arm midway between the elbow and the shoulder. Wrap the tourniquet around the patient's arm and cross the ends. Holding one end of the tourniquet against the patient's arm, stretch the other end to apply pressure against the patient's skin. Pull a loop of the stretched end under the end held tightly against the patient's skin, as shown in Figure 17-7 in the text. The				

(continued)

Procedure Steps Total Possible Points - 88 Time Limit: 10 minutes	Practice #1	Practice #2	Practice #3	Final
tourniquet should be tight enough to cause the veins to stand out but should not stop the flow of blood. You should still be able to feel the patient's radial pulse.*				
9. Palpate the proposed site and use your index finger to locate the vein, as shown in Figure 17-8 in the text. The vein will feel like a small tube with some elasticity. If you feel a pulsing beat, you have located an artery. Do not draw blood from an artery. If you cannot locate the vein within 1 minute, release the tourniquet and allow blood to flow freely for 1 to 2 minutes. Then reapply the tourniquet and try again to locate the vein.				
10. After locating the vein, clean the area with a cotton ball moistened with antiseptic or an antiseptic wipe. Use a circular motion to clean the area, starting at the center and working outward. Allow the site to air-dry.*				
11. Remove the plastic cap from the outer point of the needle cover and ask the patient to tighten the fist. Hold the patient's skin taut below the insertion site.*				
12. With a steady and quick motion, insert the needle—held at a 15-degree angle, bevel side up, and aligned parallel to the vein—into the vein. You will feel a slight resistance as the needle tip penetrates the vein wall. Penetrate to a depth of ¼ to ½ inch. Grasp the holder/adapter between your index and great (middle) fingers. Using your thumb, seat the collection tube firmly into place over the needle point, puncturing the rubber stopper. Blood will begin to flow into the collection tube.				
13. Fill each tube until the blood stops running to ensure the correct proportion of blood to additives. Switch tubes as needed by pulling one tube out of the adapter and inserting the next in a smooth and steady motion. (The soft plastic cover on the inner point of the needle retracts as each tube is inserted and recovers the needle point as each tube is removed.)				
14. Once blood is flowing steadily, ask the patient to release the fist and untie the tourniquet by pulling the end of the tucked-in loop. The tourniquet should, in general, be left on no longer than 1 minute.* You must remove the tourniquet before you withdraw the needle from the vein.*				
15. As you withdraw the needle in a smooth and steady motion, place a sterile gauze square over the insertion site. Immediately activate the safety device on the needle if it is not self-activating. Properly dispose of the needle immediately. Instruct the patient to hold the gauze pad in place with slight pressure. The patient should keep the arm straight and slightly elevated for several minutes.*				
16. If the collection tubes contain additives, you will need to invert them slowly several times.*				

(continued)

Procedure Steps Total Possible Points - 88 Time Limit: 10 minutes	Practice #1	Practice #2	Practice #3	Final
17. Label specimens and complete the paperwork.				
18. Check the patient's condition and the puncture site for bleeding. Replace the sterile gauze square with a sterile adhesive bandage.				
19. Properly dispose of used supplies and disposable instruments and disinfect the work area.				
20. Remove the gloves and wash your hands.				
21. Instruct the patient about care of the puncture site.				
22. Document the procedure in the patient's chart.				
Total Number of Points Achieved/Final Score				
Initials of Observer:				

Comments and Signatures

Reviewer's comments and signatures:

1. _____

2. _____

3. _____

Instructor's comments:

_____

CAAHEP Competency Achieved

I. P. (2) Perform venipuncture

ABHES Competencies Achieved

3. d. Recognize and identify acceptable medical abbreviations

9. f. Screen and follow up patient test results

10. c. Dispose of Biohazardous materials

10. d. Collect, label, and process specimens
    1) Perform venipuncture

PROCEDURE 17-3 PERFORMING CAPILLARY PUNCTURE

Procedure Goal

To collect a capillary blood sample using the finger puncture method

Scoring System

To score each step, use the following scoring system:
1 = poor, 2 = fair, 3 = good, 4 = excellent

A minimum score of at least a 3 must be achieved on **each** step to achieve successful completion of the technique. Detailed instructions on the scoring system are found on page 179.

Materials

Capillary puncture device (safety lancet or automatic puncture device such as Autolet or Glucolet), antiseptic and cotton balls or antiseptic wipes, sterile gauze squares, sterile adhesive bandages, reagent strips, micropipettes, smear slides

Procedure

Procedure Steps Total Possible Points - 72 Time Limit: 10 minutes	Practice #1	Practice #2	Practice #3	Final
1. Review the laboratory request form and make sure you have the necessary supplies.				
2. Greet the patient, confirm the patient's identity, and introduce yourself.				
3. Explain the purpose of the procedure and confirm that the patient has followed the pretest instructions, if indicated.*				
4. Make sure the patient is sitting in the venipuncture chair or is lying down.				
5. Wash your hands. Put on exam gloves.				
6. Examine the patient's hands to determine which finger to use for the procedure. Avoid fingers that are swollen, bruised, scarred, or calloused. Generally, the ring and great (middle) fingers are the best choices. If you notice that the patient's hands are cold, you may want to warm them between your own, have the patient put them in a warm basin of water or under warm running water, or wrap them in a warm cloth.*				
7. Prepare the patient's finger with a gentle "massaging" or rubbing motion toward the fingertip. Keep the patient's hand below heart level so that gravity helps the blood flow.				
8. Clean the area with a cotton ball moistened with antiseptic or an antiseptic wipe. Allow the site to air-dry.*				

(continued)

Procedure Steps Total Possible Points - 72 Time Limit: 10 minutes	Practice #1	Practice #2	Practice #3	Final
9. Hold the patient's finger between your thumb and forefinger. Hold the safety lancet or automatic puncture device at a right angle to the patient's fingerprint, as shown in Figure 17-14 in the text. Puncture the skin on the pad of the fingertip with a quick, sharp motion. The depth to which you puncture the skin is generally determined by the length of the lancet point. Most automatic puncturing devices are designed to penetrate to the correct depth.				
10. Allow a drop of blood to form at the end of the patient's finger. If the blood droplet is slow in forming, apply steady pressure. Avoid milking the patient's finger.*				
11. Wipe away the first droplet of blood. (This droplet is usually contaminated with tissue fluids released when the skin is punctured.) Then fill the collection devices, as described. *Micropipettes:* Hold the tip of the tube just to the edge of the blood droplet. The tube will fill through capillary action. If you are preparing microhematocrit tubes, you need to seal one end of each tube with clay sealant. *Reagent strips:* With some reagent strips (dipsticks), you must touch the strip to the blood drop but not smear it; with other strips, you must smear it. Follow the manufacturer's guidelines. *Smear slides:* Gently touch the blood droplet to the smear slide and process the slide as described in Procedure 17-4.				
12. After you have collected the required samples, dispose of the lancet immediately. Then wipe the patient's finger with a sterile gauze square. Instruct the patient to apply pressure to stop the bleeding.				
13. Label specimens and complete the paperwork. Some tests, such as glucose monitoring, must be completed immediately.				
14. Check the puncture site for bleeding. If necessary, replace the sterile gauze square with a sterile adhesive bandage.				
15. Properly dispose of used supplies and disposable instruments and disinfect the work area.				
16. Remove the gloves and wash your hands.				
17. Instruct the patient about care of the puncture site.				
18. Document the procedure in the patient's chart. (If the test has been completed, include the results.)				
Total Number of Points Achieved/Final Score				
Initials of Observer:				

(continued)

Comments and Signatures

Reviewer's comments and signatures:

1. _____

2. _____

3. _____

Instructor's comments:

_____

CAAHEP Competency Achieved

I. P. (2) Perform capillary puncture

ABHES Competencies Achieved

3. d. Recognize and identify acceptable medical abbreviations

10. c. Dispose of Biohazardous materials

10. d. Collect, label, and process specimens
    2) Perform capillary puncture

PROCEDURE 17-4 PREPARING A BLOOD SMEAR SLIDE

Procedure Goal

To prepare a blood specimen to be used in a morphologic or other study

Scoring System

To score each step, use the following scoring system:
1 = poor, 2 = fair, 3 = good, 4 = excellent

A minimum score of at least a 3 must be achieved on **each** step to achieve successful completion of the technique. Detailed instructions on the scoring system are found on page 179.

Materials

Blood specimen (either from a capillary puncture or a specimen tube containing anticoagulated blood), capillary tubes, sterile gauze squares, slide with frosted end, wooden applicator sticks

Procedure

Procedure Steps Total Possible Points - 48 Time Limit: 10 minutes	Practice #1	Practice #2	Practice #3	Final
1. Wash your hands and put on exam gloves.				
2. If you will be using blood from a capillary puncture, follow the steps in Procedure 17-3 to express a drop of blood from the patient's finger. If you will be using a venous sample, check the specimen for proper labeling, carefully uncap the specimen tube, and use wooden applicator sticks to remove any coagulated blood from the inside rim of the tube. You may use a special safety transfer device if available.*				
3. Touch the tip of the capillary tube to the blood specimen either from the patient's finger or the specimen tube. The tube will take up the correct amount through capillary action.				
4. Pull the capillary tube away from the sample, holding it carefully to prevent spillage. Wipe the outside of the capillary tube with a sterile gauze square.*				
5. With the slide on the work surface, hold the capillary tube in one hand and the frosted end of the slide against the work surface with the other.				
6. Apply a drop of blood to the slide, about ¾ inch from the frosted end, as shown in Figure 17-20 in the text. Place the capillary tube in the sharps container.				
7. Pick up the spreader slide with your dominant hand. Hold the slide at approximately a 30- to 35-degree angle. Place the edge of the spreader slide on the smear slide close to the unfrosted end. Pull the spreader slide toward the frosted end until the spreader slide touches the blood drop. Capillary action will spread the droplet along the edge of the spreader slide.*				

(continued)

Procedure Steps Total Possible Points - 48 Time Limit: 10 minutes	Practice #1	Practice #2	Practice #3	Final
8. As soon as the drop spreads out to cover most of the spreader slide edge, push the spreader slide back toward the unfrosted end of the smear slide, pulling the sample across the slide behind it, as shown in Figure 17-22 in the text. Maintain the 30- to 35-degree angle.				
9. Continue pushing the spreader until you come off the end, still maintaining the angle, as shown in Figure 17-23 in the text. The resulting smear should be approximately 1½ inches long, preferably with a margin of empty slide on all sides. The smear should be thicker on the frosted end of the slide.				
10. Properly label the slide, allow it to dry, and follow the manufacturer's directions for staining it for the required tests.				
11. Properly dispose of used supplies and disinfect the work area.				
12. Remove the gloves and wash your hands.				
Total Number of Points Achieved/Final Score				
Initials of Observer:				

Comments and Signatures

Reviewer's comments and signatures:

1. _____

2. _____

3. _____

Instructor's comments:

_____

CAAHEP Competency Achieved

I. P. (12) Perform CLIA-waived hematology testing

ABHES Competencies Achieved

10. c. Dispose of Biohazardous materials

10. d. Collect, label, and process specimens

PROCEDURE 17-5 MEASURING HEMATOCRIT PERCENTAGE AFTER CENTRIFUGE

Procedure Goal

To identify the percentage of a blood specimen represented by RBCs after the sample has been spun in a centrifuge

Scoring System

To score each step, use the following scoring system:
1 = poor, 2 = fair, 3 = good, 4 = excellent

A minimum score of at least a 3 must be achieved on **each** step to achieve successful completion of the technique. Detailed instructions on the scoring system are found on page 179.

Materials

Blood specimen (either from a capillary puncture or a specimen tube containing anticoagulated blood), microhematocrit tube, sealant tray containing sealing clay, centrifuge, hematocrit gauge, wooden applicator sticks, gauze squares

Procedure

Procedure Steps Total Possible Points - 60 Time Limit: 10 minutes	Practice #1	Practice #2	Practice #3	Final
1. Wash your hands and put on exam gloves.				
2. If you will be using blood from a capillary puncture, follow the steps in Procedure 17-3 to express a drop of blood from the patient's finger. If you will be using a venous blood sample, check the specimen for proper labeling, carefully uncap the specimen tube, and use wooden applicator sticks to remove any coagulated blood from the inside rim of the tube. Alternately, use a special safety transfer device if available.*				
3. Touch the tip of one of the microhematocrit tubes to the blood sample, as shown in Figure 17-25 in the text. The tube will take up the correct amount through capillary action.				
4. Pull the microhematocrit tube away from the sample, holding it carefully to prevent spillage. Wipe the outside of the microhematocrit tube with a gauze square.*				
5. Hold the microhematocrit tube in one hand with a gloved finger over one end to prevent leakage and press the other end of the tube gently into the clay in the sealant tray. The clay plug must completely seal the end of the tube.*				
6. Repeat the process to fill another microhematocrit tube. Tubes must be processed in pairs.*				
7. Place the tubes in the centrifuge, with the sealed ends pointing outward. If you are processing more than one sample, record the position identification number in the patient's chart to track the sample.				
8. Seal the centrifuge chamber.				

(continued)

Procedure Steps Total Possible Points - 60 Time Limit: 10 minutes	Practice #1	Practice #2	Practice #3	Final
9. Run the centrifuge for the required time, usually between 3 and 5 minutes. Allow the centrifuge to come to a complete stop before unsealing it.				
10. Determine the hematocrit percentage by comparing the column of packed RBCs in the microhematocrit tubes with the hematocrit gauge, as shown in Figure 17-28 in the text. Position each tube so that the boundary between sealing clay and RBCs is at zero on the gauge. Some centrifuges are equipped with gauges, but others require separate handheld gauges.				
11. Record the percentage value on the gauge that corresponds to the top of the column of RBCs for each tube. Compare the two results. They should not vary by more than 2%. If you record a greater variance, at least one of the tubes was filled incorrectly, and you must repeat the test.				
12. Calculate the average result by adding the two tube figures and dividing that number by 2.				
13. Properly dispose of used supplies and clean and disinfect the equipment and the area.				
14. Remove the gloves and wash your hands.				
15. Record the test result in the patient's chart. Be sure to identify abnormal results.				
Total Number of Points Achieved/Final Score				
Initials of Observer:				

Comments and Signatures

Reviewer's comments and signatures:

1. _____

2. _____

3. _____

Instructor's comments:

_____

CAAHEP Competency Achieved

I. P. (12) Perform CLIA-waived hematology testing

ABHES Competencies Achieved

3. d. Recognize and identify acceptable medical abbreviations

9. f. Screen and follow up patient test results

10. b. Perform selected CLIA-waived tests that assist with diagnosis and treatment
2) Hematology testing

10. c. Dispose of Biohazardous materials

10. d. Collect, label, and process specimens

PROCEDURE 17-6 MEASURING BLOOD GLUCOSE USING A HANDHELD GLUCOMETER

Procedure Goal

To measure the amount of glucose present in a blood sample.

Scoring System

To score each step, use the following scoring system:
1 = poor, 2 = fair, 3 = good, 4 = excellent

A minimum score of at least a 3 must be achieved on **each** step to achieve successful completion of the technique. Detailed instructions on the scoring system are found on page 179.

Materials

Safety engineered capillary puncture device (automatic puncture device or other safety lancet), antiseptic and cotton balls or antiseptic wipes, sterile gauze squares, sterile adhesive bandages, handheld glucometer, reagent strips appropriate for the device.

Procedure

Procedure Steps Total Possible Points - 56 Time Limit: 10 minutes	Practice #1	Practice #2	Practice #3	Final
1. Wash your hands and put on exam gloves.				
2. Review the manufacturer's instructions for the specific device used.				
3. Check the expiration date on the reagent strips.*				
4. Code the meter to the reagent strips if required.*				
5. Turn the device on according to the manufacturer's instructions.				
6. Perform the required quality control procedures.*				
7. Perform a capillary puncture following the steps outlined in Procedure 17-3.				
8. Touch the drop of blood to the reagent strip, allowing it to be taken up by the strip.				
9. Read the digital result after the required amount of time.				
10. Record the time of the test and result on the laboratory slip.				
11. Discard the reagent strip and used supplies according to OSHA standards.				
12. Disinfect the equipment and area.				
13. Remove the gloves and wash your hands.				
14. Document the test results in the patient's chart. Record the quality control tests in the laboratory control log.				
Total Number of Points Achieved/Final Score				
Initials of Observer:				

(continued)

Comments and Signatures

Reviewer's comments and signatures:

1. _____

2. _____

3. _____

Instructor's comments:

_____

CAAHEP Competency Achieved

I. P. (12) Perform CLIA-waived chemistry testing

ABHES Competencies Achieved

9. f. Screen and follow up patient test results

10. a. Practice quality control

10. b. Perform selected CLIA-waived tests that assist with diagnosis and treatment
     3) Chemistry testing

10. c. Dispose of Biohazardous materials

10. d. Collect, label, and process specimens

PROCEDURE 18-1 EDUCATING ADULT PATIENTS ABOUT DAILY WATER REQUIREMENTS

Procedure Goal

To teach patients how much water their bodies need to maintain health

Scoring System

To score each step, use the following scoring system:
1 = poor, 2 = fair, 3 = good, 4 = excellent

A minimum score of at least a 3 must be achieved on **each** step to achieve successful completion of the technique. Detailed instructions on the scoring system are found on page 179.

Materials

Patient education literature, patient's chart, pen

Procedure

Procedure Steps Total Possible Points - 28 Time Limit: 15 minutes	Practice #1	Practice #2	Practice #3	Final
1. Explain to patients the importance of water to the body. Point out the water content of the body and the many functions of water in the body: maintaining the body's fluid balance, lubricating the body's moving parts, transporting nutrients and secretions.				
2. Add any comments applicable to an individual patient's health status—for example, issues related to medication use, physical activity, pregnancy, fluid limitation, or increased fluid needs.*				
3. Explain that people obtain water by drinking water and other fluids and by eating water-containing foods. On average, an adult should drink six to eight glasses of water a day to maintain a healthy water balance in which intake equals excretion. People's daily need for water varies with size and age, the temperatures to which they are exposed, degree of physical exertion, and the water content of foods eaten. Make sure you reinforce the physician's or dietitian's recommendations for a particular patient's water needs.				
4. Caution patients that soft drinks, coffee, and tea are not good substitutes for water and that it would be wise to filter out any harmful chemicals contained in the local tap water or to drink bottled water, if possible.				
5. Provide patients with tips about reminders to drink the requisite amount of water. Some patients may benefit from using a water bottle of a particular size, so they know they have to drink, say, three full bottles of water each day. Another helpful tip is to make a habit of drinking a glass of water at certain points in the daily routine, such as first thing in the morning and before lunch.				

(continued)

Procedure Steps Total Possible Points - 28 Time Limit: 15 minutes	Practice #1	Practice #2	Practice #3	Final
6. Remind patients that you and the physician are available to discuss any problems or questions.				
7. Document any formal patient education sessions or significant exchanges with a patient in the patient's chart, noting whether the patient understood the information presented. Then initial the entry.*				
Total Number of Points Achieved/Final Score				
Initials of Observer:				

Comments and Signatures

Reviewer's comments and signatures:

1. _____

2. _____

3. _____

Instructor's comments:

_____

CAAHEP Competency Achieved

IV. P. (5) Instruct patients according to their needs to promote health maintenance and disease prevention

ABHES Competency Achieved

9 (r). Teach patients methods of health promotion and disease prevention

PROCEDURE 18-2 TEACHING PATIENTS HOW TO READ FOOD LABELS

Procedure Goal

To explain how patients can use food labels to plan or follow a diet

Scoring System

To score each step, use the following scoring system:
1 = poor, 2 = fair, 3 = good, 4 = excellent

A minimum score of at least a 3 must be achieved on **each** step to achieve successful completion of the technique. Detailed instructions on the scoring system are found on page 179.

Materials

Food labels from products

Procedure

Procedure Steps Total Possible Points - 28 Time Limit: 15 minutes	Practice #1	Practice #2	Practice #3	Final
1. Identify the patient and introduce yourself.				
2. Explain that food labels can be used as a valuable source of information when planning or implementing a prescribed diet.				
3. Using a label from a food package, such as the ice-cream label shown in Figure 18-16 in the text, point out the Nutrition Facts section.				
4. Describe the various elements on the label—in this case the ice-cream label. • Serving size is the basis for the nutrition information provided. One serving of the ice cream is ½ cup. There are 14 servings in the package of ice cream.* • Calories and calories from fat show the proportion of fat calories in the product. One serving of the ice cream contains 180 calories; more than 41% of the calories come from fat. • The % Daily Value section shows how many grams (g) or milligrams (mg) of a variety of nutrients are contained in one serving. Then the label shows the percentage (%) of the recommended daily intake of each given nutrient (assuming a diet of 2000 calories a day). The ice cream contains 28% of a person's recommended daily saturated fat intake and no dietary fiber. • Recommendations for total amounts of various nutrients for both a 2000-calorie and a 2500-calorie diet are shown in chart form near the bottom of the label. These numbers provide the basis for the daily value percentages. • Ingredients are listed in order from largest quantity to smallest quantity. In this half-gallon of ice cream, skim milk, cream, and cookie dough are the most abundant ingredients.				

(continued)

Procedure Steps Total Possible Points - 28 Time Limit: 15 minutes	Practice #1	Practice #2	Practice #3	Final
5. Inform the patient that a variety of similar products with significantly different nutritional values are often available. Explain that patients can use nutrition labels, such as those shown in Figures 18-16 and 18-17 in the text, to evaluate and compare such similar products. Patients must consider what a product contributes to their diets, not simply what it lacks. To do this, patients must read the entire label. Compared with the regular ice cream, the "light, no sugar added" ice cream contains less fat, fewer carbohydrates, and two grams of dietary fiber, but it contributes an additional 25 milligrams of sodium and contains sugar alcohol, which is an artificial sweetner.				
6. Ask the patient to compare two other similar products and determine which would fit in better as part of a healthy, nutritious diet that meets that patient's individual needs.				
7. Document the patient education session in the patient's chart, indicate the patient's understanding, and initial the entry. Use Progress Notes on page 503.*				
Total Number of Points Achieved/Final Score				
Initials of Observer:				

Comments and Signatures

Reviewer's comments and signatures:

1. _____

2. _____

3. _____

Instructor's comments:

_____

CAAHEP Competency Achieved

IV. P. (5) Instruct patients according to their needs to promote health maintenance and disease prevention

ABHES Competency Achieved

9 (r). Teach patients methods of health promotion and disease prevention

PROCEDURE 18-3 ALERTING PATIENTS WITH FOOD ALLERGIES TO THE DANGERS OF COMMON FOODS

Procedure Goal

To explain how patients can eliminate allergy-causing foods from their diets

Scoring System

To score each step, use the following scoring system:
1 = poor, 2 = fair, 3 = good, 4 = excellent

A minimum score of at least a 3 must be achieved on **each** step to achieve successful completion of the technique. Detailed instructions on the scoring system are found on page 179.

Materials

Results of the patient's allergy tests, patient's chart, pen, patient education materials

Procedure

Procedure Steps Total Possible Points - 36 Time Limit: 15 minutes	Practice #1	Practice #2	Practice #3	Final
1. Identify the patient and introduce yourself.				
2. Discuss the results of the patient's allergy tests (if available), reinforcing the physician's instructions. Provide the patient with a checklist of the foods that the patient has been found to be allergic to and review this list with the patient.				
3. Discuss with the patient the possible allergic reactions those foods can cause.*				
4. Discuss with the patient the need to avoid or eliminate those foods from the diet. Point out that the patient needs to be alert to avoid the allergy-causing foods not only in their basic forms but also as ingredients in prepared dishes and packaged foods. (Patients allergic to peanuts, for example, should avoid products containing peanut oil as well as peanuts.)				
5. Tell the patient to read labels carefully and to inquire at restaurants about the use of those ingredients in dishes listed on the menu.				
6. With the physician's or dietitian's consent, talk with the patient about the possibility of finding adequate substitutes for the foods if they are among the patient's favorites. Also discuss, if necessary, how the patient can obtain the nutrients in those foods from other sources (for example, the need for extra calcium sources if the patient is allergic to dairy products). Provide these explanations to the patient in writing, if appropriate, along with supplementary materials such as recipe pamphlets, a list of resources for obtaining food substitutes, and so on.				
7. Discuss with the patient the procedures to follow if the allergy-causing foods are accidentally ingested.*				

(continued)

Procedure Steps Total Possible Points - 36 Time Limit: 15 minutes	Practice #1	Practice #2	Practice #3	Final
8. Answer the patient's questions and remind the patient that you and the rest of the medical team are available if any questions or problems arise later on.				
9. Document the patient education session or interchange in the patient's chart, indicate the patient's understanding, and initial the entry. Use Progress Notes on page 505.*				
Total Number of Points Achieved/Final Score				
Initials of Observer:				

Comments and Signatures

Reviewer's comments and signatures:

1. _____

2. _____

3. _____

Instructor's comments:

_____

CAAHEP Competency Achieved

IV. P. (5) Instruct patients according to their needs to promote health maintenance and disease prevention

ABHES Competency Achieved

9 (r). Teach patients methods of health promotion and disease prevention

Name_____ Date_____

Evaluated by_____ Score_____

PROCEDURE 19-1 HELPING THE PHYSICIAN COMPLY WITH THE CONTROLLED SUBSTANCES ACT OF 1970

Procedure Goal

To comply with the Controlled Substances Act of 1970

Scoring System

To score each step, use the following scoring system:
1 = poor, 2 = fair, 3 = good, 4 = excellent

A minimum score of at least a 3 must be achieved on **each** step to achieve successful completion of the technique. Detailed instructions on the scoring system are found on page 179.

Materials

DEA Form 224, DEA Form 222, DEA Form 41, pen

Procedure

Procedure Steps Total Possible Points - 28 Time Limit: 10 minutes	Practice #1	Practice #2	Practice #3	Final
1. Use DEA Form 224 to register the physician with the Drug Enforcement Administration, found on page 507 of this workbook. Be sure to register each office location at which the physician administers or dispenses drugs covered under Schedules II through V. Renew all registrations every 3 years using DEA Form 224a. Form 224 can be printed from the U.S. Department of Justice website. Renewal applications (Form 224a) can be completed through registration at this site.				
2. Order Schedule II drugs using DEA Form 222, found on page 509 of this workbook, as instructed by the physician. (Stocks of these drugs should be kept to a minimum.)*				
3. Include the physician's DEA registration number on every prescription for a drug in Schedules II through V.*				
4. Complete an inventory of all drugs in Schedules II through V every 2 years (as permitted in your state; this task may be reserved to other health-care professionals).				
5. Store all drugs in Schedules II through V in a secure, locked safe or cabinet (as permitted in your state).*				
6. Keep accurate dispensing and inventory records for at least 2 years.				
7. Dispose of expired or unused drugs according to the DEA regulations. Always complete DEA Form 41 when disposing of controlled drugs.				
Total Number of Points Achieved/Final Score				
Initials of Observer:				

(continued)

Comments and Signatures

Reviewer's comments and signatures:

1. _____

2. _____

3. _____

Instructor's comments:

_____

CAAHEP Competency Achieved

IX. C. (13) Discuss all levels of governmental legislation and regulation as they apply to medical assisting practice, including FDA and DEA regulations

ABHES Competency Achieved

6 (e) Comply with federal, state, and local health laws and regulations

PROCEDURE 19-2 RENEWING THE PHYSICIAN'S DEA REGISTRATION

Procedure Goal

To accurately complete DEA Form 224a to renew the physician's DEA registration on time

Scoring System

To score each step, use the following scoring system:
1 = poor, 2 = fair, 3 = good, 4 = excellent

A minimum score of at least a 3 must be achieved on **each** step to achieve successful completion of the technique. Detailed instructions on the scoring system are found on page 179.

Materials

Calendar, tickler file (optional), pen, DEA Form 224a on page 511 of this workbook, or Internet connection for electronic renewal

Procedure

Procedure Steps Total Possible Points - 24 Time Limit: 10 minutes	Practice #1	Practice #2	Practice #3	Final
1. Calculate a period of 3 years from the date of the original registration or the most recent renewal. Note that date as the expiration date of the physician's DEA registration.				
2. Subtract 45 days from the expiration date and mark this date on the calendar or create a reminder in your electronic calendar program. You also might put a reminder to submit renewal forms in the physician's tickler file for that date.*				
3. If you receive registration renewal paperwork (DEA Form 224a) from the DEA well before the submission date, put it in a safe place until you can complete it and have the physician sign it.				
4. Before the expiration deadline, complete DEA Form 224a as instructed on the form and have the physician sign it. Prepare or request a check for the fee.				
5. Submit the original and one copy of the completed form with the appropriate fee to the DEA so that it will arrive before the deadline. Keep one copy for the office records.				
6. Applicants are encouraged to use the online forms system for electronic renewal. Search the Internet for DEA Form 224A. Note: The DEA form website is for renewals only and Internet renewals should not be done if you have already sent a paper renewal. Update and complete the areas of the form including Personal Information, Activity, State License(s), Background Information, Payment, and Confirmation. You will be able to print copies of the form once completed.*				
Total Number of Points Achieved/Final Score				
Initials of Observer:				

(continued)

Comments and Signatures

Reviewer's comments and signatures:

1. _____

2. _____

3. _____

Instructor's comments:

_____

CAAHEP Competency Achieved

IX. C. (13) Discuss all levels of governmental legislation and regulation as they apply to medical assisting practice, including FDA and DEA regulations

ABHES Competency Achieved

6 (e) Comply with federal, state, and local health laws and regulations

PROCEDURE 19-3 RENEWING A PRESCRIPTION BY TELEPHONE

Procedure Goal

To ensure a complete and accurate prescription is received by the patient

Scoring System

To score each step, use the following scoring system:
1 = poor, 2 = fair, 3 = good, 4 = excellent

A minimum score of at least a 3 must be achieved on **each** step to achieve successful completion of the technique. Detailed instructions on the scoring system are found on page 179.

Materials

Telephone, appropriate phone numbers, message pad or prescription refill request form, pen and patient chart with prescription order

Procedure

Procedure Steps Total Possible Points - 52 Time Limit: 10 minutes	Practice #1	Practice #2	Practice #3	Final
1. Take the message from the call or the message system. For the prescription to be complete, you must obtain the patient's name, date of birth, phone number, pharmacy name and/or phone number, medication, and dosage.				
2. Follow your facility policy regarding prescription renewals. Typically, the prescription is usually called into the pharmacy the day it is requested. An example policy may be posted at the facility and may state, "Nonemergency prescription refill requests must be made during regular business hours. Please allow 24 hours for processing."				
3. Communicate the policy to the patient. You should know the policy and the time when the refills will be reviewed. For example, you might state, "Dr. Alexander will review the prescription between patients and it will be telephoned within one hour to the pharmacy. I will call you back if there is a problem."*				
4. Obtain the patient's chart or reference the electronic chart to verify you have the correct patient and that the patient is currently taking the medication. Check the patient's list of medications, which are usually part of the chart.				
5. Give the prescription refill request and the chart to the physician or prescriber. Do not give a prescription refill request to the physician without the chart or chart access information. Wait for an authorization from the physician before you proceed.*				
6. Once the physician authorizes the prescription, prepare to call the pharmacy with the renewal information. You cannot call in Schedule II or III medications. However, renewals can be called in for Schedule IV and V medications. Be				

(continued)

Procedure Steps Total Possible Points - 52 Time Limit: 10 minutes	Practice #1	Practice #2	Practice #3	Final
certain to have the physician order, the patient's chart, and the refill request in front of you when you make the call. The request should include the name of the drug, the drug dosage, the frequency and mode of administration, the number of refills authorized, and the name and phone number of the pharmacy.				
7. Telephone the pharmacy. Identify yourself by name, the practice name, and the doctor's name.*				
8. State the purpose of the call. (Example: "I am calling to request a prescription refill for a patient.")				
9. Identify the patient. Include the patient's name, date of birth, address, and phone number.*				
10. Identify the drug (spelling the name when necessary), the dosage, the frequency and mode of administration, and any other special instructions or changes for administration (such as "take at bedtime").*				
11. State the number of refills authorized.				
12. If leaving a message on a pharmacy voicemail system set up for physicians, state your name, the name of the doctor you represent, and your phone number before you hang up.*				
13. Document the prescription renewal in the chart after the medication has been called into the pharmacy. Include the date, the time, the name of pharmacy, and the person taking your call. Also include the medication, dose, amount, directions, and number of refills. Sign your first initial, last name, and title.				
Total Number of Points Achieved/Final Score				
Initials of Observer:				

Comments and Signatures

Reviewer's comments and signatures:

1. _____

2. _____

3. _____

Instructor's comments:

_____

CAAHEP Competency Achieved

IV. P. (7) Demonstrate telephone techniques

ABHES Competency Achieved

8 (ee) Use proper telephone techniques

PROCEDURE 20-1 ADMINISTERING ORAL DRUGS

Procedure Goal

To safely administer an oral drug to a patient

Scoring System

To score each step, use the following scoring system:
1 = poor, 2 = fair, 3 = good, 4 = excellent

A minimum score of at least a 3 must be achieved on **each** step to achieve successful completion of the technique. Detailed instructions on the scoring system are found on page 179.

Materials

Drug order (in patient chart), container of oral drug, small paper cup (for tablets, capsules, or caplets) or plastic calibrated medicine cup (for liquids), glass of water or juice, straw (optional), package insert or drug information sheet

Procedure

Procedure Steps Total Possible Points - 52 Time Limit: 10 minutes	Practice #1	Practice #2	Practice #3	Final
1. Identify the patient and wash your hands.				
2. Select the ordered drug (tablet, capsule, or liquid).				
3. Check the rights, comparing information against the drug order.*				
4. If you are unfamiliar with the drug, check the *PDR* or other drug reference, read the package insert, or speak with the physician. Determine whether the drug may be taken with or followed by water or juice.				
5. Ask the patient about any drug or food allergies. If the patient is not allergic to the ordered drug or other ingredients used to prepare it, proceed.*				
6. Perform any calculations needed to provide the prescribed dose. If you are unsure of your calculations, check them with a coworker or the physician.				
If You Are Giving Tablets or Capsules				
7. Open the container and tap the correct number into the cap. Do not touch the inside of the cap because it is sterile. If you pour out too many tablets or capsules and you have not touched them, tap the excess back into the container.				
8. Tap the tablets or capsules from the cap into the paper cup.				
9. Recap the container immediately.*				
10. Give the patient the cup along with a glass of water or juice. If the patient finds it easier to drink with a straw, unwrap the straw and place it in the fluid. If patients have difficulty swallowing pills, have them drink some water or juice before putting the pills in the mouth.*				

(continued)

Procedure Steps Total Possible Points - 52 Time Limit: 10 minutes	Practice #1	Practice #2	Practice #3	Final
If You Are Giving a Liquid Drug				
11. If the liquid is a suspension, shake it well.				
12. Locate the mark on the medicine cup for the prescribed dose. Keeping your thumbnail on the mark, hold the cup at eye level and pour the correct amount of the drug. Keep the label side of the bottle on top as you pour, or put your palm over it.*				
13. After pouring the drug, place the cup on a flat surface and check the drug level again. At eye level the base of the meniscus (the crescent-shaped form at the top of the liquid) should align with the mark that indicates the prescribed dose. If you poured out too much, discard it.*				
14. Give the medicine cup to the patient with instructions to drink the liquid. If appropriate, offer a glass of water or juice to wash down the drug.				
After You Have Given an Oral Drug				
15. Wash your hands.				
16. Give the patient an information sheet about the drug. Discuss the information with the patient and answer any questions she may have. If the patient has questions you cannot answer, refer her to the physician.				
17. Document the drug administration with the date, time, drug name, dosage, expiration date, lot number, manufacturer, route, site, significant patient reactions, and any patient education in the patient's chart.				
Total Number of Points Achieved/Final Score				
Initials of Observer:				

Comments and Signatures

Reviewer's comments and signatures:

1. _____

2. _____

3. _____

Instructor's comments:

_____

CAAHEP Competencies Achieved

I. P. (8) Administer oral medications

II. P. (1) Prepare proper dosages of medication for administration

II. A. (1) Verify ordered doses/dosages prior to administration

ABHES Competency Achieved

9 (j) Prepare and administer oral and parenteral medications as directed by physicians

Name_____ Date_____

Evaluated by_____ Score_____

PROCEDURE 20-2 ADMINISTERING BUCCAL OR SUBLINGUAL DRUGS

Procedure Goal

To safely administer a buccal or sublingual drug to a patient

Scoring System

To score each step, use the following scoring system:
1 = poor, 2 = fair, 3 = good, 4 = excellent

A minimum score of at least a 3 must be achieved on **each** step to achieve successful completion of the technique. Detailed instructions on the scoring system are found on page 179.

Materials

Drug order (in patient chart), container of buccal or sublingual drug, small paper cup, package insert or drug information sheet

Procedure

Procedure Steps Total Possible Points - 56 Time Limit: 10 minutes	Practice #1	Practice #2	Practice #3	Final
1. Identify the patient and wash your hands.				
2. Select the ordered drug.				
3. Check the rights, comparing information against the drug order.*				
4. If you are unfamiliar with the drug, check the *PDR* or other drug reference, read the package insert, or speak with the physician.				
5. Ask the patient about any drug or food allergies. If the patient is not allergic to the ordered drug or other ingredients used to prepare it, proceed.*				
6. Perform any calculations needed to provide the prescribed dose. If you are unsure of your calculations, check them with a coworker or the physician.				
7. Open the container and tap the correct number into the cap. Do not touch the inside of the cap because it is sterile. If you pour out too many tablets or capsules and you have not touched them, tap the excess back into the container.				
8. Tap the tablets or capsules from the cap into the paper cup.				
9. Recap the container immediately.*				
If You Are Giving Buccal Medication 10. Provide patient instruction, including • Tell the patient not to chew or swallow the tablet. • Place the medication between the cheek and gum until it dissolves.* • Instruct the patient not to eat, drink, or smoke until the tablet is completely dissolved.*				

(continued)

Procedure Steps Total Possible Points - 56 Time Limit: 10 minutes	Practice #1	Practice #2	Practice #3	Final
If You Are Giving a Sublingual Drug				
10. Provide patient instruction, including • Tell the patient not to chew or swallow the tablet. • Place the medication under the tongue until it dissolves.* • Instruct the patient not to eat, drink, or smoke until the tablet is completely dissolved.*				
After You Have Given a Buccal or Sublingual Medication				
11. Remain with patients until their tablet dissolves to monitor for possible adverse reaction and to ensure that patients have allowed the tablet to dissolve in the mouth instead of chewing or swallowing it.				
12. Wash your hands.				
13. Give the patient an information sheet about the drug. Discuss the information with the patient and answer any questions she may have. If the patient has questions you cannot answer, refer her to the physician.				
14. Document the drug administration with the date, time, drug name, dosage, expiration date, lot number, manufacturer, route, site, significant patient reactions, and any patient education in the patient's chart.				
Total Number of Points Achieved/Final Score				
Initials of Observer:				

Comments and Signatures

Reviewer's comments and signatures:

1. _____

2. _____

3. _____

Instructor's comments:

_____

CAAHEP Competencies Achieved

I. P. (7) Select proper sites for administering parenteral medication

I. P. (9) Administer parenteral (excluding IV) medications

II. P. (1) Prepare proper dosages of medication for administration

II. A. (1) Verify ordered doses/dosages prior to administration

ABHES Competency Achieved

9 (j) Prepare and administer oral and parenteral medications as directed by physicians

PROCEDURE 20-3 DRAWING A DRUG FROM AN AMPULE

Procedure Goal

To safely open an ampule and draw a drug, using sterile technique

Scoring System

To score each step, use the following scoring system:
1 = poor, 2 = fair, 3 = good, 4 = excellent

A minimum score of at least a 3 must be achieved on **each** step to achieve successful completion of the technique. Detailed instructions on the scoring system are found on page 179.

Materials

Ampule of drug, alcohol swab, 2-by-2-inch gauze square, small file (provided by the drug manufacturer), sterile filtered needle, sterile needle, and a syringe of the appropriate size

Procedure

Procedure Steps Total Possible Points - 28 Time Limit: 10 minutes	Practice #1	Practice #2	Practice #3	Final
1. Wash your hands and put on exam gloves.				
2. Gently tap the top of the ampule with your forefinger to settle the liquid to the bottom of the ampule.				
3. Wipe the ampule's neck with an alcohol swab.				
4. Wrap the 2-by-2-inch gauze square around the ampule's neck. Then snap the neck away from you. If it does not snap easily, score the neck with the small file and snap it again.				
5. Insert the filtered needle into the ampule without touching the side of the ampule.*				
6. Pull back on the plunger to aspirate (remove by vacuum or suction) the liquid completely into the syringe.				
7. Replace with the regular needle and push the plunger on the syringe until the medication just reaches the tip of the needle. The drug is now ready for injection.				
Total Number of Points Achieved/Final Score				
Initials of Observer:				

Comments and Signatures

Reviewer's comments and signatures:

1. _____

2. _____

3. _____

Instructor's comments:

_____

(continued)

CAAHEP Competencies Achieved

II. P. (1) Prepare proper dosages of medication for administration

II. A. (1) Verify ordered doses/dosages prior to administration

ABHES Competency Achieved

9 (j) Prepare and administer oral and parenteral medications as directed by physicians

PROCEDURE 20-4 RECONSTITUTING AND DRAWING A DRUG FOR INJECTION

Procedure Goal

To reconstitute and draw a drug for injection, using sterile technique

Scoring System

To score each step, use the following scoring system:
1 = poor, 2 = fair, 3 = good, 4 = excellent

A minimum score of at least a 3 must be achieved on **each** step to achieve successful completion of the technique. Detailed instructions on the scoring system are found on page 179.

Materials

Vial of drug, vial of diluent, alcohol swabs, two disposable sterile needle and syringe sets of appropriate size, sharps container

Procedure

Procedure Steps Total Possible Points - 40 Time Limit: 15 minutes	Practice #1	Practice #2	Practice #3	Final
1. Wash your hands and put on exam gloves.				
2. Place the drug vial and diluent vial on the countertop. Wipe the rubber diaphragm of each with an alcohol swab.				
3. Remove the cap from the needle and the guard from the syringe. Pull the plunger back to the mark that equals the amount of diluent needed to reconstitute the drug ordered.*				
4. Puncture the diaphragm of the vial of diluent with the needle and inject the air into the diluent.*				
5. Invert the vial and aspirate the diluent.				
6. Remove the needle from the diluent vial, inject the diluent into the drug vial, and withdraw the needle. Properly dispose of this needle and syringe.				
7. Roll the vial between your hands to mix the drug and diluent thoroughly. Do not shake the vial unless so directed on the drug label. When completely mixed, the solution in the vial should have no flakes. The solution will be clear or cloudy when completely mixed (depending on the drug).				
8. Remove the cap and guard from the second needle and syringe.				
9. Pull back the plunger to the mark that reflects the amount of drug ordered. Inject the air into the drug vial.				
10. Invert the vial and aspirate the proper amount of the drug into the syringe. The drug is now ready for injection.				
Total Number of Points Achieved/Final Score				
Initials of Observer:				

(continued)

Comments and Signatures

Reviewer's comments and signatures:

1. _____

2. _____

3. _____

Instructor's comments:

_____

CAAHEP Competencies Achieved

II. P. (1) Prepare proper dosages of medication for administration

II. A. (1) Verify ordered doses/dosages prior to administration

ABHES Competency Achieved

9 (j) Prepare and administer oral and parenteral medications as directed by physicians

Procedure 20-5 Giving an Intradermal Injection

Procedure Goal

To administer an intradermal injection safely and effectively, using sterile technique

Scoring System

To score each step, use the following scoring system:
1 = poor, 2 = fair, 3 = good, 4 = excellent

A minimum score of at least a 3 must be achieved on **each** step to achieve successful completion of the technique. Detailed instructions on the scoring system are found on page 179.

Materials

Drug order (in patient's chart), alcohol swab, disposable needle and syringe of the appropriate size filled with the ordered dose of drug, sharps container

Procedure

Procedure Steps Total Possible Points - 48 Time Limit: 15 minutes	Practice #1	Practice #2	Practice #3	Final
1. Identify the patient. Wash your hands and put on exam gloves.				
2. Check the rights, comparing information against the drug order.*				
3. Identify the injection site on the patient's forearm. To do so, rest the patient's arm on a table with the palm up. Measure two to three finger-widths below the antecubital space and a hand-width above the wrist. The space between is available for the injection.				
4. Prepare the skin with the alcohol swab, moving in a circle from the center out.				
5. Let the skin dry before giving the injection.*				
6. Hold the patient's forearm and stretch the skin taut with one hand.				
7. With the other hand, place the needle—bevel up—almost flat against the patient's skin. Press the needle against the skin and insert it.				
8. Inject the drug slowly and gently. You should see the needle through the skin and feel resistance. As the drug enters the upper layer of skin, a wheal (raised area of the skin) will form.				
9. After the full dose of the drug has been injected, withdraw the needle. Properly dispose of used materials and the needle and syringe immediately.				
10. Remove the gloves and wash your hands.				
11. Stay with the patient to monitor for unexpected reactions.				
12. Document the injection with the date, time, drug name, dosage, expiration date, lot number, manufacturer, route, site, significant patient reactions, and any patient education in the patient's chart.				

(continued)

Procedure Steps Total Possible Points - 48 Time Limit: 15 minutes	Practice #1	Practice #2	Practice #3	Final
Total Number of Points Achieved/Final Score				
Initials of Observer:				

Comments and Signatures

Reviewer's comments and signatures:

1. _____

2. _____

3. _____

Instructor's comments:

_____

CAAHEP Competencies Achieved

I. P. (7) Select proper sites for administering parenteral medication

I. P. (9) Administer parenteral (excluding IV) medications

II. P. (1) Prepare proper dosages of medication for administration

II. A. (1) Verify ordered doses/dosages prior to administration

ABHES Competency Achieved

9 (j) Prepare and administer oral and parenteral medications as directed by physicians

PROCEDURE 20-6 GIVING A SUBCUTANEOUS (SUB-Q) INJECTION

Procedure Goal

To administer a subcutaneous injection safely and effectively, using sterile technique

Scoring System

To score each step, use the following scoring system:
1 = poor, 2 = fair, 3 = good, 4 = excellent

A minimum score of at least a 3 must be achieved on **each** step to achieve successful completion of the technique. Detailed instructions on the scoring system are found on page 179.

Materials

Drug order (in patient's chart), alcohol swabs, sterile 2 × 2 gauze or cotton ball, container of the ordered drug, disposable needle and syringe of the appropriate size, sharps container

Procedure

Procedure Steps Total Possible Points - 56 Time Limit: 15 minutes	Practice #1	Practice #2	Practice #3	Final
1. Identify the patient. Wash your hands and put on exam gloves.				
2. Check the rights, comparing information against the drug order.*				
3. Prepare the drug and draw it up to the mark on the syringe that matches the ordered dose.				
4. Choose a site and clean it with an alcohol swab, moving in a circle from the center out. Let the area dry.				
5. Pinch the skin firmly to lift the subcutaneous tissue.				
6. Position the needle—bevel up—at a 45-degree angle to the skin.*				
7. Insert the needle in one quick motion. Then release the skin and inject the drug slowly. With some medications you will check the placement of the needle by pulling back on the plunger before injecting. If blood is seen in the hub, you should withdraw the needle and start with a fresh needle and syringe. If no blood is seen, inject the medication slowly.				
8. After the full dose of the drug has been injected, place a 2 × 2 gauze or cotton ball over the site and withdraw the needle at the same angle you inserted it.				
9. Apply pressure at the puncture site with the gauze or cotton ball.				
10. Massage the site gently to help distribute the drug, if indicated. Do not massage insulin, heparin, or other anticoagulant medications.*				
11. Properly dispose of the used materials and the needle and syringe.				
12. Remove the gloves and wash your hands.				

(continued)

Procedure Steps Total Possible Points - 56 Time Limit: 15 minutes	Practice #1	Practice #2	Practice #3	Final
13. Stay with the patient to monitor for unexpected reactions.				
14. Document the injection with the date, time, drug name, dosage, expiration date, lot number, manufacturer, route, site, significant patient reactions, and any patient education in the patient's chart.				
Total Number of Points Achieved/Final Score				
Initials of Observer:				

Comments and Signatures

Reviewer's comments and signatures:

1. _____

2. _____

3. _____

Instructor's comments:

_____

CAAHEP Competencies Achieved

I. P. (7) Select proper sites for administering parenteral medication

I. P. (9) Administer parenteral (excluding IV) medications

II. P. (1) Prepare proper dosages of medication for administration

II. A. (1) Verify ordered doses/dosages prior to administration

ABHES Competency Achieved

9 (j) Prepare and administer oral and parenteral medications as directed by physicians

PROCEDURE 20-7 GIVING AN INTRAMUSCULAR INJECTION

Procedure Goal

To administer an intramuscular injection safely and effectively, using sterile technique

Scoring System

To score each step, use the following scoring system:
1 = poor, 2 = fair, 3 = good, 4 = excellent

A minimum score of at least a 3 must be achieved on **each** step to achieve successful completion of the technique. Detailed instructions on the scoring system are found on page 179.

Materials

Drug order (in patient's chart), alcohol swabs, sterile 2 × 2 gauze or cotton ball, container of the ordered drug, disposable needle and syringe of the appropriate size, sharps container

Procedure

Procedure Steps Total Possible Points - 56 Time Limit: 15 minutes	Practice #1	Practice #2	Practice #3	Final
1. Identify the patient. Wash your hands and put on exam gloves.				
2. Check the rights, comparing information against the drug order.*				
3. Prepare the drug and draw it up to the mark on the syringe that matches the ordered dose.				
4. Choose a site and gently tap it. Tapping stimulates the nerve endings and reduces pain caused by the needle insertion.				
5. Clean the site with an alcohol swab, moving in a circle from the center out. Let the site dry.				
6. Stretch the skin taut over the injection site.				
7. Hold the needle and syringe at a 90-degree angle to the skin. Then insert the needle with a quick, dart-like thrust.*				
8. Release the skin and aspirate by pulling back slightly on the plunger to check the needle placement. If pulling back on the plunger produces blood, placement is incorrect and you must begin again with a fresh needle and syringe. If pulling back on the plunger produces no blood, placement is correct. Inject the drug slowly.*				
9. After the full dose of the drug has been injected, place a 2 × 2 gauze or cotton ball over the site. Then quickly remove the needle at a 90-degree angle.				
10. Use the 2 × 2 gauze or cotton ball to apply pressure to the site and massage it, if indicated.				
11. Properly dispose of used materials and the needle and syringe.				
12. Remove the gloves and wash your hands.				
13. Stay with the patient to monitor for unexpected reactions.				

(continued)

Procedure Steps Total Possible Points - 56 Time Limit: 15 minutes	Practice #1	Practice #2	Practice #3	Final
14. Document the injection with the date, time, drug name, dosage, expiration date, lot number, manufacturer, route, site, significant patient reactions, and any patient education in the patient's chart.				
Total Number of Points Achieved/Final Score				
Initials of Observer:				

Comments and Signatures

Reviewer's comments and signatures:

1. _____

2. _____

3. _____

Instructor's comments:

_____

CAAHEP Competencies Achieved

I. P. (7) Select proper sites for administering parenteral medication

I. P. (9) Administer parenteral (excluding IV) medications

II. P. (1) Prepare proper dosages of medication for administration

II. A. (1) Verify ordered doses/dosages prior to administration

ABHES Competency Achieved

9 (j) Prepare and administer oral and parenteral medications as directed by physicians

PROCEDURE 20-8 ADMINISTERING INHALATION THERAPY

Procedure Goal

To administer inhalation therapy safely and effectively

Scoring System

To score each step, use the following scoring system:
1 = poor, 2 = fair, 3 = good, 4 = excellent

A minimum score of at least a 3 must be achieved on **each** step to achieve successful completion of the technique. Detailed instructions on the scoring system are found on page 179.

Materials

Drug order (in patient's chart), container of the ordered drug, tissues, package insert or patient education sheet about medication

Procedure

Procedure Steps Total Possible Points - 40 Time Limit: 20 minutes	Practice #1	Practice #2	Practice #3	Final
1. Identify the patient. Wash your hands.				
2. Check the rights, comparing information against the drug order. Make sure you have the correct type of inhaler based upon the order (oral or nasal).*				
3. Prepare the container of medication as directed. Use the package insert and show the directions to the patient.				
4. Shake the container as directed and stress this step to the patient.*				
For a Nasal Inhaler 5. Instruct the patient to complete the following steps: • Have the patient blow the nose to clear the nostrils. • Tilt the head back, and with one hand, place the inhaler tip about ½ inch into the nostril. • Point the tip straight up toward the inner corner of the eye.* • Use the opposite hand to block the other nostril. • Inhale gently while quickly and firmly squeezing the inhaler. • Remove the inhaler tip and exhale through the mouth. • Shake the inhaler and repeat the process in the other nostril. • If indicated in the package insert, instruct patients to keep the head tilted back and not to blow their nose for several minutes.				
For an Oral Inhaler 5. Instruct the patient to complete the following steps: • Warm the canister by rolling it between the palms of your hands. • Uncap the mouthpiece and assemble the inhaler as directed on the package insert. • Hold the mouth open and place the canister in the mouth or about 1 inch from the mouth.				

(continued)

Procedure Steps Total Possible Points - 40 Time Limit: 20 minutes	Practice #1	Practice #2	Practice #3	Final
• Check the package insert for the proper placement. • Exhale normally and inhale through the canister as he or she depresses it. The medication must be inhaled. • Breathe in until the lungs are full and hold the breath for 10 seconds. • Breathe out normally.				
After You Have Given an Inhalation Medication				
6. Remain with the patient to monitor for changes and possible adverse reaction.				
7. Recap and secure the medication container. Instruct the patient in this procedure.				
8. Wash your hands.				
9. Give the patient an information sheet about the drug. Discuss the information with the patient and answer any questions she may have. If the patient has questions you cannot answer, refer her to the physician.				
10. Document the drug administration with the date, time, drug name, dosage, expiration date, lot number, manufacturer, route, site, significant patient reactions, and any patient education in the patient's chart.				
Total Number of Points Achieved/Final Score				
Initials of Observer:				

Comments and Signatures

Reviewer's comments and signatures:

1. _____

2. _____

3. _____

Instructor's comments:

_____

CAAHEP Competencies Achieved

I. P. (7) Select proper sites for administering parenteral medication

I. P. (9) Administer parenteral (excluding IV) medications

II. P. (1) Prepare proper dosages of medication for administration

II. A. (1) Verify ordered doses/dosages prior to administration

ABHES Competency Achieved

9 (j) Prepare and administer oral and parenteral medications as directed by physicians

PROCEDURE 20-9 ADMINISTERING AND REMOVING A TRANSDERMAL PATCH AND PROVIDING PATIENT INSTRUCTION

Procedure Goal

To safely administer and remove a transdermal patch drug to a patient

Scoring System

To score each step, use the following scoring system:

1 = poor, 2 = fair, 3 = good, 4 = excellent

A minimum score of at least a 3 must be achieved on **each** step to achieve successful completion of the technique. Detailed instructions on the scoring system are found on page 179.

Materials

Drug order (in patient chart), transdermal patch medication, gloves, package insert or drug information sheet, patient chart

Procedure

Procedure Steps Total Possible Points - 76 Time Limit: 10 minutes	Practice #1	Practice #2	Practice #3	Final
1. Identify the patient, wash your hands, and put on gloves.*				
2. Select the ordered transdermal patch and check the rights, comparing information against the drug order.*				
3. Ask the patient about any drug or food allergies. If the patient is not allergic to the ordered drug or other ingredients used to prepare it, proceed.*				
4. If you are unfamiliar with the drug, check the *PDR* or other drug reference, read the package insert, or speak with the physician. The package insert is extremely detailed for transdermal medications and should be used when applying the medication and/or doing patient teaching.				
5. Perform any calculations needed to provide the prescribed dose. If you are unsure of your calculations, check them with a coworker or the physician.				
Applying the Transdermal Medication				
6. Remove the patch from its pouch. The plastic backing is easily peeled off once the patch is removed from the pouch. For patches without a protective pouch, bend the sides of the transdermal unit back and forth until the clear plastic backing snaps down the middle.				
7. For either type of patch, demonstrate how to peel off the clear plastic backing to expose the sticky side of the patch.				
8. Apply the patch to a reasonably hair-free site, such as the abdomen. Note that estrogen patches are usually placed on the hip.				

(continued)

Procedure Steps Total Possible Points - 76 Time Limit: 10 minutes	Practice #1	Practice #2	Practice #3	Final
9. Instruct the patient how to apply the patch. Advise the patient to avoid using the extremities below the knee or elbow, skin folds, scar tissue, or burned or irritated areas.*				
Removing the Transdermal Patch				
6. Gently lift and slowly peel the patch back from the skin. Wash the area with soap and dry it with a towel. Instruct the patient on this technique.				
7. Explain to the patient that the skin may appear red and warm, which is normal. Reassure the patient that the redness will disappear. In some cases, lotion may be applied to the skin if it feels dry.				
8. Instruct the patient to notify the doctor if the redness does not disappear in several days or if a rash develops.				
9. *Never* apply a new patch to the site just used. It is best to allow each site to rest between applications. Some transdermal systems call for waiting 7 days before using a site again. Be sure to check the package directions regarding site rotation.				
After You Have Applied and/or Removed the Transdermal Patch				
10. Wash your hands and instruct the patient they should do the same after applying or removing a transdermal system at home.				
11. Give the patient an information sheet about the drug. Discuss the information with the patient and answer any questions she may have. If the patient has questions you cannot answer, refer her to the physician.				
12. Document the drug administration with the date, time, drug name, dosage, expiration date, lot number, manufacturer, route, site, significant patient reactions, and any patient education in the patient's chart.				
Total Number of Points Achieved/Final Score				
Initials of Observer:				

Comments and Signatures

Reviewer's comments and signatures:

1. _____

2. _____

3. _____

Instructor's comments:

_____

CAAHEP Competencies Achieved

I. P. (7) Select proper sites for administering parenteral medication

I. P. (9) Administer parenteral (excluding IV) medications

II. P. (1) Prepare proper dosages of medication for administration

II. A. (1) Verify ordered doses/dosages prior to administration

ABHES Competency Achieved

9 (j) Prepare and administer oral and parenteral medications as directed by physicians

PROCEDURE 20-10 ASSISTING WITH ADMINISTRATION OF A URETHRAL DRUG

Procedure Goal

To assist with a urethral administration

Scoring System

To score each step, use the following scoring system:
1 = poor, 2 = fair, 3 = good, 4 = excellent

A minimum score of at least a 3 must be achieved on **each** step to achieve successful completion of the technique. Detailed instructions on the scoring system are found on page 179.

Materials

Urinary catheter kit, either a syringe without a needle or tubing and a bag (depending on the amount of drug to be administered), sterile gloves, the prescribed drug, a drape, and a bedsaver pad

Procedure

Procedure Steps Total Possible Points - 48 Time Limit: 10 minutes	Practice #1	Practice #2	Practice #3	Final
1. Wash your hands and use sterile technique to assemble the equipment.				
2. Check the rights, comparing information against the drug order, and explain the procedure and the drug order to the patient.*				
3. Assist the patient into the lithotomy position and drape her to preserve her modesty while exposing the vulva.				
4. Place a bedsaver pad under the buttocks.				
5. Open the catheter kit.				
6. Put on sterile gloves.				
7. Cleanse the vulva as you would to perform catheterization, using the materials in the kit. As you sweep down with the antiseptic swab, watch for the urethral opening to "wink."*				
8. The physician or nurse will insert the lubricated catheter. Tell the patient that she should feel pressure, not pain, and that the physician or nurse is going to attach the syringe to the catheter and insert the drug (or attach the tubing and bag to the catheter and let the drug run in by gravity).				
9. After instilling the drug, the physician or nurse will clamp the catheter and leave the drug in place for the ordered amount of time.				
10. Stay with the patient not only to ensure that she remains still but also to reassure her that the full feeling in the bladder is normal. She also may say she feels the need to urinate. Advise her that this feeling, too, is normal and is caused by the catheter.				

(continued)

Procedure Steps Total Possible Points - 48 Time Limit: 10 minutes	Practice #1	Practice #2	Practice #3	Final
11. When the time is up, unclamp the catheter, gently remove it, and allow the patient to urinate. Assist the patient as needed.				
12. While the patient is dressing, immediately document the drug instillation with date, time, drug, dose, route, and any significant patient reactions.				
Total Number of Points Achieved/Final Score				
Initials of Observer:				

Comments and Signatures

Reviewer's comments and signatures:

1. _____

2. _____

3. _____

Instructor's comments:

_____

CAAHEP Competencies Achieved

I. P. (7) Select proper sites for administering parenteral medication

I. P. (9) Administer parenteral (excluding IV) medications

II. P. (1) Prepare proper dosages of medication for administration

II. A. (1) Verify ordered doses/dosages prior to administration

ABHES Competency Achieved

9 (j) Prepare and administer oral and parenteral medications as directed by physicians

PROCEDURE 20-11 ADMINISTERING A VAGINAL MEDICATION

Procedure Goal

To safely administer a vaginal medication with patient instruction

Scoring System

To score each step, use the following scoring system:
1 = poor, 2 = fair, 3 = good, 4 = excellent

A minimum score of at least a 3 must be achieved on **each** step to achieve successful completion of the technique. Detailed instructions on the scoring system are found on page 179.

Materials

Prescription or drug order in the patient's chart, a cloth or paper drape, a bedsaver pad, gloves, cotton balls, water-soluble lubricant, and the prescribed drug

Procedure

Procedure Steps Total Possible Points - 52 Time Limit: 15 minutes	Practice #1	Practice #2	Practice #3	Final
1. Wash your hands.				
2. Check the rights, comparing information against the drug order, and explain the procedure and the drug order to the patient.*				
3. Give the patient the opportunity to empty her bladder before beginning.				
4. Assist the patient into the lithotomy position and drape her.*				
5. Place a bedsaver pad under the buttocks.				
6. Put on gloves.				
7. Cleanse the perineum with soap and water, using one cotton ball per stroke, and cleanse the center last, while spreading the labia.*				
8. Lubricate the vaginal suppository applicator in lubricant spread on a paper towel. For vaginal drugs in the forms of creams, ointments, gels, and tablets, use the appropriate applicator, preparing it according to the package insert.				
9. While spreading the labia with one hand, insert the applicator with the other (the applicator should be about 2 inches into the vagina and angled toward the sacrum).				
10. Release the labia and push the applicator's plunger to release the suppository into the vagina.				
11. Remove the applicator and wipe any excess lubricant off the patient.				
12. Help her to a sitting position and assist with dressing if needed.				

(continued)

Procedure Steps Total Possible Points - 52 Time Limit: 15 minutes	Practice #1	Practice #2	Practice #3	Final
13. Document the administration with date, time, drug, dose, route, and any significant patient reactions.				
Total Number of Points Achieved/Final Score				
Initials of Observer:				

Comments and Signatures

Reviewer's comments and signatures:

1. _____

2. _____

3. _____

Instructor's comments:

_____

CAAHEP Competencies Achieved

I. P. (7) Select proper sites for administering parenteral medication

I. P. (9) Administer parenteral (excluding IV) medications

II. P. (1) Prepare proper dosages of medication for administration

II. A. (1) Verify ordered doses/dosages prior to administration

ABHES Competency Achieved

9 (j) Prepare and administer oral and parenteral medications as directed by physicians

Procedure 20-12 Administering a Rectal Medication

Procedure Goal

To safely administer a rectal medication

Scoring System

To score each step, use the following scoring system:
1 = poor, 2 = fair, 3 = good, 4 = excellent

A minimum score of at least a 3 must be achieved on **each** step to achieve successful completion of the technique. Detailed instructions on the scoring system are found on page 179.

Materials

Prescription or drug order in the patient's chart, a cloth or paper drape, a bedsaver pad, gloves, water-soluble lubricant, and the prescribed drug

Procedure

Procedure Steps Total Possible Points - 52 Time Limit: 15 minutes	Practice #1	Practice #2	Practice #3	Final
1. Check the rights, comparing information against the drug order.*				
2. Explain the procedure and the drug order to the patient.				
3. Give the patient the opportunity to empty the bladder before beginning.				
4. Help the patient into Sims' position. Place a bedsaver pad under the patient.				
5. Lift the patient's gown to expose the anus.				
6. Put on gloves and prepare the medication.				
When Administering a Suppository				
7. Lubricate the tapered end of the suppository with about 1 tsp of lubricant.				
8. While spreading the patient's buttocks with one hand, insert the suppository—tapered end first—into the anus with the other hand.				
9. Gently advance the suppository past the sphincter with your index finger. Before it passes the sphincter, the suppository may feel as if it is being pushed back out the anus. When it passes the sphincter, it seems to disappear.				
10. Use tissues to remove excess lubricant from the area.				
11. Remove your gloves and ask the patient to lie quietly and retain the suppository for at least 20 minutes. When the treatment is completed, help the patient to a sitting, then standing, position.*				
When Administering a Retention Enema 7. Place the tip of a syringe into a rectal tube. Let a little rectal solution flow through the syringe and tube. While holding the tip up, clamp the tubing.				

(continued)

Procedure Steps Total Possible Points - 52 Time Limit: 15 minutes	Practice #1	Practice #2	Practice #3	Final
8. Lubricate the end of the tube, spread the patient's buttocks, and slide the tube into the rectum about 4 inches.				
9. Slowly pour the rectal solution into the syringe, release the clamp, and let gravity move the solution into the patient. When you have administered the ordered amount of solution, clamp the tube and then remove it.				
10. Using tissues, apply pressure over the anus for 20 seconds to stifle the patient's urge to defecate and then wipe any excess lubricant or solution from the area. Encourage the patient to retain the enema for the time ordered.*				
11. When the time has passed, help the patient use a bedpan or direct the patient to a toilet to expel the solution.				
After the Administration Is Complete				
12. Remove your gloves and wash your hands.				
13. Immediately document the drug administration with date, time, drug, dose, route, and any significant patient reactions.				
Total Number of Points Achieved/Final Score				
Initials of Observer:				

Comments and Signatures

Reviewer's comments and signatures:

1. _____

2. _____

3. _____

Instructor's comments:

_____

CAAHEP Competencies Achieved

I. P. (7) Select proper sites for administering parenteral medication

I. P. (9) Administer parenteral (excluding IV) medications

II. P. (1) Prepare proper dosages of medication for administration

II. A. (1) Verify ordered doses/dosages prior to administration

ABHES Competency Achieved

9 (j) Prepare and administer oral and parenteral medications as directed by physicians

PROCEDURE 20-13 ADMINISTERING EYE MEDICATIONS

Procedure Goal

To instill medication into the eye for treatment of certain eye disorders

Scoring System

To score each step, use the following scoring system:
1 = poor, 2 = fair, 3 = good, 4 = excellent

A minimum score of at least a 3 must be achieved on **each** step to achieve successful completion of the technique. Detailed instructions on the scoring system are found on page 179.

Materials

Medication (drops, cream, or ointment), tissues, eye patch (if applicable)

Procedure

Procedure Steps Total Possible Points - 96 Time Limit: 15 minutes	Practice #1	Practice #2	Practice #3	Final
1. Identify the patient, introduce yourself, and explain the procedure.				
2. Review the doctor's medication order. This should include the patient's name, drug name, concentration, number of drops (if a liquid), into which eye(s) the medication is to be administered, and the frequency of administration.*				
3. Compare the drug with the medication order three times, checking the rights of medication administration.*				
4. Ask whether the patient has any known allergies to substances contained in the medication.				
5. Wash your hands and put on gloves.				
6. Assemble the supplies.				
7. Ask the patient to lie down or to sit back in a chair with the head tilted back.				
8. Give the patient a tissue to blot excess medication as needed.				
9. Remove an eye patch, if present.				
10. Ask the patient to look at the ceiling. Instruct the patient to keep both eyes open during the procedure.				
11. With a tissue, gently pull the lower eyelid down by pressing downward on the patient's cheekbone just below the eyelid with your nondominant hand. This pressure will open a pocket of space between the eyelid and the eye.				
Eyedrops 12. Resting your dominant hand on the patient's forehead, hold the filled eyedropper or bottle approximately ½ inch from the conjunctiva.*				

(continued)

Procedure Steps Total Possible Points - 96 Time Limit: 15 minutes	Practice #1	Practice #2	Practice #3	Final
13. Drop the prescribed number of drops into the pocket. If any drops land outside the eye, repeat instilling the drops that missed the eye.				
Creams or Ointments				
12. Rest your dominant hand on the patient's forehead and hold the tube or applicator above the conjunctiva.				
13. Without touching the eyelid or conjunctiva with the applicator, evenly apply a thin ribbon of cream or ointment along the inside edge of the lower eyelid on the conjunctiva, working from the medial (inner) to the lateral (outer) side.*				
All Medications				
14. Release the lower lid and instruct the patient to gently close the eyes.				
15. Repeat the procedure for the other eye as necessary.				
16. Remove any excess medication by wiping each eyelid gently with a fresh tissue from the medial to the lateral side.				
17. Apply a clean eye patch to cover the entire eye as necessary.				
18. Ask whether the patient felt any discomfort and observe for any adverse reactions. Notify the doctor as necessary.				
19. Instruct the patient on self-administration of medication and patch application as necessary.				
20. Ask the patient to repeat the instructions.				
21. Provide written instructions.				
22. Properly dispose of used disposable materials.				
23. Remove gloves and wash your hands.				
24. Document administration in the patient's chart. Include the drug, concentration, the number of drops, the time of administration, and the eye(s) that received the medication.				
Total Number of Points Achieved/Final Score				
Initials of Observer:				

Comments and Signatures

Reviewer's comments and signatures:

1. _____

2. _____

3. _____

Instructor's comments:

_____

CAAHEP Competencies Achieved

I. P. (7) Select proper sites for administering parenteral medication

I. P. (9) Administer parenteral (excluding IV) medications

II. P. (1) Prepare proper dosages of medication for administration

II. A. (1) Verify ordered doses/dosages prior to administration

ABHES Competency Achieved

9 (j) Prepare and administer oral and parenteral medications as directed by physicians

PROCEDURE 20-14 PERFORMING EYE IRRIGATION

Procedure Goal

To flush the eye to remove foreign particles or relieve eye irritation

Scoring System

To score each step, use the following scoring system:
1 = poor, 2 = fair, 3 = good, 4 = excellent

A minimum score of at least a 3 must be achieved on **each** step to achieve successful completion of the technique. Detailed instructions on the scoring system are found on page 179.

Materials

Sterile irrigating solution, sterile basin, sterile irrigating syringe and kidney-shaped basin, tissues

Procedure

Procedure Steps Total Possible Points - 68 Time Limit: 20 minutes	Practice #1	Practice #2	Practice #3	Final
1. Identify the patient, introduce yourself, and explain the procedure.				
2. Review the physician's order. This should include the patient's name, the irrigating solution, the volume of solution, and for which eye(s) the irrigation is to be performed.				
3. Compare the solution with the instructions three times, checking the rights of medication administration.*				
4. Wash your hands and put on gloves, a gown, and a face shield.*				
5. Assemble supplies.				
6. Ask the patient to lie down or to sit with the head tilted back and to the side that is being irrigated. The solution should not spill over into the other eye.*				
7. Place a towel over the patient's shoulder (or under the head and shoulder, if the patient is lying down). Have the patient hold the kidney-shaped basin at the side of the head next to the eye to be irrigated.				
8. Pour the solution into the sterile basin.				
9. Fill the irrigating syringe with solution (approximately 50 mL).				
10. Hold a tissue on the patient's cheekbone below the lower eyelid with your nondominant hand, and press downward to expose the eye socket.				
11. Holding the tip of the syringe ½ inch away from the eye, direct the solution onto the lower conjunctiva from the inner to the outer aspect of the eye. (Avoid directing the solution against the cornea because it is sensitive; do not use excessive force.)*				

(continued)

Procedure Steps Total Possible Points - 68 Time Limit: 20 minutes	Practice #1	Practice #2	Practice #3	Final
12. Refill the syringe and continue irrigation until the prescribed volume of solution is used or until the solution is used up.				
13. Dry the area around the eye with tissues.				
14. Properly dispose of used disposable materials.				
15. Remove your gloves, gown, and face shield and wash your hands.				
16. Record in the patient's chart the procedure, the amount of solution used, the time of administration, and the eye(s) irrigated.				
17. Put on gloves and clean the equipment and room according to OSHA guidelines.				
Total Number of Points Achieved/Final Score				
Initials of Observer:				

Comments and Signatures

Reviewer's comments and signatures:

1. _____

2. _____

3. _____

Instructor's comments:

_____

CAAHEP Competencies Achieved

I. P. (7) Select proper sites for administering parenteral medication

I. P. (9) Administer parenteral (excluding IV) medications

II. P. (1) Prepare proper dosages of medication for administration

II. A. (1) Verify ordered doses/dosages prior to administration

ABHES Competency Achieved

9 (j) Prepare and administer oral and parenteral medications as directed by physicians

PROCEDURE 20-15 ADMINISTERING EARDROPS

Procedure Goal

To instill medication into the ear to treat certain ear disorders

Scoring System

To score each step, use the following scoring system:
1 = poor, 2 = fair, 3 = good, 4 = excellent

A minimum score of at least a 3 must be achieved on **each** step to achieve successful completion of the technique. Detailed instructions on the scoring system are found on page 179.

Materials

Liquid medication, cotton balls

Procedure

Procedure Steps Total Possible Points - 88 Time Limit: 6 minutes	Practice #1	Practice #2	Practice #3	Final
1. Identify the patient, introduce yourself, and explain the procedure.				
2. Check the physician's medication order. It should include the patient's name, drug name, concentration, the number of drops, into which ear(s) the medication is to be administered, and the frequency of administration.				
3. Compare the drug with the instructions three times, checking the rights of medication administration.*				
4. Ask whether the patient has any allergies to ear medications.				
5. Wash your hands and put on gloves.				
6. Assemble supplies.				
7. If the medication is cold, warm it to room temperature with your hands or by placing the bottle in a pan of warm water.*				
8. Have the patient lie on the side with the ear to be treated facing up.				
9. Straighten the ear canal by pulling the auricle upward and outward for adults, down and back for infants and children.*				
10. Hold the dropper ½ inch above the ear canal.*				
11. Gently squeeze the bottle or dropper bulb to administer the correct number of drops.				
12. Have the patient remain in this position for 10 minutes.				
13. If ordered, loosely place a small wad of cotton in the outermost part of the ear canal.				
14. Note any adverse reaction, notifying the physician as necessary.				
15. Repeat the procedure for the other ear if ordered.				
16. Instruct the patient on how to administer the drops at home.				
17. Ask the patient to repeat the instructions.*				

(continued)

Procedure Steps Total Possible Points - 88 Time Limit: 6 minutes	Practice #1	Practice #2	Practice #3	Final
18. Provide written instructions.				
19. Remove the cotton after 15 minutes.				
20. Properly dispose of used disposable materials.				
21. Remove gloves and wash your hands.				
22. Record in the patient's chart the medication, concentration, the number of drops, the time of administration, and which ear(s) received the medication.				
Total Number of Points Achieved/Final Score				
Initials of Observer:				

Comments and Signatures

Reviewer's comments and signatures:

1. _____

2. _____

3. _____

Instructor's comments:

_____

CAAHEP Competencies Achieved

I. P. (7) Select proper sites for administering parenteral medication

I. P. (9) Administer parenteral (excluding IV) medications

II. P. (1) Prepare proper dosages of medication for administration

II. A. (1) Verify ordered doses/dosages prior to administration

ABHES Competency Achieved

9 (j) Prepare and administer oral and parenteral medications as directed by physicians

PROCEDURE 20-16 PERFORMING EAR IRRIGATION

Procedure Goal

To wash out the ear canal to remove impacted cerumen, relieve inflammation, or remove a foreign body

Scoring System

To score each step, use the following scoring system:
1 = poor, 2 = fair, 3 = good, 4 = excellent

A minimum score of at least a 3 must be achieved on **each** step to achieve successful completion of the technique. Detailed instructions on the scoring system are found on page 179.

Materials

Fresh irrigating solution, clean basin, clean irrigating syringe, towel or absorbent pad, kidney-shaped basin, cotton balls

Procedure

Procedure Steps Total Possible Points - 84 Time Limit: 15 minutes	Practice #1	Practice #2	Practice #3	Final
1. Identify the patient, introduce yourself, and explain the procedure.				
2. Check the doctor's order. It should include the patient's name, the irrigating solution, the volume of solution, and for which ear(s) the irrigation is to be performed. If the doctor has not specified the volume of solution, use the amount needed to remove the wax.				
3. Compare the solution with the instructions three times, checking the rights of medication administration.*				
4. Wash your hands and put on gloves, a gown, and a face shield.*				
5. Look into the patient's ear to identify if cerumen or a foreign body needs to be removed. You will know when you have completed the irrigation when the cerumen or foreign body is removed.				
6. Assemble the supplies.				
7. If the solution is cold, warm it to room temperature by placing the bottle in a pan of warm water.*				
8. Have the patient sit or lie on her back with the ear to be treated facing you.				
9. Place a towel over the patient's shoulder (or under the head and shoulder if she is lying down) and have her hold the kidney-shaped basin under her ear.				
10. Pour the solution into the other basin.				
11. If necessary, gently clean the external ear with cotton moistened with the solution.				
12. Fill the irrigating syringe with solution (approximately 50 mL).				

(continued)

Procedure Steps Total Possible Points - 84 Time Limit: 15 minutes	Practice #1	Practice #2	Practice #3	Final
13. Straighten the ear canal by pulling the auricle upward and outward for adults, down and back for infants and children.*				
14. Holding the tip of the syringe ½ inch above the opening of the ear, slowly instill the solution into the ear. Allow the fluid to drain out during the process.*				
15. Refill the syringe and continue irrigation until the canal is cleaned or the solution is used up.				
16. Dry the external ear with a cotton ball and leave a clean cotton ball loosely in place for 5–10 minutes.				
17. If the patient becomes dizzy or nauseated, allow her time to regain balance before standing up. Assist her as needed.				
18. Properly dispose of used disposable materials.				
19. Remove your gloves, gown, and face shield and wash your hands.				
20. Record in the patient's chart the procedure and result, the amount of solution used, the time of administration, and the ear(s) irrigated.				
21. Put on gloves and clean the equipment and room according to OSHA guidelines.				
Total Number of Points Achieved/Final Score				
Initials of Observer:				

Comments and Signatures

Reviewer's comments and signatures:

1. _____

2. _____

3. _____

Instructor's comments:

_____

CAAHEP Competencies Achieved

I. P. (7) Select proper sites for administering parenteral medication

I. P. (9) Administer parenteral (excluding IV) medications

II. P. (1) Prepare proper dosages of medication for administration

II. A. (1) Verify ordered doses/dosages prior to administration

ABHES Competency Achieved

9 (j) Prepare and administer oral and parenteral medications as directed by physicians

PROCEDURE 21-1 OBTAINING AN ECG

Procedure Goal

To obtain a graphic representation of the electrical activity of a patient's heart

Scoring System

To score each step, use the following scoring system:
1 = poor, 2 = fair, 3 = good, 4 = excellent

A minimum score of at least a 3 must be achieved on **each** step to achieve successful completion of the technique. Detailed instructions on the scoring system are found on page 179.

Materials

Electrocardiograph, ECG paper, electrodes, electrolyte preparation, wires, patient gown, drape, blanket, pillows, gauze pads, alcohol, moist towel, small scissors for trimming hair (if needed)

Procedure

Procedure Steps Total Possible Points - 108 Time Limit: 15 minutes	Practice #1	Practice #2	Practice #3	Final
1. Turn on the electrocardiograph and, if necessary, allow the stylus to heat up.				
2. Identify the patient, introduce yourself, and explain the procedure.				
3. Wash your hands.				
4. Ask the patient to disrobe from the waist up and remove jewelry, socks or stockings, bra, and shoes. If the electrodes will be placed on the patient's legs, have the patient roll up his or her pant legs. Sometimes the electrodes are placed on the sides of the lower abdomen—check the manufacturer's instructions. Provide a gown if the patient is female and instruct her to wear the gown with the opening in front.*				
5. Assist the patient onto the table and into a supine position. Cover the patient with a drape (and a blanket if the room is cool). If the patient experiences difficulty breathing or cannot tolerate lying flat, use a Fowler's or semi-Fowler's position, adjusting with pillows under the head and knees for comfort if needed.				
6. Tell the patient to rest quietly and breathe normally. Explain the importance of lying still to prevent false readings.				
7. Wash the patient's skin, using gauze pads moistened with alcohol. Then rub it vigorously with dry gauze pads to promote better contact of the electrodes.*				
8. If the patient's leg or chest hair is dense, use a small pair of scissors to closely trim the hair where you will attach the electrode.				

(continued)

Procedure Steps Total Possible Points - 108 Time Limit: 15 minutes	Practice #1	Practice #2	Practice #3	Final
9. Apply electrodes to fleshy portions of the limbs, making sure that the electrodes on one arm and leg are placed similarly to those on the other arm and leg. Attach electrodes to areas that are not bony or muscular. The arm lead tabs on the electrode point downward and the electrode tabs for the leg leads point upward. Peel off the backings of the disposable electrodes and press them into place.*				
10. Apply the precordial electrodes at specified locations on the chest. Precordial electrode tabs point downward.				
11. Attach wires and cables, making sure all wire tips follow the patient's body contours.				
12. Check all electrodes and wires for proper placement and connection; drape wires over the patient to avoid creating tension on the electrodes that could result in artifacts.				
13. Enter the patient data into the electrocardiograph. Press the on, run, or record button. Standardize the machine, if necessary, by following these steps: a. Set the paper speed to 25 mm per second or as instructed. b. Set the sensitivity setting to 1 or as instructed. c. Turn the lead selector to standardization mode. d. Adjust the stylus so the baseline is centered. e. Press the standardization button. The stylus should move upward above the baseline 10 mm (two large squares).				
14. Run the ECG. a. If the machine has an automatic feature, set the lead selector to automatic. b. For manual tracings, turn the lead selector to standby mode. Select the first lead (I) and record the tracing. Switch the machine to standby and then repeat the procedure for all 12 leads.				
15. Check tracings for artifacts.				
16. Correct problems and repeat any tracings that are not clear.				
17. Disconnect the patient from the machine.				
18. Remove the tracing from the machine and label it with the patient's name, the date, and your initials.				
19. Disconnect the wires from the electrodes and remove the electrodes from the patient.				
20. Clean the patient's skin with a moist towel.				
21. Assist the patient into a sitting position.				
22. Allow a moment for rest and then assist the patient from the table.*				
23. Assist the patient in dressing if necessary, or allow the patient privacy to dress.				
24. Wash your hands.				
25. Record the procedure in the patient's chart.				

Procedure Steps Total Possible Points - 108 Time Limit: 15 minutes	Practice #1	Practice #2	Practice #3	Final
26. Properly dispose of used materials and disposable electrodes.				
27. Clean and disinfect the equipment and the room according to OSHA guidelines.				
Total Number of Points Achieved/Final Score				
Initials of Observer:				

Comments and Signatures

Reviewer's comments and signatures:

1. _____

2. _____

3. _____

Instructor's comments:

_____

CAAHEP Competency Achieved

I. P. (5) Perform electrocardiography

ABHES Competencies Achieved

2 (c) Assist the physician with the regimen of diagnostic and treatment modalities as they relate to each body system

9 (o) Perform: 1) Electrocardiograms

PROCEDURE 21-2 HOLTER MONITORING

Procedure Goal

To monitor the electrical activity of a patient's heart over a 24-hour period to detect cardiac abnormalities that may go undetected during routine electrocardiography or stress testing

Scoring System

To score each step, use the following scoring system:
1 = poor, 2 = fair, 3 = good, 4 = excellent

A minimum score of at least a 3 must be achieved on **each** step to achieve successful completion of the technique. Detailed instructions on the scoring system are found on page 179.

Materials

Holter monitor, battery, cassette tape, patient diary or log, alcohol, gauze pads, small scissors for trimming hair, disposable electrodes, hypoallergenic tape, drape, electrocardiograph

Procedure

Procedure Steps Total Possible Points - 72 Time Limit: 15 minutes	Practice #1	Practice #2	Practice #3	Final
1. Identify the patient, introduce yourself, and explain the procedure.				
2. Ask the patient to remove clothing from the waist up; provide a drape if necessary.				
3. Wash your hands and assemble the equipment.				
4. Assist the patient into a comfortable position (sitting or supine).				
5. If the patient's body hair is particularly dense, put on exam gloves and trim the areas where the electrodes will be attached.*				
6. Clean the electrode sites with alcohol and gauze.				
7. Rub each electrode site vigorously with a dry gauze square.*				
8. Attach wires to the electrodes and peel off the paper backing on the electrodes. Apply as indicated, pressing firmly to ensure that each electrode is securely attached and is making good contact with the skin.*				
9. Attach the patient cable.				
10. Insert a fresh battery and position the unit.				
11. Tape wires, cable, and electrodes as necessary to avoid tension on the wires as the patient moves.				
12. Insert the cassette tape and turn on the unit.				
13. Confirm that the cassette tape is actually running. Indicate the start time in the patient's chart.*				
14. Instruct the patient on proper use of the monitor and how to enter information in the diary. Caution the patient not to alter any diary entries; it is crucial to know what the patient is doing at all times.				

(continued)

Procedure Steps Total Possible Points - 72 Time Limit: 15 minutes	Practice #1	Practice #2	Practice #3	Final
15. Schedule the patient's return visit for the same time on the following day.				
16. On the following day, remove the electrodes, discard them, and clean the electrode sites.				
17. Wash your hands.				
18. Remove the cassette and obtain a printout of the tracing according to office procedure. Document all parts of the procedure.				
Total Number of Points Achieved/Final Score				
Initials of Observer:				

Comments and Signatures

Reviewer's comments and signatures:

1. _____

2. _____

3. _____

Instructor's comments:

_____

CAAHEP Competency Achieved

I. P. (5) Perform electrocardiography

ABHES Competencies Achieved

2 (c) Assist the physician with the regimen of diagnostic and treatment modalities as they relate to each body system

9 (o) Perform: 1) Electrocardiograms

PROCEDURE 21-3 MEASURING FORCED VITAL CAPACITY USING SPIROMETRY

Procedure Goal

To determine a patient's forced vital capacity using a volume-displacing spirometer

Scoring System

To score each step, use the following scoring system:
1 = poor, 2 = fair, 3 = good, 4 = excellent

A minimum score of at least a 3 must be achieved on **each** step to achieve successful completion of the technique. Detailed instructions on the scoring system are found on page 179.

Materials

Adult scale with height bar, spirometer, patient tubing (tubing that runs from the mouthpiece to the machine), mouthpiece, nose clip, disinfectant

Procedure

Procedure Steps Total Possible Points - 84 Time Limit: 10 minutes	Practice #1	Practice #2	Practice #3	Final
1. Prepare the equipment. Ensure that the paper supply in the machine is adequate.				
2. Calibrate the machine as necessary.				
3. Identify the patient and introduce yourself.				
4. Check the patient's chart to see whether there are special instructions to follow.				
5. Ask whether the patient has followed instructions.				
6. Wash your hands and put on exam gloves.				
7. Measure and record the patient's height and weight.				
8. Explain the proper positioning.				
9. Explain the procedure.				
10. Demonstrate the procedure.*				
11. Turn on the spirometer and enter applicable patient data and the number of tests to be performed.				
12. Ensure that the patient has loosened any tight clothing, is comfortable, and is in the proper position. Apply the nose clip.				
13. Have the patient perform the first maneuver, coaching when necessary.				
14. Determine whether the maneuver is acceptable.				
15. Offer feedback to the patient and recommendations for improvement if necessary.				
16. Have the patient perform additional maneuvers until three acceptable maneuvers are obtained.				

(continued)

Procedure Steps Total Possible Points - 84 Time Limit: 10 minutes	Practice #1	Practice #2	Practice #3	Final
17. Record the procedure in the patient's chart and place the chart and the test results on the physician's desk for interpretation.				
18. Ask the patient to remain until the physician reviews the results.*				
19. Properly dispose of used materials and disposable instruments.				
20. Sanitize and disinfect patient tubing and reusable mouthpiece and nose clip.				
21. Clean and disinfect the equipment and room according to OSHA guidelines.				
Total Number of Points Achieved/Final Score				
Initials of Observer:				

Comments and Signatures

Reviewer's comments and signatures:

1. _____

2. _____

3. _____

Instructor's comments:

_____

CAAHEP Competency Achieved

I. P. (4) Perform pulmonary function testing

ABHES Competencies Achieved

2 (c) Assist the physician with the regimen of diagnostic and treatment modalities as they relate to each body system

9 (o) Perform: 2) Respiratory testing

PROCEDURE 21-4 OBTAINING A PEAK EXPIRATORY FLOW RATE

Procedure Goal

To determine a patient's peak expiratory flow rate

Scoring System

To score each step, use the following scoring system:
1 = poor, 2 = fair, 3 = good, 4 = excellent

A minimum score of at least a 3 must be achieved on **each** step to achieve successful completion of the technique. Detailed instructions on the scoring system are found on page 179.

Materials

Peak flow meter, disposable mouthpiece

Procedure

Procedure Steps Total Possible Points - 64 Time Limit: 10 minutes	Practice #1	Practice #2	Practice #3	Final
1. Assemble all necessary equipment and supplies for the test.				
2. Wash your hands and identify the patient.				
3. Explain and demonstrate the procedure to the patient.*				
4. Position the patient in a sitting or standing position with good posture. Make sure that any chewing gum or food is removed from the patient's mouth.				
5. Set the indicator to zero.*				
6. Ensure that the disposable mouthpiece is securely placed onto the peak flow meter.				
7. Hold the peak flow meter with the gauge uppermost and ensure that your fingers are away from the gauge.				
8. Instruct patient to take as deep a breath as possible.				
9. Instruct the patient to place the mouthpiece into her mouth and close her lips tightly around the mouthpiece, sealing her lips around the mouthpiece.				
10. Instruct the patient to blow out as fast and as hard as possible.*				
11. Observe the reading where the arrowhead is on the indicator.				
12. Reset the indicator to zero and repeat the procedure two times, for a total of three readings. You will know the technique is correct if the reading results are close. If coughing occurs during the procedures, repeat the step.				
13. Document the readings into the patient's chart. The highest reading will be peak flow rate.*				

(continued)

Procedure Steps Total Possible Points - 64 Time Limit: 10 minutes	Practice #1	Practice #2	Practice #3	Final
14. Dispose of mouthpiece in a biohazardous waste container.				
15. Disinfect or dispose of the peak flow meter per office policy.				
16. Wash your hands.				
Total Number of Points Achieved/Final Score				
Initials of Observer:				

Comments and Signatures

Reviewer's comments and signatures:

1. _____

2. _____

3. _____

Instructor's comments:

_____

CAAHEP Competency Achieved

I. P. (4) Perform pulmonary function testing

ABHES Competencies Achieved

2 (c) Assist the physician with the regimen of diagnostic and treatment modalities as they relate to each body system

9 (o) Perform: 2) Respiratory testing

PROCEDURE 21-5 OBTAINING A PULSE OXIMETRY READING

Procedure Goal

To obtain a pulse oximetry reading

Scoring System

To score each step, use the following scoring system:
1 = poor, 2 = fair, 3 = good, 4 = excellent

A minimum score of at least a 3 must be achieved on **each** step to achieve successful completion of the technique. Detailed instructions on the scoring system are found on page 179.

Materials

Pulse oximeter

Procedure

Procedure Steps Total Possible Points - 44 Time Limit: 5 minutes	Practice #1	Practice #2	Practice #3	Final
1. Assemble all the necessary equipment and supplies.				
2. Wash your hands and correctly identify the patient.				
3. Select the appropriate site to apply the sensor to by assessing capillary refill in the patient's toe or finger.*				
4. Prepare the selected site, removing nail polish or earrings if necessary. Wipe the selected site with alcohol and allow it to air-dry.*				
5. Attach the sensor to the site (if a finger is used, placed in the clip).				
6. Instruct the patient to breathe normally.				
7. Attach the sensor cable to the oximeter. Turn on the oximeter and listen to the tone.				
8. Set the alarm limits for high and low oxygen saturations and high and low pulse rates as directed by the physician's order.				
9. Read the saturation level and document it in the patient's chart. Report to the physician readings that are less than 95%. Manually check the patient's pulse and compare it to the pulse oximeter. Document all the readings and the application site in the patient's medical chart.				
10. Wash your hands.				
11. Rotate the patient's finger sites every four hours if using a pulse oximeter long-term.				
Total Number of Points Achieved/Final Score				
Initials of Observer:				

(continued)

Comments and Signatures

Reviewer's comments and signatures:

1. _____

2. _____

3. _____

Instructor's comments:

_____

CAAHEP Competencies Achieved

I. P. (4) Perform pulmonary function testing

I. P. (1) Obtain Vital Signs

ABHES Competencies Achieved

2 (c) Assist the physician with the regimen of diagnostic and treatment modalities as they relate to each body system

9 (o) Perform: 2) Respiratory testing

PROCEDURE 22-1 ASSISTING WITH AN X-RAY EXAM

Procedure Goal

To assist with a radiologic procedure under the supervision of a radiologic technologist

Scoring System

To score each step, use the following scoring system:
1 = poor, 2 = fair, 3 = good, 4 = excellent

A minimum score of at least a 3 must be achieved on **each** step to achieve successful completion of the technique. Detailed instructions on the scoring system are found on page 179.

Materials

X-ray exam order, x-ray machine, x-ray film and holder, x-ray film developer, drape, patient shield

Procedure

Procedure Steps Total Possible Points - 60 Time Limit: 10 minutes	Practice #1	Practice #2	Practice #3	Final
1. Check the x-ray exam order and equipment needed.				
2. Identify the patient and introduce yourself.				
3. Determine whether the patient has complied with the preprocedure instructions. Do not depend on the patient to inform you, but ask the patient if and how he prepped for the procedure.*				
4. Explain the procedure and the purpose of the exam to the patient.				
5. Instruct the patient to remove clothing and all metals (including jewelry) as needed, according to body area to be examined, and to put on a gown. Explain that metals may interfere with the image. Ask whether the patient has any surgical metal or a pacemaker and report this information to the radiologic technologist. Leave the room to ensure patient privacy.				
Note: Steps 6 through 11 are nearly always performed by a radiologic technologist.				
6. Position the patient according to the x-ray view ordered.				
7. Drape the patient and place the patient shield appropriately.				
8. Instruct the patient about the need to remain still and to hold his breath when requested.				
9. Leave the room or stand behind a lead shield during the exposure.				
10. Ask the patient to assume a comfortable position while the films are developed. Explain that x-rays sometimes must be repeated.				
11. Develop the films.				
12. Determine if the x-ray films are satisfactory by allowing the radiologist to review the films.*				

(continued)

Procedure Steps Total Possible Points - 60 Time Limit: 10 minutes	Practice #1	Practice #2	Practice #3	Final
13. Instruct the patient to dress and tell the patient when to contact the physician's office for the results.				
14. Label the dry, finished x-ray films; place them in a properly labeled envelope; and file them according to the policies of your office.				
15. Record the x-ray exam, along with the final written findings, in the patient's chart.				
Total Number of Points Achieved/Final Score				
Initials of Observer:				

Comments and Signatures

Reviewer's comments and signatures:

1. _____

2. _____

3. _____

Instructor's comments:

_____

CAAHEP Competencies Achieved

IV. P. (6) Prepare a patient for procedures and/or treatments

III. A. (2) Explain the rationale for performance of a procedure to the patient

III. A (3) Show awareness of patient's concerns regarding their perceptions related to the procedure being performed

ABHES Competencies Achieved

2 (c) Assist the physician with the regimen of diagnostic and treatment modalities as they relate to each body system

9 (m) Assist physician with routine and specialty examinations and treatments

PROCEDURE 22-2 DOCUMENTATION AND FILING TECHNIQUES FOR X-RAYS

Procedure Goal

To document x-ray information and file x-ray films properly

Scoring System

To score each step, use the following scoring system:
1 = poor, 2 = fair, 3 = good, 4 = excellent

A minimum score of at least a 3 must be achieved on **each** step to achieve successful completion of the technique. Detailed instructions on the scoring system are found on page 179.

Materials

X-ray film(s), patient x-ray record card or book, label, film-filing envelopes, film-filing cabinet, inserts, marking pen

Procedure

Procedure Steps Total Possible Points - 16 Time Limit: 10 minutes	Practice #1	Practice #2	Practice #3	Final
1. Document the patient's x-ray information on the patient record card or in the record book. Include the patient's name, the date, the type of x-ray, and the number of x-rays taken.				
2. Verify that the film is properly labeled with the referring doctor's name, the date, and the patient's name. To note corrections or unusual positions or to identify a film that does not include labeling, attach the appropriate label and complete the necessary information. Some facilities also record the name of the radiologist who interpreted the x-ray.*				
3. Place the processed film in a film-filing envelope. File the envelope alphabetically or chronologically (or according to your office's protocol) in the filing cabinet.				
4. If you remove an envelope for any reason, put an insert or an "out card" in its place until it is returned to the cabinet.*				
Total Number of Points Achieved/Final Score				
Initials of Observer:				

(continued)

Comments and Signatures

Reviewer's comments and signatures:

1. _____

2. _____

3. _____

Instructor's comments:

_____

CAAHEP Competencies Achieved

IV. P. (3) Use medical terminology, pronouncing medical terms correctly, to communicate information, patient history, data, and observation

IV. P. (8) Document Patient Care

ABHES Competencies Achieved

8 (jj) Perform fundamental writing skills including correct grammar, spelling, and formatting techniques when writing prescriptions, documenting medical records, etc.

8. II. Apply electronic technology

PROCEDURE 23-1 RÉSUMÉ WRITING

Objective

To write a résumé that reflects a defined career objective and highlights your skills

Scoring System

To score each step, use the following scoring system:
1 = poor, 2 = fair, 3 = good, 4 = excellent

A minimum score of at least a 3 must be achieved on **each** step to achieve successful completion of the technique. Detailed instructions on the scoring system are found on page 179.

Materials

Paper; pen; dictionary; thesaurus; computer

Procedure

Procedure Steps Total Possible Points - 32 Time Limit: 20 minutes	Practice #1	Practice #2	Practice #3	Final
1. Write your full name, address (temporary and permanent, if you have both), telephone number with area code, and e-mail address (if you have one).				
2. List your general career objective. You also may choose to summarize your skills. If you want to phrase your objective to fit a specific position, you should include that information in a cover letter to accompany the résumé.				
3. List the highest level of education or the most recently obtained degree first. Include the school name, degree earned, and date of graduation. Be sure to list any special projects, courses, or participation in overseas study programs.				
4. Summarize your work experience. List your most recent or most relevant employment first. Describe your responsibilities and list job titles, company names, and dates of employment. Summer employment, volunteer work, and student externships also may be included. Use short sentences with strong action words such as *directed, designed, developed,* and *organized.* For example, condense a responsibility into "Handled insurance and billing" or "Drafted correspondence as requested."*				
5. List any memberships and affiliations with professional organizations. List them alphabetically or by order of importance.				
6. Do not list references on your résumé.*				
7. Do not list the salary you wish to receive in a medical assisting position. Salary requirements should not be discussed until a job offer is received. If the ad you are answering requests that you include a required salary, it is best to state a range (no broader than $5,000 from lowest to highest point in the range for an annual salary).				

(continued)

Procedure Steps Total Possible Points - 32 Time Limit: 20 minutes	Practice #1	Practice #2	Practice #3	Final
8. Print your résumé on an 8½- by 11-inch sheet of high-quality white, off-white, or pastel bond paper. Carefully check your résumé for spelling, punctuation, and grammatical errors. Have someone else double-check your résumé whenever possible.*				
Total Number of Points Achieved/Final Score				
Initials of Observer:				

Comments and Signatures

Reviewer's comments and signatures:

1. _____

2. _____

3. _____

Instructor's comments:

_____

CAAHEP Competencies Achieved

IV. C. (8) Recognize elements of fundamental writing skills

IV. P. (10) Compose professional/business letters

ABHES Competency Achieved

11 (a) Perform the essential requirements for employment such as résumé writing, effective interviewing, dressing professionally, and following up appropriately

PROCEDURE 23-2 WRITING THANK-YOU NOTES

Objective

To write an appropriate, professional thank-you note after an interview or externship

Scoring System

To score each step, use the following scoring system:
1 = poor, 2 = fair, 3 = good, 4 = excellent

A minimum score of at least a 3 must be achieved on **each** step to achieve successful completion of the technique. Detailed instructions on the scoring system are found on page 179.

Materials

Paper; pen; dictionary; thesaurus; computer; #10 business envelope

Procedure

Procedure Steps Total Possible Points - 32 Time Limit: 10 minutes	Practice #1	Practice #2	Practice #3	Final
1. Complete the letter within 2 days of the interview or completion of the externship. Begin by typing the date at the top of the letter.*				
2. Type the name of the person who interviewed you (or who was your mentor in the externship). Include credentials and title, such as Dr. or Director of Client Services. Include the complete address of the office or organization.				
3. Start the letter with "Dear Dr., Mr., Mrs., Miss, or Ms. _____:"				
4. In the first paragraph, thank the interviewer for his time and for granting the interview. Discuss some specific impressions, for example, "I found the interview and tour of the facilities an enjoyable experience. I would welcome the opportunity to work in such a state-of-the-art medical setting." If you are writing to thank your mentor for her time during your externship and for allowing you to perform your externship at her office, practice, or clinic, discuss the knowledge and experience you gained during the externship.				
5. In the second paragraph, mention the aspects of the job or externship that you found most interesting or challenging. For a job interview thank-you note, state how your skills and qualifications will make you an asset to the staff. When preparing an externship thank-you letter, mention interest in any future positions.				
6. In the last paragraph, thank the interviewer for considering you for the position. Ask to be contacted at his earliest convenience regarding his employment decision.				
7. Close the letter with "Sincerely" and type your name. Leave enough space above your typewritten name to sign your name.				

(continued)

Procedure Steps Total Possible Points - 32 Time Limit: 10 minutes	Practice #1	Practice #2	Practice #3	Final
8. Type your return address in the upper-left corner of the #10 business envelope. Then type the interviewer's name and address in the envelope's center, apply the proper postage, and mail the letter. You also can e-mail your thank-you letter. Proper letter format and professional tone and appearance still apply. Send the thank-you letter as an attachment.				
Total Number of Points Achieved/Final Score				
Initials of Observer:				

Comments and Signatures

Reviewer's comments and signatures:

1. _____

2. _____

3. _____

Instructor's comments:

_____

CAAHEP Competencies Achieved

IV. C. (8) Recognize elements of fundamental writing skills

IV. P. (10) Compose professional/business letters

ABHES Competency Achieved

11 (a) Perform the essential requirements for employment such as resume writing, effective interviewing, dressing professionally, and following up appropriately

Work Product Documentation/Forms

Use these forms while performing procedures that include a work product icon.

WORK // PRODUCT **PROCEDURE WORK PRODUCT FORMS**

PROCEDURE 3-2 NOTIFYING STATE AND COUNTY AGENCIES ABOUT REPORTABLE DISEASES

Name _____ Class _____ Date _____

MICHIGAN DEPARTMENT OF PUBLIC HEALTH
Division of Disease Surveillance

ENTERIC ILLNESS CASE INVESTIGATION
(Please check appropriate illness)

_____ Shigellosis   _____ Giardiasis
_____ Non-typhoid Salmonellosis   _____ Amebiasis
_____ Campylobacter enteritis

CASE INFORMATION

Name: _____ Age or Birthdate: _____ Sex: _____ Race: _____

Address: _____ Phone: _____
       (Street)   (City)   (County)   (Zip)

Occupation: _____ *High Risk: Y N
         (What)   (Where)
    (If infant or student list school, nursery or day care center)

Attending   Address or   Was the patient
Physician: _____ Phone: _____ hospitalized: Y N

Hospital: _____ Dates: _____
                                 (Admission)   (Discharge)

Onset: _____ Date recovered: _____ Symptom Summary: _____

_____

_____

Suspected Causative Agent: _____
(include species or serotype if known)

HOUSEHOLD CONTACTS INFORMATION

Name	Age	Family Relationship	Occupation	*High Risk Y N	Provide date of onset for all household members with concurrent similar illness
1)					
2)					
3)					
4)					
5)					
6)					
7)					
8)					
9)					
10)					

*"High Risk" = occupation as food handler, direct patient care worker, day care center worker or person attending day care or who is institutionalized. Stool specimens should be obtained on "high risk" cases and "high risk" household contacts as appropriate for the illness. Results may be recorded in Laboratory Information Section of this form (see over).

Name of the person who completed this form: _____ County: _____

Information obtained from: _____ Date: _____

Telephone Interview: _____ Home Visit: _____ Outbreak Investigation: _____

C-30 Rev. 10/83   AUTH: Act 368, P.A. 1978

PROCEDURE 3-2 NOTIFYING STATE AND COUNTY AGENCIES ABOUT REPORTABLE DISEASES (*concluded*)

Name _____ Class _____ Date _____

NON-HOUSEHOLD CONTACTS WITH A CONCURRENT SIMILAR ILLNESS

Name	Approximate date of onset of symptoms	Address and/or Phone	Relationship to case (Nature of contact)
1)			
2)			
3)			
4)			
5)			

ADDITIONAL EXPOSURES OR COMMENTS

Home Sewage System: Municipal   Septic Tank   Other_____

Home drinking Water Type: Municipal   Private Well   Other_____

As appropriate for the illness, ask about meals eaten away from home, stores where groceries bought, brand of poultry, meat, dairy products consumed, overnight travel, recent foreign travel, group functions, exposure to raw milk, untreated water, animals, etc. within one incubation period before onset.

(shigellosis to 7 days, salmonellosis - up to 3 days, Campylobacter enteritis - up to 10 days)

Be specific, provide place name(s) and date(s).

FOLLOW-UP FECAL CULTURE RESULTS FOR "HIGH RISK" CASE AND/OR CONTACTS.

Name or Initials	Date(s) Obtained and Findings
1)	
2)	
3)	
4)	
5)	

ARIZONA DEPARTMENT OF HEALTH SERVICES
COMMUNICABLE DISEASE REPORT
Important Instructions on Reverse Side
PLEASE PRINT OR TYPE

County/IHS ID Number/Chapter   State ID Number

PATIENT'S NAME (Last)   (First)   DATE OF BIRTH   SEX ☐ Male ☐ Female   ETHNICITY ☐ Hispanic ☐ Non-Hispanic

STREET ADDRESS   CENSUS TRACT   CITY   RACE ☐ White ☐ Am. Indian ☐ Asian ☐ Black ☐ Other ☐ Unknown

COUNTY   STATE   ZIP CODE   PHONE NO.

DIAGNOSIS OR SUSPECT REPORTABLE CONDITION

DATE ONSET   DATE OF DIAGNOSIS   LAB RESULTS

COUNTY USE ONLY:
LAB CONFIRMATION DATE:_____
☐ Negative
☐ Positive
☐ Not Done
☐ Unknown

PATIENT OCCUPATION OR SCHOOL

PHYSICIAN OR OTHER REPORTING SOURCE   PHONE NUMBER

COUNTY USE ONLY:
☐ Confirmed case
☐ Probable case
☐ Outbreak Associated
☐ Ruled Out

STREET ADDRESS   CITY   STATE   ZIP CODE

Original and 1st copy to County Health Department   ☐ CHECK IF ADDITIONAL FORMS ARE NEEDED (Quantity)_____

PROCEDURE 5-2 USING A PROGRESS NOTE

Name _____ Class _____ Date _____

Total Care Clinic
Progress Notes

Name: _____ Chart #: _____

DATE	

Name _____ Class _____ Date _____

Name _____ DOB _____ Date _____

ALLERGIES: _____ Note

Review of Systems

Systems	NL	Note	Systems	NL	Note
Constitutional			Musculoskeletal		
Eyes			Skin/breasts		
ENT/mouth			Neurologic		
Cardiovascular			Psychiatric		
Respiratory			Endocrine		
GI			Hem/lymph		
GU			Allergy/immun		

Current Medicines	Date	Current Diagnosis

H: _____ W: _____ T: _____ P: _____ R: _____

B/P Sitting _____ or Standing _____ Supine _____

Last Tetanus _____

L.M.P. _____

Social Habits Yes No

Tobacco ___ ___

Alcohol ___ ___

O2 Sat: _____ Pain Scale: _____ | Rec. Drugs ___ ___

CC:

HPI:

PROCEDURE 5-3 OBTAINING A MEDICAL HISTORY

Name _____ Class _____ Date _____

Total Care Clinic
Medical History Form

Name _____
Age _____ Date of birth _____ Sex _____ Marital status _____
Place of birth _____ Occupation _____ Blood type _____
Reason for visit _____
Are you seeing another doctor, health practitioner or therapist? If yes, Who? _____

Medications _____
Allergies to medications _____
Supplements _____
Surgeries _____
Injuries _____
Have you ever had the following problems? When? _____

Weight loss _____ Kidney disease _____
Weight gain _____ Frequent urination _____
Fevers _____ Chills _____
Arthritis _____ Muscle cramps _____
Blurred vision _____ Dizziness _____
Ringing in the ears _____ Thyroid disease _____
Hearing loss _____ Chest pain _____
Swollen glands _____ HIV positive _____
Pneumonia _____ Gall bladder disease _____
Difficulty breathing _____ Diverticulitis _____
Heart attack _____ Back pain _____
Ankle swelling _____ Depression _____
Sinusitis _____ Fibromyalgia _____
Peptic ulcers _____ Tuberculosis _____
Pancreatitis _____ Mononucleosis _____
Hepatitis type? _____ Hemorrhoids _____
Food allergies _____
Varicose veins _____
Anxiety _____
Fatigue _____
Epstein Barr _____
Hypertension _____
Diabetes _____
Insomnia _____
Numbness _____
Anemia _____
Yeast infections _____
Memory loss _____

Social Habits:

Do you smoke cigarettes? _____ How many per day? _____ How long? _____
Do you drink caffeinated beverages? _____ How many per day? _____
Do you drink alcohol? _____ How often? _____ What type? _____
Do you use recreational drugs? _____ How often? _____ What type? _____
How many sexual partners? _____ Have you had unprotected sex? _____
Do you exercise? _____ What type? _____ How often? _____
Do you have any dietary restrictions? _____

Family History:

Age of mother _____ Age of father _____ Siblings _____
If deceased mark age of death _____
Has any of your family had the following diseases (please mark who)
Cancer _____ Arthritis _____ High blood pressure _____
Heart disease _____ Stroke _____ Diabetes _____
Allergies/Asthma _____ Emphysema _____
Mental disorders _____ Tuberculosis _____
Other _____

Preventative Health

Mammogram _____ Chest X-ray _____
Pap smear _____ Sigmoid/Colonoscopy _____
Blood chemistry _____ Pneumovax _____
Hemmocult _____ TB _____ Other immunizations _____
Tetanus _____
Flu shot _____

For Women Only

Age of onset of first menses _____ Are your periods regular? _____
Length of time between cycles? _____ How many days? _____
No. of pregnancies _____ Miscarriages? _____ No. of living children? _____
What form of birth control do you use? _____ Have you had an abnormal pap? _____
If yes, describe type of problem and treatment _____

For Men Only

Have you ever had prostate problems? _____
Have you had any of the symptoms listed below? _____
Frequent urination _____
Waking more than once at night to urinate _____
Decrease in urine flow or dribbling _____
Burning or discharge from the penis _____
Testicular swelling or lumps _____
Sexual problems _____
Have you had a PSA? _____ Was it normal? _____

Patient Signature _____
Date _____

Name _____ Class _____ Date _____

(All information is strictly confidential)

FAMILY HISTORY — Fill in health information about your family.

Check (✓) if your blood relatives had any of the following:

Relation	Age	State of Health	Age at Death	Cause of Death	Disease	Relationship to you
Father					Arthritis, Gout	
Mother					Asthma, Hay Fever	
Brothers					Cancer	
					Chemical Dependency	
					Diabetes	
Sisters					Heart Disease, Strokes	
					High Blood Pressure	
					Kidney Disease	
					Tuberculosis	
					Other	

HOSPITALIZATIONS

Year	Hospital	Reason for Hospitalization and Outcome

Have you ever had a blood transfusion? ☐ Yes ☐ No
If yes, please give approximate dates.

SERIOUS ILLNESS/INJURIES	DATE	OUTCOME

PREGNANCY HISTORY

Year of Birth	Sex of Birth	Complications if any

HEALTH HABITS Check (✓) which substances you use and describe how much you use.

Caffeine	
Tobacco	
Drugs	
Other	

OCCUPATIONAL CONCERNS Check (✓) if your work exposes you to the following:

Stress	
Hazardous Substances	
Heavy Lifting	
Other	

Your occupation: _____

I certify that the above information is correct to the best of my knowledge. I will not hold my doctor or any members of his/her staff responsible for any errors or omissions that I may have made in the completion of this form.

Signature _____ Date _____

Reviewed By _____ Date _____

HEALTH HISTORY
(Confidential)

Name _____ Today's Date _____

Age _____ Birthdate _____ Date of last physical examination _____

What is your reason for visit? _____

SYMPTOMS Check (✓) symptoms you currently have or have had in the past year.

GENERAL
☐ Chills
☐ Depression
☐ Dizziness
☐ Fainting
☐ Fever
☐ Forgetfulness
☐ Headache
☐ Loss of sleep
☐ Loss of weight
☐ Nervousness
☐ Numbness
☐ Sweats

MUSCLE/JOINT/BONE
Pain, weakness, numbness in:
☐ Arms ☐ Hips
☐ Back ☐ Legs
☐ Feet ☐ Neck
☐ Hands ☐ Shoulders

GENITO-URINARY
☐ Blood in urine
☐ Frequent urination
☐ Lack of bladder control
☐ Painful urination

GASTROINTESTINAL
☐ Appetite poor
☐ Bloating
☐ Bowel changes
☐ Constipation
☐ Diarrhea
☐ Excessive hunger
☐ Excessive thirst
☐ Gas
☐ Hemorrhoids
☐ Indigestion
☐ Nausea
☐ Rectal bleeding
☐ Stomach pain
☐ Vomiting
☐ Vomiting blood

CARDIOVASCULAR
☐ Chest pain
☐ High blood pressure
☐ Irregular heart beat
☐ Low blood pressure
☐ Poor circulation
☐ Rapid heart beat
☐ Swelling of ankles
☐ Varicose veins

EYE, EAR, NOSE, THROAT
☐ Bleeding gums
☐ Blurred vision
☐ Crossed eyes
☐ Difficulty swallowing
☐ Double vision
☐ Earache
☐ Ear discharge
☐ Hay fever
☐ Hoarseness
☐ Loss of hearing
☐ Nosebleeds
☐ Persistent cough
☐ Ringing in ears
☐ Sinus problems
☐ Vision – Flashes
☐ Vision – Halos

SKIN
☐ Bruise easily
☐ Hives
☐ Itching
☐ Change in moles
☐ Rash
☐ Scars
☐ Sore that won't heal

MEN only
☐ Breast lump
☐ Erection difficulties
☐ Lump in testicles
☐ Penis discharge
☐ Sore on penis
☐ Other

WOMEN only
☐ Abnormal Pap smear
☐ Bleeding between periods
☐ Breast lump
☐ Extreme menstrual pain
☐ Hot flashes
☐ Nipple discharge
☐ Painful intercourse
☐ Vaginal discharge
☐ Other

Date of last menstrual period _____
Date of last Pap smear _____
Have you had a mammogram? _____
Are you pregnant? _____
Number of children _____

CONDITIONS Check (✓) conditions you have or have had in the past.

☐ AIDS
☐ Alcoholism
☐ Anemia
☐ Anorexia
☐ Appendicitis
☐ Arthritis
☐ Asthma
☐ Bleeding Disorders
☐ Breast Lump
☐ Bronchitis
☐ Bulimia
☐ Cancer
☐ Cataracts

☐ Chemical Dependency
☐ Chicken Pox
☐ Diabetes
☐ Emphysema
☐ Epilepsy
☐ Glaucoma
☐ Goiter
☐ Gonorrhea
☐ Gout
☐ Heart Disease
☐ Hepatitis
☐ Hernia
☐ Herpes

☐ High Cholesterol
☐ HIV Positive
☐ Kidney Disease
☐ Liver Disease
☐ Measles
☐ Migraine Headaches
☐ Miscarriage
☐ Mononucleosis
☐ Multiple Sclerosis
☐ Mumps
☐ Pacemaker
☐ Pneumonia
☐ Polio

☐ Prostate Problem
☐ Psychiatric Care
☐ Rheumatic Fever
☐ Scarlet Fever
☐ Stroke
☐ Suicide Attempt
☐ Thyroid Problems
☐ Tonsillitis
☐ Tuberculosis
☐ Typhoid Fever
☐ Ulcers
☐ Vaginal Infections
☐ Venereal Disease

MEDICATIONS List medications you are currently taking.

ALLERGIES To medications or substances

Pharmacy Name _____ Phone _____

PROCEDURE 6-1 MEASURING AND RECORDING TEMPERATURE

Name _____ Class _____ Date _____

TOTAL CARE CLINIC
Facility _____

DATE	TIME	T	P	R	BP		DATE	TIME	T	P	R	BP	

Patient Name:	Last:	First:	Middle:	Physician:

VITAL SIGN CHART # _____

PROCEDURE 6-2 MEASURING AND RECORDING PULSE AND RESPIRATIONS

Name _____ Class _____ Date _____

TOTAL CARE CLINIC
Facility _____

DATE	TIME	T	P	R	BP		DATE	TIME	T	P	R	BP	

Patient Name:	Last:	First:	Middle:	Physician:

VITAL SIGN CHART # _____

PROCEDURE 6-3 TAKING THE BLOOD PRESSURE OF ADULTS AND OLDER CHILDREN

Name _____ Class _____ Date _____

TOTAL CARE CLINIC
Facility _____

DATE	TIME	T	P	R	BP		DATE	TIME	T	P	R	BP	

Patient Name:	Last:	First:	Middle:	Physician:

VITAL SIGN CHART # _____

PROCEDURE 6-4 MEASURING ADULTS AND CHILDREN

Name _____ Class _____ Date _____

TOTAL CARE CLINIC

Facility _____

MONTH:_____ YEAR:_____

DATE	WEIGHT	HEIGHT

MONTH:_____ YEAR:_____

DATE	WEIGHT	HEIGHT

MONTH:_____ YEAR:_____

DATE	WEIGHT	HEIGHT

MONTH:_____ YEAR:_____

DATE	WEIGHT	HEIGHT

MONTH:_____ YEAR:_____

DATE	WEIGHT	HEIGHT

MONTH:_____ YEAR:_____

DATE	WEIGHT	HEIGHT

MONTH:_____ YEAR:_____

DATE	WEIGHT	HEIGHT

MONTH:_____ YEAR:_____

DATE	WEIGHT	HEIGHT

MONTH:_____ YEAR:_____

DATE	WEIGHT	HEIGHT

MONTH:_____ YEAR:_____

DATE	WEIGHT	HEIGHT

MONTH:_____ YEAR:_____

DATE	WEIGHT	HEIGHT

MONTH:_____ YEAR:_____

DATE	WEIGHT	HEIGHT

Patient Name:	Last:	First:	Middle:	Admin. Number:
Physician:				

WEIGHT RECORD

Name _____ Class _____ Date _____

2 to 20 years: Boys
Body mass index-for-age percentiles

NAME _____

RECORD # _____

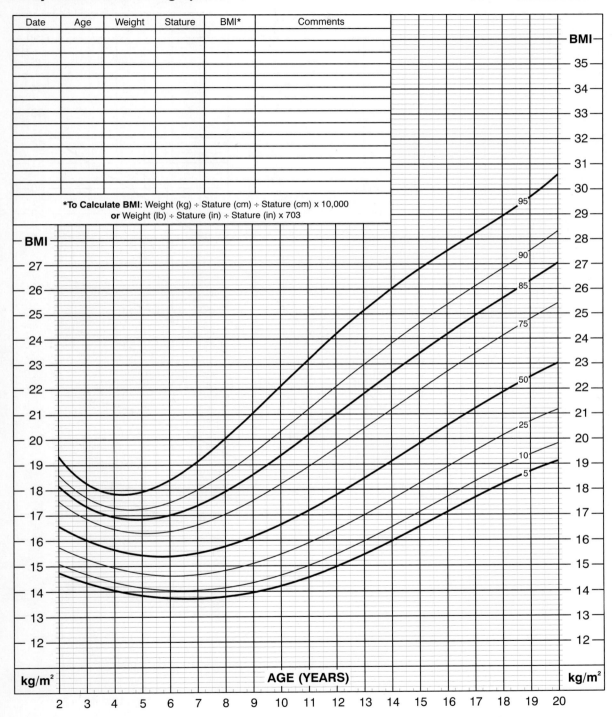

Date	Age	Weight	Stature	BMI*	Comments

*To Calculate BMI: Weight (kg) ÷ Stature (cm) ÷ Stature (cm) x 10,000
or Weight (lb) ÷ Stature (in) ÷ Stature (in) x 703

AGE (YEARS)

Published May 30, 2000 (modified 10/16/00).
SOURCE: Developed by the National Center for Health Statistics in collaboration with
the National Center for Chronic Disease Prevention and Health Promotion (2000).
http://www.cdc.gov/growthcharts

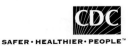

SAFER · HEALTHIER · PEOPLE™

Name _____ Class _____ Date _____

2 to 20 years: Girls
Body mass index-for-age percentiles

NAME _____

RECORD # _____

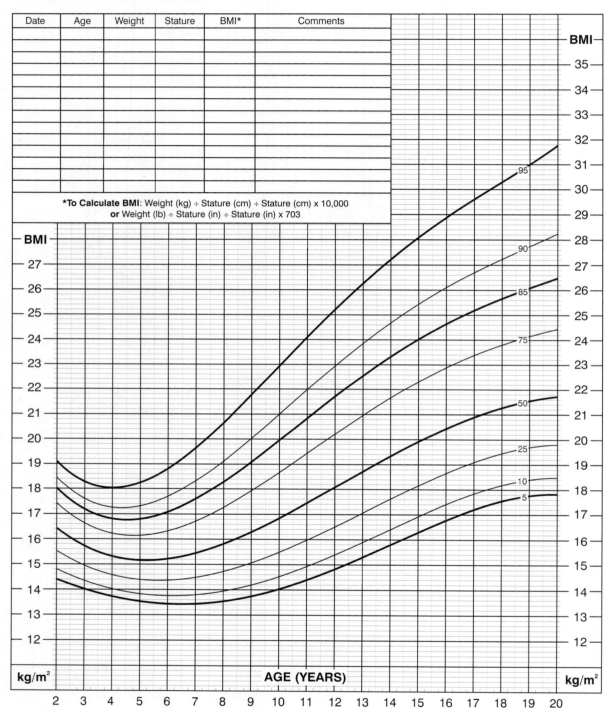

*To Calculate BMI: Weight (kg) ÷ Stature (cm) ÷ Stature (cm) x 10,000
or Weight (lb) ÷ Stature (in) ÷ Stature (in) x 703

Date	Age	Weight	Stature	BMI*	Comments

AGE (YEARS)

Published May 30, 2000 (modified 10/16/00).
SOURCE: Developed by the National Center for Health Statistics in collaboration with
the National Center for Chronic Disease Prevention and Health Promotion (2000).
http://www.cdc.gov/growthcharts

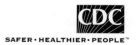

SAFER·HEALTHIER·PEOPLE™

Name _____ Class _____ Date _____

2 to 20 years: Boys
Stature-for-age and Weight-for-age percentiles

NAME _____

RECORD # _____

Mother's Stature _____		Father's Stature _____		
Date	Age	Weight	Stature	BMI*

To Calculate BMI: Weight (kg) ÷ Stature (cm) ÷ Stature (cm) x 10,000
or Weight (lb) ÷ Stature (in) ÷ Stature (in) x 703

AGE (YEARS)

STATURE

WEIGHT

Published May 30, 2000 (modified 11/21/00).
SOURCE: Developed by the National Center for Health Statistics in collaboration with
the National Center for Chronic Disease Prevention and Health Promotion (2000).
http://www.cdc.gov/growthcharts

CDC
SAFER · HEALTHIER · PEOPLE™

Procedure 6-4 **441**

PROCEDURE 6-4 MEASURING ADULTS AND CHILDREN *(concluded)*

Name _____ Class _____ Date _____

2 to 20 years: Girls
Stature-for-age and Weight-for-age percentiles

NAME _____

RECORD # _____

Mother's Stature		Father's Stature		
Date	Age	Weight	Stature	BMI*

*To Calculate BMI: Weight (kg) ÷ Stature (cm) ÷ Stature (cm) x 10,000
or Weight (lb) ÷ Stature (in) ÷ Stature (in) x 703

Published May 30, 2000 (modified 11/21/00).
SOURCE: Developed by the National Center for Health Statistics in collaboration with
the National Center for Chronic Disease Prevention and Health Promotion (2000).
http://www.cdc.gov/growthcharts

SAFER·HEALTHIER·PEOPLE™

PROCEDURE 6-5 MEASURING INFANTS

Name _____ Class _____ Date _____

TOTAL CARE CLINIC

Facility _____

MONTH:_____ YEAR:_____

DATE	WEIGHT	HEIGHT

MONTH:_____ YEAR:_____

DATE	WEIGHT	HEIGHT

MONTH:_____ YEAR:_____

DATE	WEIGHT	HEIGHT

MONTH:_____ YEAR:_____

DATE	WEIGHT	HEIGHT

MONTH:_____ YEAR:_____

DATE	WEIGHT	HEIGHT

MONTH:_____ YEAR:_____

DATE	WEIGHT	HEIGHT

MONTH:_____ YEAR:_____

DATE	WEIGHT	HEIGHT

MONTH:_____ YEAR:_____

DATE	WEIGHT	HEIGHT

MONTH:_____ YEAR:_____

DATE	WEIGHT	HEIGHT

MONTH:_____ YEAR:_____

DATE	WEIGHT	HEIGHT

MONTH:_____ YEAR:_____

DATE	WEIGHT	HEIGHT

MONTH:_____ YEAR:_____

DATE	WEIGHT	HEIGHT

Patient Name: Last: First: Middle:	Admin. Number:
Physician:	

WEIGHT RECORD

PROCEDURE 6-5 MEASURING INFANTS *(continued)*

Name _____ Class _____ Date _____

Birth to 36 months: Girls
Head circumference-for-age and
Weight-for-length percentiles

NAME _____

RECORD # _____

[Growth chart: CDC Birth to 36 months Girls — Head circumference-for-age and Weight-for-length percentiles]

AGE (MONTHS): Birth 3 6 9 12 15 18 21 24 27 30 33 36

HEAD CIRCUMFERENCE (in/cm, percentiles 95, 90, 75, 50, 25, 10, 5)

WEIGHT (kg/lb)

LENGTH (cm 64–100 / in 26–41)

Date	Age	Weight	Length	Head Circ.	Comment

Published May 30, 2000 (modified 10/16/00).
SOURCE: Developed by the National Center for Health Statistics in collaboration with
the National Center for Chronic Disease Prevention and Health Promotion (2000).
http://www.cdc.gov/growthcharts

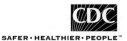

CDC
SAFER · HEALTHIER · PEOPLE™

Name _____ Class _____ Date _____

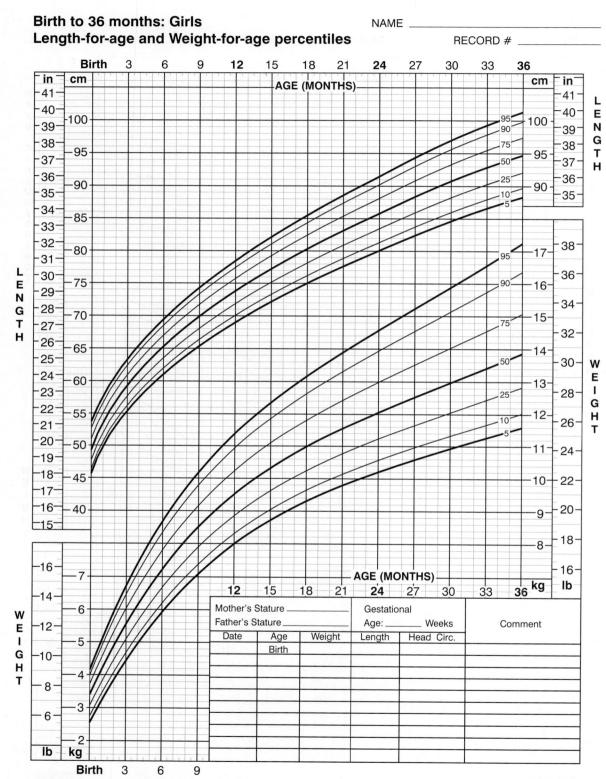

Birth to 36 months: Girls
Length-for-age and Weight-for-age percentiles

NAME _____

RECORD # _____

Mother's Stature _____
Father's Stature _____

Gestational
Age: _____ Weeks

Comment

Date	Age	Weight	Length	Head Circ.
Birth				

Published May 30, 2000 (modified 4/20/01).
SOURCE: Developed by the National Center for Health Statistics in collaboration with
the National Center for Chronic Disease Prevention and Health Promotion (2000).
http://www.cdc.gov/growthcharts

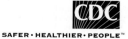

SAFER · HEALTHIER · PEOPLE™

Name _____ Class _____ Date _____

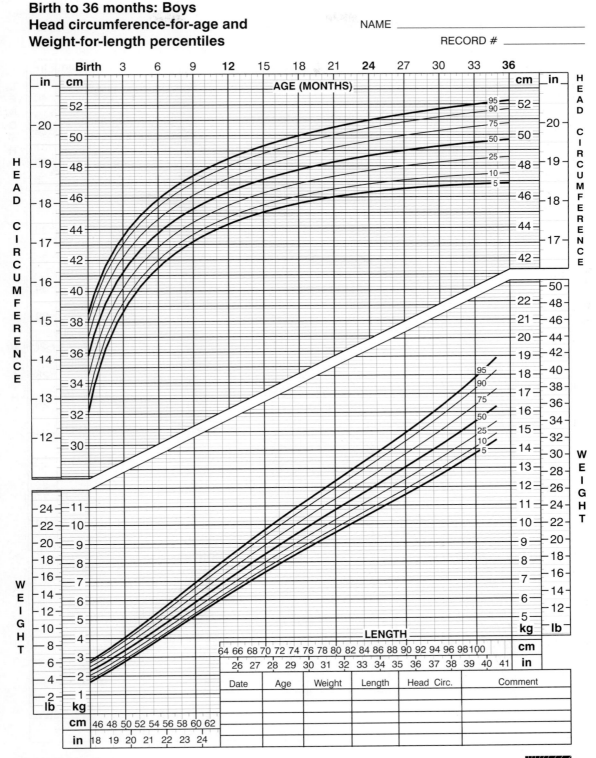

Birth to 36 months: Boys
Head circumference-for-age and
Weight-for-length percentiles

NAME _____

RECORD # _____

Published May 30, 2000 (modified 10/16/00).
SOURCE: Developed by the National Center for Health Statistics in collaboration with
the National Center for Chronic Disease Prevention and Health Promotion (2000).
http://www.cdc.gov/growthcharts

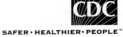

SAFER · HEALTHIER · PEOPLE™

Name _____ Class _____ Date _____

Birth to 36 months: Boys
Length-for-age and Weight-for-age percentiles

NAME _____

RECORD # _____

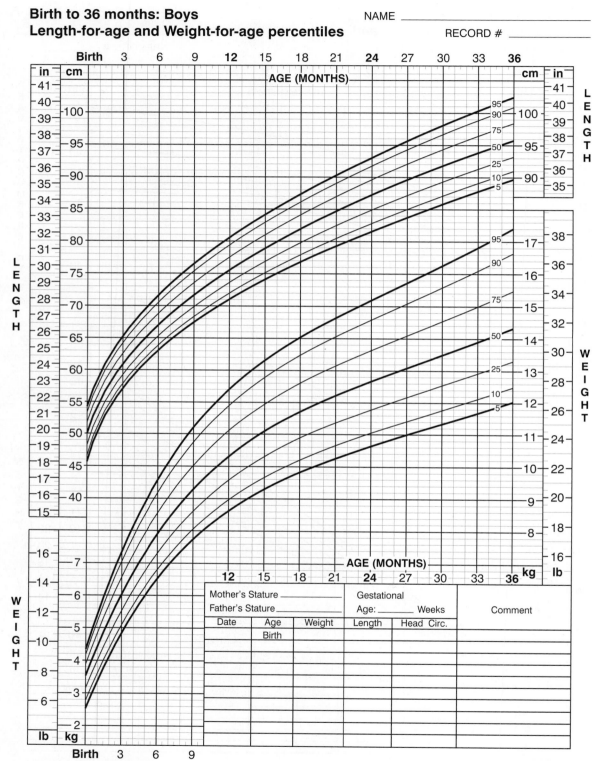

Published May 30, 2000 (modified 4/20/01).
SOURCE: Developed by the National Center for Health Statistics in collaboration with
the National Center for Chronic Disease Prevention and Health Promotion (2000).
http://www.cdc.gov/growthcharts

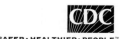

SAFER·HEALTHIER·PEOPLE™

PROCEDURE 7-5 PERFORMING VISION SCREENING TESTS

Name _____ Class _____ Date _____

Total Care Clinic
Progress Notes

Name: _____ Chart #: _____

DATE	

PROCEDURE 7-6 MEASURING AUDITORY ACTIVITY

Name _____ Class _____ Date _____

Total Care Clinic
Progress Notes

Name: _____ Chart #: _____

DATE	

PROCEDURE 9-1 ASSISTING WITH A SCRATCH TEST EXAMINATION

Name _____ Class _____ Date _____

Total Care Clinic
Progress Notes

Name: _____ Chart #: _____

DATE	

PROCEDURE 10-4 ASSISTING AS A FLOATER (UNSTERILE ASSISTANT) DURING MINOR SURGICAL PROCEDURES

Name _____ Class _____ Date _____

‖‖‖‖‖‖‖‖‖‖
70Y

Account No.

Specimen Date			Specimen Time		Patient Name (Last)		(First, MI)		Sex	Date of Birth			Age	
Mo	Day	Yr	Hr	Min						Mo	Day	Yr	Yrs	Mos

50 8649 9000 4

Patient I.D. #   Physician I.D.   Patient/Resp. Party's Phone #

* I certify that I have read the informed consent on the back and understand its content.

Responsible Party or Insured's Name (Last, First)   Patient's SS #

Patient's Signature

Address   City   State   Zip Code

Resp. Party's Employer   Medicaid Number/HMO #   Medicare #

Physician Name   UPIN #   Physician's Signature   Provider #

Diagnosis Code (ICD-9)   Insurance Code or Company Name and Address   Insurance I.D. #   Workers Comp. Yes No

Group # or Name   Relationship to Insured (Circle One) 1-Self 2-Spouse 3-Other

REV. 6/95

Urine Random   † Ⓤ Total 24hr. Vol. _____ Ht. _____ Wt. _____

| ✱ = EDTA Plasma | Ⓢ = Serum | Ⓡ = Red | Ⓖ = Gray | Ⓑ = Light Blue |
| AF = Amniotic Fluid | Ⓕ = Frozen Specimen | Ⓛ = Lavender | GN = Green | RB = Royal Blue |

Apply Labels to Patient Specimens Only
Patient Control No.

50 8649 9000 4   50 8649 9000 4   50 8649 9000 4

50 8649 9000 4   50 8649 9000 4   50 8649 9000 4   50 8649 9000 4

CHEMISTRY REQUEST

Code	Test		Code	Test		Code	Test	
58867	☐ Basic Chemistry	Ⓢ	1693	☐ Glycohemoglobin, Total	Ⓛ	4465	☐ Prolactin	Ⓢ
1396	☐ Amylase, Serum	Ⓢ	4416	☐ HCG, Beta Chain, Quant	Ⓢ	4747	☐ Prostatic Acid Phosphatase (EIA)	Ⓢ
6254	☐ Antinuclear Antibody (ANA), Qnt.	Ⓢ	1453	☐ Hemoglobin A1C	Ⓛ	10322	☐ Prostate-Specific Antigen (PSA)	Ⓢ
1040	☐ BUN	Ⓢ	6510	☐ Hepatitis B Surf Antigen (HBsAg)	Ⓢ	5199	☐ Prothrombin Time	Ⓑ
7419	☐ Carbamazepine (Tegretol)	Ⓢ	6395	☐ Hepatitis B Surf Antibody (Anti HBs)	Ⓢ	6502	☐ Ra Latex Screen	Ⓢ
5009	☐ CBC With Differential	Ⓛ	58560	☐ Hepatitis Profile I (Diagnostic)	Ⓢ	5215	☐ Sedimentation Rate	Ⓛ
2139	☐ CEA-EIA Roche	△ ✱	46938	☐ Hepatitis Profile II (Follow up)	Ⓢ	6072	☐ STS	Ⓢ
98012	☐ Chlamydia by DNA Probe	△	58552	☐ Hepatitis Profile VII (A and B)	Ⓢ	1149	☐ T₄ (Thyroxine)	Ⓢ
96479	☐ Chlamydia/GC, DNA Probe	△	83824	☐ HIV-1 ABS-EIA	Ⓢ	7336	☐ Theophylline (Theo-Dur)	Ⓢ
1065	☐ Cholesterol, Total	Ⓢ	7625	☐ Lead, Blood	RB	620	☐ Thyroid Profile I	Ⓢ
1370	☐ Creatinine, Serum	Ⓢ	235002	☐ Lipid Profile I (Lipoprotein Analysis)	Ⓢ	27011	☐ Thyroid Profile II	Ⓢ
7385	☐ Digoxin (Lanoxin)	Ⓢ	235028	☐ Lipid Profile III (incl Apolipoproteins)	Ⓢ	4259	☐ TSH, 3rd Generation	Ⓢ
604	☐ Electrolytes (Na, K, Cl)	Ⓢ	7708	☐ Lithium	Ⓢ	810	☐ Vitamin B-12 and Folate	Ⓢ
4598	☐ Ferritin	Ⓢ	505	☐ Liver Profile A	Ⓢ			
4309	☐ Follicle Stim. Hormone (FSH)	Ⓢ	7401	☐ Phenytoin (Dilantin)	Ⓢ		**URINE CHEMISTRY**	
1818	☐ Glucose	Ⓖ	1180	☐ Potassium	Ⓢ	3038	☐ Urinalysis (Microscopic if indicated)	Ⓤ
	☐ Glucose Tolerance	Ⓖ	4556	☐ Pregnancy, Serum, Ql.	Ⓢ	3772	☐ Urinalysis, Complete	Ⓤ
	Indicate No. Of Tubes _____		53520	☐ Prenatal Profile B with HBsAG	2-L Ⓡ			

ADDITIONAL TESTS

Test #   Name

☐ 1375 24 Hr Urine for Protein Ⓤ

☐ 4550 Pregnancy, Urine, Qul Ⓤ

PROCEDURE 10-7 SUTURE REMOVAL

Name _____ Class _____ Date _____

<table>
<tr><td colspan="2" align="center">**Total Care Clinic**
Progress Notes</td></tr>
<tr><td colspan="2">Name: _____ Chart #: _____</td></tr>
<tr><td>DATE</td><td></td></tr>
<tr><td></td><td></td></tr>
<tr><td></td><td></td></tr>
<tr><td></td><td></td></tr>
<tr><td></td><td></td></tr>
<tr><td></td><td></td></tr>
<tr><td></td><td></td></tr>
<tr><td></td><td></td></tr>
<tr><td></td><td></td></tr>
<tr><td></td><td></td></tr>
<tr><td></td><td></td></tr>
<tr><td></td><td></td></tr>
<tr><td></td><td></td></tr>
<tr><td></td><td></td></tr>
<tr><td></td><td></td></tr>
<tr><td></td><td></td></tr>
<tr><td></td><td></td></tr>
<tr><td></td><td></td></tr>
<tr><td></td><td></td></tr>
</table>

PROCEDURE 11-1 ADMINISTERING CRYOTHERAPY

Name _____ Class _____ Date _____

Total Care Clinic
Progress Notes

Name: _____ Chart #: _____

DATE	

Procedure 11-2 Administering Thermotherapy

Name _____ Class _____ Date _____

Total Care Clinic
Progress Notes

Name: _____ Chart #: _____

DATE	

Procedure 12-2 Performing an Emergency Assessment

Name _____ Class _____ Date _____

Total Care Clinic
Progress Notes

Name: _____ Chart #: _____

DATE	

Procedure 12-5 Controlling Bleeding

Name _____ Class _____ Date _____

<table>
<tr><td colspan="2" align="center">**Total Care Clinic**
Progress Notes</td></tr>
<tr><td colspan="2">Name: _____ Chart #: _____</td></tr>
<tr><td>DATE</td><td></td></tr>
<tr><td></td><td></td></tr>
<tr><td></td><td></td></tr>
<tr><td></td><td></td></tr>
<tr><td></td><td></td></tr>
<tr><td></td><td></td></tr>
<tr><td></td><td></td></tr>
<tr><td></td><td></td></tr>
<tr><td></td><td></td></tr>
<tr><td></td><td></td></tr>
<tr><td></td><td></td></tr>
<tr><td></td><td></td></tr>
<tr><td></td><td></td></tr>
<tr><td></td><td></td></tr>
<tr><td></td><td></td></tr>
<tr><td></td><td></td></tr>
<tr><td></td><td></td></tr>
<tr><td></td><td></td></tr>
<tr><td></td><td></td></tr>
<tr><td></td><td></td></tr>
</table>

Procedure 12-6 Cleaning Minor Wounds

Name _____ Class _____ Date _____

Total Care Clinic
Progress Notes

Name: _____ Chart #: _____

DATE	

PROCEDURE 15-1 OBTAINING A THROAT CULTURE SPECIMEN

Name _____ Class _____ Date _____

Total Care Clinic
Progress Notes

Name: _____ Chart #:_____

DATE	

PROCEDURE 15-2 PREPARING MICROBIOLOGICAL SPECIMENS FOR TRANSPORT TO AN OUTPATIENT LABORATORY

Name _____ Class _____ Date _____

Significant Clinical Information

_____ Fasting   _____ Non-Fasting

CHEMISTRY REQUEST

(EMBOSSING AREA)

Submit Separate Specimens (Not Request Forms) for each Frozen Test Requested.

Account No.

Specimen Date Mo Day Yr	Specimen Time Hr Min	Patient Name (Last)	(First, MI)	Sex	Date of Birth Mo Day Yr	Age Yrs Mos

50 8649 9000 4

* I certify that I have read the informed consent on the back and understand its content.

REV. 6/95

Patient's Signature

	Patient I.D. #	Physician I.D.	Patient/Resp. Party's Phone #
	Responsible Party or Insured's Name (Last, First)		Patient's SS #
Resp. Party's Employer	Address	City	State Zip Code
Physician Name	Medicaid Number/HMO #	Medicare #	
Diagnosis Code (ICD-9)	UPIN #	Physician's Signature	Provider #
Group # or Name	Insurance Code or Company Name and Address	Insurance I.D. #	Workers Comp. Yes No
	Relationship to Insured (Circle One) 1-Self 2-Spouse 3-Other		

Urine Random   † Ⓤ Total 24hr. Vol. _____ Ht. _____ Wt. _____

✪ = EDTA Plasma	Ⓢ = Serum	Ⓡ = Red	Ⓖ = Gray	Ⓑ = Light Blue
AF = Amniotic Fluid	Ⓕ = Frozen Specimen	Ⓛ = Lavender	GN = Green	RB = Royal Blue

Apply Labels to Patient Specimens Only
Patient Control No

50 8649 9000 4

50 8649 9000 4   50 8649 9000 4   50 8649 9000 4

CHEMISTRY REQUEST

58867	☐ Basic Chemistry	Ⓢ	1693	☐ Glycohemoglobin, Total	Ⓛ	4465	☐ Prolactin Ⓢ
1396	☐ Amylase, Serum	Ⓢ	4416	☐ HCG, Beta Chain, Quant	Ⓢ	4747	☐ Prostatic Acid Phosphatase (EIA) Ⓢ
6254	☐ Antinuclear Antibody (ANA), Qnt.	Ⓢ	1453	☐ Hemoglobin A1C	Ⓛ	10322	☐ Prostate-Specific Antigen (PSA) Ⓢ
1040	☐ BUN	Ⓢ	6510	☐ Hepatitis B Surf Antigen (HBsAg)	Ⓢ	5199	☐ Prothrombin Time Ⓑ
7419	☐ Carbamazepine (Tegretol)	Ⓢ	6395	☐ Hepatitis B Surf Antibody (Anti HBs)	Ⓢ	6502	☐ Ra Latex Screen Ⓢ
5009	☐ CBC With Differential	Ⓛ	58560	☐ Hepatitis Profile I (Diagnostic)	Ⓢ	5215	☐ Sedimentation Rate Ⓛ
2139	☐ CEA-EIA Roche	△ ✪	46938	☐ Hepatitis Profile II (Follow up)	Ⓢ	6072	☐ STS Ⓢ
98012	☐ Chlamydia by DNA Probe	△	58552	☐ Hepatitis Profile VII (A and B)	Ⓢ	1149	☐ T₄ (Thyroxine) Ⓢ
96479	☐ Chlamydia/GC, DNA Probe	△	83824	☐ HIV-1 ABS-EIA	Ⓢ	7336	☐ Theophylline (Theo-Dur) Ⓢ
1065	☐ Cholesterol, Total	Ⓢ	7625	☐ Lead, Blood	RB	620	☐ Thyroid Profile I Ⓢ
1370	☐ Creatinine, Serum	Ⓢ	235002	☐ Lipid Profile I (Lipoprotein Analysis)	Ⓢ	27011	☐ Thyroid Profile II Ⓢ
7385	☐ Digoxin (Lanoxin)	Ⓢ	235028	☐ Lipid Profile III (incl Apolipoproteins)	Ⓢ	4259	☐ TSH, 3rd Generation Ⓢ
604	☐ Electrolytes (Na, K, Cl)	Ⓢ	7708	☐ Lithium	Ⓢ	810	☐ Vitamin B-12 and Folate Ⓢ
4598	☐ Ferritin	Ⓢ	505	☐ Liver Profile A	Ⓢ		
4309	☐ Follicle Stim. Hormone (FSH)	Ⓢ	7401	☐ Phenytoin (Dilantin)	Ⓢ		
1818	☐ Glucose	Ⓖ	1180	☐ Potassium	Ⓢ		
	☐ Glucose Tolerance	Ⓖ	4556	☐ Pregnancy, Serum, Ql.	Ⓢ		
	Indicate No. Of Tubes _____		53520	☐ Prenatal Profile B with HBsAG	2-L Ⓡ		

ADDITIONAL TESTS

Test #	Name
☐ 1375	24 Hr Urine for Protein Ⓤ
☐ 4550	Pregnancy, Urine, Qul Ⓤ

URINE CHEMISTRY

3038	☐ Urinalysis (Microscopic if indicated) Ⓤ
3772	☐ Urinalysis, Complete Ⓤ

PROCEDURE 16-1 COLLECTING A CLEAN-CATCH MIDSTREAM URINE SPECIMEN

Name _____ Class _____ Date _____

⊔ ||||||||||||||||||
70Y

┌─────────────────────────────────────┐
│ Significant Clinical Information   │
│   │
│ _____ Fasting   _____ Non-Fasting │
│   │
│   CHEMISTRY   │
│   REQUEST   │
│   │
│   (EMBOSSING AREA)   │
└─────────────────────────────────────┘

Submit Separate Specimens (Not Request Forms) for each Frozen Test Requested.

Account No.

REV. 6/95

Specimen Date Mo Day Yr	Specimen Time Hr Min	Patient Name (Last)	(First, MI)	Sex	Date of Birth Mo Day Yr	Age Yrs Mos

50 8649 9000 4

* I certify that I have read the informed consent on the back and understand its content.

_____
Patient's Signature

Patient I.D. #	Physician I.D.	Patient/Resp. Party's Phone #
Responsible Party or Insured's Name (Last, First)		Patient's SS #
Address	City	State Zip Code

Resp. Party's Employer | Medicaid Number/HMO # | Medicare #

Physician Name | UPIN # | Physician's Signature | Provider #

Diagnosis Code (ICD-9) | Insurance Code or Company Name and Address | Insurance I.D. # | Workers Comp. Yes No

Group # or Name | Relationship to Insured (Circle One) 1-Self 2-Spouse 3-Other

---

Urine Random	† Ⓤ Total 24hr. Vol. _____ Ht. _____ Wt. _____

| (✱) = EDTA Plasma | Ⓢ = Serum | Ⓡ = Red | Ⓖ = Gray | Ⓑ = Light Blue |
| (AF) = Amniotic Fluid | Ⓕ = Frozen Specimen | Ⓛ = Lavender | (GN) = Green | (RB) = Royal Blue |

■ Apply Labels to Patient Specimens Only
Patient Control No. ➡

50 8649 9000 4   50 8649 9000 4   50 8649 9000 4

50 8649 9000 4

50 8649 9000 4   50 8649 9000 4   50 8649 9000 4

CHEMISTRY REQUEST

Code	Test		Code	Test		Code	Test	
58867	☐ Basic Chemistry	Ⓢ	1693	☐ Glycohemoglobin, Total	Ⓛ	4465	☐ Prolactin	Ⓢ
1396	☐ Amylase, Serum	Ⓢ	4416	☐ HCG, Beta Chain, Quant	Ⓢ	4747	☐ Prostatic Acid Phosphatase (EIA)	Ⓢ
6254	☐ Antinuclear Antibody (ANA), Qnt.	Ⓢ	1453	☐ Hemoglobin A1C	Ⓛ	10322	☐ Prostate-Specific Antigen (PSA)	Ⓢ
1040	☐ BUN	Ⓢ	6510	☐ Hepatitis B Surf Antigen (HBsAg)	Ⓢ	5199	☐ Prothrombin Time	Ⓑ
7419	☐ Carbamazepine (Tegretol)	Ⓢ	6395	☐ Hepatitis B Surf Antibody (Anti HBs)	Ⓢ	6502	☐ Ra Latex Screen	Ⓢ
5009	☐ CBC With Differential	Ⓛ	58560	☐ Hepatitis Profile I (Diagnostic)	Ⓢ	5215	☐ Sedimentation Rate	Ⓛ
2139	☐ CEA-EIA Roche	△ (✱)	46938	☐ Hepatitis Profile II (Follow up)	Ⓢ	6072	☐ STS	Ⓢ
98012	☐ Chlamydia by DNA Probe	△	58552	☐ Hepatitis Profile VII (A and B)	Ⓢ	1149	☐ T₄ (Thyroxine)	Ⓢ
96479	☐ Chlamydia/GC, DNA Probe	△	83824	☐ HIV-1 ABS-EIA	Ⓢ	7336	☐ Theophylline (Theo-Dur)	Ⓢ
1065	☐ Cholesterol, Total	Ⓢ	7625	☐ Lead, Blood	(RB)	620	☐ Thyroid Profile I	Ⓢ
1370	☐ Creatinine, Serum	Ⓢ	235002	☐ Lipid Profile I (Lipoprotein Analysis)	Ⓢ	27011	☐ Thyroid Profile II	Ⓢ
7385	☐ Digoxin (Lanoxin)	Ⓢ	235028	☐ Lipid Profile III (incl Apolipoproteins)	Ⓢ	4259	☐ TSH, 3rd Generation	Ⓢ
604	☐ Electrolytes (Na, K, Cl)	Ⓢ	7708	☐ Lithium	Ⓢ	810	☐ Vitamin B-12 and Folate	Ⓢ
4598	☐ Ferritin	Ⓢ	505	☐ Liver Profile A	Ⓢ			
4309	☐ Follicle Stim. Hormone (FSH)	Ⓢ	7401	☐ Phenytoin (Dilantin)	Ⓢ	**URINE CHEMISTRY**		
1818	☐ Glucose	Ⓖ	1180	☐ Potassium	Ⓢ	3038	☐ Urinalysis (Microscopic if indicated)	Ⓤ
	☐ Glucose Tolerance	Ⓖ	4556	☐ Pregnancy, Serum, Ql.	Ⓢ	3772	☐ Urinalysis, Complete	Ⓤ
	Indicate No. Of Tubes _____		53520	☐ Prenatal Profile B with HBsAG	(2-L)(Ⓡ)			

ADDITIONAL TESTS

Test #	Name
☐ 1375	24 Hr Urine for Protein Ⓤ
☐ 4550	Pregnancy, Urine, Qul Ⓤ

PROCEDURE 16-2 COLLECTING A URINE SPECIMEN FROM A PEDIATRIC PATIENT

Name _____ Class _____ Date _____

Total Care Clinic
Progress Notes

Name: _____ Chart #: _____

DATE	

PROCEDURE 16-3 ESTABLISHING A CHAIN OF CUSTODY FOR A URINE SPECIMEN

Name _____ Class _____ Date _____

Total Care Clinic
Newfield, New Jersey 07655-3213
201-555-4000

Drug Screen Consent Form

A urine drug test is required by_____ as part of your pre-employment screening. Please provide us with a list of all medications that you are presently taking.

_____

_____

_____

_____

_____

I understand that my prospective or continued employment is contingent on a successful screening.

Date: _____ Signature:_____

Witness: _____

PROCEDURE 16-3 ESTABLISHING A CHAIN OF CUSTODY FOR A URINE SPECIMEN *(continued)*

Name _____ Class _____ Date _____

Total Care Clinic
Progress Notes

Name: _____ Chart #: _____

DATE	

PROCEDURE 16-3 ESTABLISHING A CHAIN OF CUSTODY FOR A URINE SPECIMEN *(concluded)*

Name _____ Class _____ Date _____

CHAIN OF CUSTODY FORM

TOTAL CARE LABORATORY

542 East Park Boulevard
Funton, XY 12345-6789
(521) 234-0001

SPECIMEN I.D. NO:

STEP 1—TO BE COMPLETED BY COLLECTOR OR EMPLOYER REPRESENTATIVE.

Employer Name, Address, and I.D. No.:   OR   Medical Review Officer Name and Address:

_____   _____

_____   _____

_____   _____

Donor Social Security No. or Employee I.D. No.: _____

Donor I.D. verified: ❏ Photo I.D.   ❏ Employer Representative _____
Signature

Reason for test: (check one)   ❏ Preemployment   ❏ Random   ❏ Postaccident

❏ Periodic   ❏ Reasonable suspicion/cause

❏ Return to duty   ❏ Other (specify)

Test(s) to be performed: _____   Total tests ordered: [   ]

Type of specimen obtained: ❏ Urine   ❏ Blood   ❏ Semen   ❏ Other (specify)

Submit only one specimen with each requisition.

STEP 2—TO BE COMPLETED BY COLLECTOR.

For urine specimens, read temperature within 4 minutes of collection.
Check here if specimen temperature is within range.   ❏ Yes, 90°–100°F/32°–38°C
Or record actual temperature here: _____

STEP 3—TO BE COMPLETED BY COLLECTOR.

Collection site: _____   Address _____

City _____   State _____   Zip _____   Phone _____

Collection date: _____   Time: _____   ❏ a.m.   ❏ p.m.

I certify that the specimen identified on this form is the specimen presented to me by the donor identified in step 1 above, and that it was collected, labeled, and sealed in the donor's presence.

Collector's name: _____   Signature of collector _____

STEP 4—TO BE INITIATED BY DONOR AND COMPLETED AS NECESSARY THEREAFTER.

Purpose of change	Released by Signature	Received by Signature	Date
A. Provide specimen for testing			
B. Shipment to Laboratory			
C.			

Comments:

STEP 5—TO BE COMPLETED BY THE LABORATORY:

Specimen package seal(s) intact when received in lab?   ❏ Yes   ❏ No. If no, explain.

Laboratory receiver's initials _____

Copy 1 - Original - Must accompany specimen to laboratory.

PROCEDURE 16-4 MEASURING SPECIFIC GRAVITY WITH A REFRACTOMETER

Name _____ Class _____ Date _____

Total Care Clinic
Laboratory Report Form

Patient Name _____Medical Record # _____ Age _____ Sex_____

Address _____ Phone _____

Referring Physician _____

Laboratory Findings:

Date	Blood Test	Patient Result	Normal Value/Range

Date	Urinalysis	Patient Result	Normal Value/Range

Test completed by: _____ _____
                        (Print name)   (Signature)

PROCEDURE 16-5 PERFORMING A REAGENT STRIP TEST

Name _____ Class _____ Date _____

Total Care Clinic
Laboratory Report Form

Patient Name _____Medical Record # _____ Age _____ Sex_____

Address _____ Phone _____

Referring Physician _____

Laboratory Findings:

Date	Blood Test	Patient Result	Normal Value/Range

Date	Urinalysis	Patient Result	Normal Value/Range

Test completed by: _____   _____
                         (Print name)   (Signature)

PROCEDURE 16-6 PREGNANCY TESTING USING THE EIA METHOD

Total Care Clinic
Progress Notes

Name: _____ Chart #:_____

DATE	

Name _____ Class _____ Date _____

Quality Control Daily Log

Name of Unit	Glucose Control Solution	Strip Lot No./ Exp. Date	Low Control Value 35–65 mg/dL	High Control Value 175–235 mg/dL	Analyzed By	Date	Remedial Action Taken If Control Values Abnormal	Retest After Remedial Action Taken

PROCEDURE 16-7 PROCESSING A URINE SPECIMEN FOR MICROSCOPIC EXAMINATION OF SEDIMENT

Name _____ Class _____ Date _____

Total Care Clinic
Laboratory Report Form

Patient Name _____ Medical Record # _____ Age _____ Sex_____

Address _____ Phone _____

Referring Physician _____

Laboratory Findings:

Date	Blood Test	Patient Result	Normal Value/Range

Date	Urinalysis	Patient Result	Normal Value/Range

Test completed by: _____   _____
                          (Print name)   (Signature)

PROCEDURE 16-7 PROCESSING A URINE SPECIMEN FOR MICROSCOPIC EXAMINATION OF SEDIMENT *(concluded)*

Name _____ Class _____ Date _____

Total Care Clinic
Progress Notes

Name: _____ Chart #: _____

DATE	

PROCEDURE 17-1 QUALITY CONTROL PROCEDURES FOR BLOOD SPECIMEN COLLECTION

Name _____ Class _____ Date _____

Significant Clinical Information

_____ Fasting   _____ Non-Fasting

CHEMISTRY REQUEST

(EMBOSSING AREA)

Submit Separate Specimens (Not Request Forms) for each Frozen Test Requested.

Account No.

Specimen Date Mo Day Yr	Specimen Time Hr Min	Patient Name (Last)	(First, MI)	Sex	Date of Birth Mo Day Yr	Age Yrs Mos

| **50 8649 9000 4** | Patient I.D. # | Physician I.D. | Patient/Resp. Party's Phone # |

* I certify that I have read the informed consent on the back and understand its content.

Patient's Signature

| Responsible Party or Insured's Name (Last, First) | | Patient's SS # |

REV. 6/95

| Address | City | State | Zip Code |

| Resp. Party's Employer | Medicaid Number/HMO # | Medicare # |

| Physician Name | UPIN # | Physician's Signature | Provider # |

| Diagnosis Code (ICD-9) | Insurance Code or Company Name and Address | Insurance I.D. # | Workers Comp. Yes No |

| Group # or Name | Relationship to Insured (Circle One) 1-Self 2-Spouse 3-Other |

Urine Random   † Ⓤ Total 24hr. Vol. _____ Ht. _____ Wt. _____

| ✷ = EDTA Plasma | Ⓢ = Serum | Ⓡ = Red | Ⓖ = Gray | Ⓑ = Light Blue |
| AF = Amniotic Fluid | Ⓕ = Frozen Specimen | Ⓛ = Lavender | GN = Green | RB = Royal Blue |

Apply Labels to Patient Specimens Only
Patient Control No. ➡

50 8649 9000 4
50 8649 9000 4

50 8649 9000 4
50 8649 9000 4

50 8649 9000 4
50 8649 9000 4

50 8649 9000 4

CHEMISTRY REQUEST

58867	☐ Basic Chemistry	Ⓢ	1693	☐ Glycohemoglobin, Total	Ⓛ	4465	☐ Prolactin	Ⓢ	
1396	☐ Amylase, Serum	Ⓢ	4416	☐ HCG, Beta Chain, Quant	Ⓢ	4747	☐ Prostatic Acid Phosphatase (EIA)	Ⓢ	
6254	☐ Antinuclear Antibody (ANA), Qnt.	Ⓢ	1453	☐ Hemoglobin A1C	Ⓛ	10322	☐ Prostate-Specific Antigen (PSA)	Ⓢ	
1040	☐ BUN	Ⓢ	6510	☐ Hepatitis B Surf Antigen (HBsAg)	Ⓢ	5199	☐ Prothrombin Time	Ⓑ	
7419	☐ Carbamazepine (Tegretol)	Ⓢ	6395	☐ Hepatitis B Surf Antibody (Anti HBs)	Ⓢ	6502	☐ Ra Latex Screen	Ⓢ	
5009	☐ CBC With Differential	Ⓛ	58560	☐ Hepatitis Profile I (Diagnostic)	Ⓢ	5215	☐ Sedimentation Rate	Ⓛ	
2139	☐ CEA-EIA Roche	△ ✷	46938	☐ Hepatitis Profile II (Follow up)	Ⓢ	6072	☐ STS	Ⓢ	
98012	☐ Chlamydia by DNA Probe	△	58552	☐ Hepatitis Profile VII (A and B)	Ⓢ	1149	☐ T₄ (Thyroxine)	Ⓢ	
96479	☐ Chlamydia/GC, DNA Probe	△	83824	☐ HIV-1 ABS-EIA	Ⓢ	7336	☐ Theophylline (Theo-Dur)	Ⓢ	
1065	☐ Cholesterol, Total	Ⓢ	7625	☐ Lead, Blood	RB	620	☐ Thyroid Profile I	Ⓢ	
1370	☐ Creatinine, Serum	Ⓢ	235002	☐ Lipid Profile I (Lipoprotein Analysis)	Ⓢ	27011	☐ Thyroid Profile II	Ⓢ	
7385	☐ Digoxin (Lanoxin)	Ⓢ	235028	☐ Lipid Profile III (incl Apolipoproteins)	Ⓢ	4259	☐ TSH, 3rd Generation	Ⓢ	
604	☐ Electrolytes (Na, K, Cl)	Ⓢ	7708	☐ Lithium	Ⓢ	810	☐ Vitamin B-12 and Folate	Ⓢ	
4598	☐ Ferritin	Ⓢ	505	☐ Liver Profile A					
4309	☐ Follicle Stim. Hormone (FSH)	Ⓢ	7401	☐ Phenytoin (Dilantin)	Ⓢ		**URINE CHEMISTRY**		
1818	☐ Glucose	Ⓖ	1180	☐ Potassium	Ⓢ	3038	☐ Urinalysis (Microscopic if indicated)	Ⓤ	
	☐ Glucose Tolerance	Ⓖ	4556	☐ Pregnancy, Serum, Ql.	Ⓢ	3772	☐ Urinalysis, Complete	Ⓤ	
	Indicate No. Of Tubes _____		53520	☐ Prenatal Profile B with HBsAG	2-L Ⓡ				

ADDITIONAL TESTS

Test #	Name
☐ 1375	24 Hr Urine for Protein Ⓤ
☐ 4550	Pregnancy, Urine, Qul Ⓤ

PROCEDURE 17-2 PERFORMING VENIPUNCTURE USING AN EVACUATION SYSTEM

Name _____ Class _____ Date _____

<table>
<tr><td colspan="2" align="center">**Total Care Clinic**
Progress Notes</td></tr>
<tr><td colspan="2">Name: _____ Chart #: _____</td></tr>
<tr><td>DATE</td><td></td></tr>
<tr><td></td><td></td></tr>
<tr><td></td><td></td></tr>
<tr><td></td><td></td></tr>
<tr><td></td><td></td></tr>
<tr><td></td><td></td></tr>
<tr><td></td><td></td></tr>
<tr><td></td><td></td></tr>
<tr><td></td><td></td></tr>
<tr><td></td><td></td></tr>
<tr><td></td><td></td></tr>
<tr><td></td><td></td></tr>
<tr><td></td><td></td></tr>
<tr><td></td><td></td></tr>
<tr><td></td><td></td></tr>
<tr><td></td><td></td></tr>
<tr><td></td><td></td></tr>
<tr><td></td><td></td></tr>
<tr><td></td><td></td></tr>
</table>

Name _____ Class _____ Date _____

70Y

Account No.

Specimen Date Mo Day Yr	Specimen Time Hr Min	Patient Name (Last)	(First, MI)	Sex	Date of Birth Mo Day Yr	Age Yrs Mos

50 8649 9000 4

Patient I.D. #	Physician I.D.	Patient/Resp. Party's Phone #

* I certify that I have read the informed consent on the back and understand its content.

Responsible Party or Insured's Name (Last, First)	Patient's SS #

Patient's Signature

Address	City	State	Zip Code

REV. 6/95

Resp. Party's Employer	Medicaid Number/HMO #	Medicare #

Physician Name	UPIN #	Physician's Signature	Provider #

Diagnosis Code (ICD-9)	Insurance Code or Company Name and Address	Insurance I.D. #	Workers Comp. Yes No

Group # or Name	Relationship to Insured (Circle One) 1-Self 2-Spouse 3-Other

Urine Random   † Ⓤ Total 24hr. Vol. _____ Ht. _____ Wt. _____

✸ EDTA Plasma	Ⓢ = Serum	Ⓡ = Red	Ⓖ = Gray	Ⓑ = Light Blue
AF = Amniotic Fluid	Ⓕ = Frozen Specimen	Ⓛ = Lavender	GN = Green	RB = Royal Blue

Apply Labels to Patient Specimens Only Patient Control No.

50 8649 9000 4

50 8649 9000 4   50 8649 9000 4   50 8649 9000 4

CHEMISTRY REQUEST

#	Test		#	Test		#	Test	
58867	☐ Basic Chemistry	Ⓢ	1693	☐ Glycohemoglobin, Total	Ⓛ	4465	☐ Prolactin	Ⓢ
1396	☐ Amylase, Serum	Ⓢ	4416	☐ HCG, Beta Chain, Quant	Ⓢ	4747	☐ Prostatic Acid Phosphatase (EIA)	Ⓢ
6254	☐ Antinuclear Antibody (ANA), Qnt.	Ⓢ	1453	☐ Hemoglobin A1C	Ⓛ	10322	☐ Prostate-Specific Antigen (PSA)	Ⓢ
1040	☐ BUN	Ⓢ	6510	☐ Hepatitis B Surf Antigen (HBsAg)	Ⓢ	5199	☐ Prothrombin Time	Ⓑ
7419	☐ Carbamazepine (Tegretol)	Ⓢ	6395	☐ Hepatitis B Surf Antibody (Anti HBs)	Ⓢ	6502	☐ Ra Latex Screen	Ⓢ
5009	☐ CBC With Differential	Ⓛ	58560	☐ Hepatitis Profile I (Diagnostic)	Ⓢ	5215	☐ Sedimentation Rate	Ⓛ
2139	☐ CEA-EIA Roche	△ ✸	46938	☐ Hepatitis Profile II (Follow up)	Ⓢ	6072	☐ STS	Ⓢ
98012	☐ Chlamydia by DNA Probe	△	58552	☐ Hepatitis Profile VII (A and B)	Ⓢ	1149	☐ T₄ (Thyroxine)	Ⓢ
96479	☐ Chlamydia/GC, DNA Probe	△	83824	☐ HIV-1 ABS-EIA	Ⓢ	7336	☐ Theophylline (Theo-Dur)	Ⓢ
1065	☐ Cholesterol, Total	Ⓢ	7625	☐ Lead, Blood	RB	620	☐ Thyroid Profile I	Ⓢ
1370	☐ Creatinine, Serum	Ⓢ	235002	☐ Lipid Profile I (Lipoprotein Analysis)	Ⓢ	27011	☐ Thyroid Profile II	Ⓢ
7385	☐ Digoxin (Lanoxin)	Ⓢ	235028	☐ Lipid Profile III (incl Apolipoproteins)	Ⓢ	4259	☐ TSH, 3rd Generation	Ⓢ
604	☐ Electrolytes (Na, K, Cl)	Ⓢ	7708	☐ Lithium	Ⓢ	810	☐ Vitamin B-12 and Folate	Ⓢ
4598	☐ Ferritin	Ⓢ	505	☐ Liver Profile A	Ⓢ			
4309	☐ Follicle Stim. Hormone (FSH)	Ⓢ	7401	☐ Phenytoin (Dilantin)	Ⓢ	**URINE CHEMISTRY**		
1818	☐ Glucose	Ⓖ	1180	☐ Potassium	Ⓢ	3038	☐ Urinalysis (Microscopic if indicated)	Ⓤ
	☐ Glucose Tolerance	Ⓖ	4556	☐ Pregnancy, Serum, Ql.	Ⓢ	3772	☐ Urinalysis, Complete	Ⓤ
	Indicate No. Of Tubes _____		53520	☐ Prenatal Profile B with HBsAG	2-L Ⓡ			

ADDITIONAL TESTS

Test # | Name

☐ 1375 24 Hr Urine for Protein Ⓤ

☐ 4550 Pregnancy, Urine, Qul Ⓤ

PROCEDURE 17-2 PERFORMING VENIPUNCTURE USING AN EVACUATION SYSTEM (concluded)

Name _____ Class _____ Date _____

Total Care Clinic
Laboratory Report Form

Patient Name _____ Medical Record # _____ Age _____ Sex_____

Address _____ Phone _____

Referring Physician _____

Laboratory Findings:

Date	Blood Test	Patient Result	Normal Value/Range

Date	Urinalysis	Patient Result	Normal Value/Range

Test completed by: _____ _____
              (Print name)   (Signature)

Procedure 17-3 Performing Capillary Puncture

Name _____ Class _____ Date _____

Total Care Clinic
Progress Notes

Name: _____ Chart #: _____

DATE	

Name _____ Class _____ Date _____

||||70Y

Significant Clinical Information

_____ Fasting   _____ Non-Fasting

CHEMISTRY REQUEST

(EMBOSSING AREA)

Submit Separate Specimens (Not Request Forms) for each Frozen Test Requested.

Account No.

Specimen Date Mo Day Yr	Specimen Time Hr Min	Patient Name (Last)	(First, MI)	Sex	Date of Birth Mo Day Yr	Age Yrs Mos

50 8649 9000 4

* I certify that I have read the informed consent on the back and understand its content.

Patient I.D. #   Physician I.D.   Patient/Resp. Party's Phone #

Responsible Party or Insured's Name (Last, First)   Patient's SS #

Patient's Signature

Address   City   State   Zip Code

Resp. Party's Employer   Medicaid Number/HMO #   Medicare #

Physician Name   UPIN #   Physician's Signature   Provider #

Diagnosis Code (ICD-9)   Insurance Code or Company Name and Address   Insurance I.D. #   Workers Comp. Yes No

Group # or Name   Relationship to Insured (Circle One) 1-Self 2-Spouse 3-Other

REV. 6/95

Urine Random   † Ⓤ Total 24hr. Vol. _____ Ht. _____ Wt. _____

| ✱ = EDTA Plasma | Ⓢ = Serum | Ⓡ = Red | Ⓖ = Gray | Ⓑ = Light Blue |
| AF = Amniotic Fluid | Ⓕ = Frozen Specimen | Ⓛ = Lavender | GN = Green | RB = Royal Blue |

Apply Labels to Patient Specimens Only   Patient Control No.

50 8649 9000 4

CHEMISTRY REQUEST

58867	☐ Basic Chemistry Ⓢ	1693	☐ Glycohemoglobin, Total Ⓛ	4465	☐ Prolactin Ⓢ	**ADDITIONAL TESTS**	
1396	☐ Amylase, Serum Ⓢ	4416	☐ HCG, Beta Chain, Quant Ⓢ	4747	☐ Prostatic Acid Phosphatase (EIA) Ⓢ	Test #	Name
6254	☐ Antinuclear Antibody (ANA), Qnt. Ⓢ	1453	☐ Hemoglobin A1C Ⓛ	10322	☐ Prostate-Specific Antigen (PSA) Ⓢ		
1040	☐ BUN Ⓢ	6510	☐ Hepatitis B Surf Antigen (HBsAg) Ⓢ	5199	☐ Prothrombin Time Ⓑ	☐ 1375 24 Hr Urine for Protein Ⓤ	
7419	☐ Carbamazepine (Tegretol) Ⓢ	6395	☐ Hepatitis B Surf Antibody (Anti HBs) Ⓢ	6502	☐ Ra Latex Screen Ⓢ		
5009	☐ CBC With Differential Ⓛ	58560	☐ Hepatitis Profile I (Diagnostic) Ⓢ	5215	☐ Sedimentation Rate Ⓛ	☐ 4550 Pregnancy, Urine, Qul Ⓤ	
2139	☐ CEA-EIA Roche △ ✱	46938	☐ Hepatitis Profile II (Follow up) Ⓢ	6072	☐ STS Ⓢ		
98012	☐ Chlamydia by DNA Probe △	58552	☐ Hepatitis Profile VII (A and B) Ⓢ	1149	☐ T₄ (Thyroxine) Ⓢ		
96479	☐ Chlamydia/GC, DNA Probe △	83824	☐ HIV-1 ABS-EIA Ⓢ	7336	☐ Theophylline (Theo-Dur) Ⓢ		
1065	☐ Cholesterol, Total Ⓢ	7625	☐ Lead, Blood RB	620	☐ Thyroid Profile I Ⓢ		
1370	☐ Creatinine, Serum Ⓢ	235002	☐ Lipid Profile I (Lipoprotein Analysis) Ⓢ	27011	☐ Thyroid Profile II Ⓢ		
7385	☐ Digoxin (Lanoxin) Ⓢ	235028	☐ Lipid Profile III (incl Apolipoproteins) Ⓢ	4259	☐ TSH, 3rd Generation Ⓢ		
604	☐ Electrolytes (Na, K, Cl) Ⓢ	7708	☐ Lithium Ⓢ	810	☐ Vitamin B-12 and Folate Ⓢ		
4598	☐ Ferritin Ⓢ	505	☐ Liver Profile A Ⓢ	**URINE CHEMISTRY**			
4309	☐ Follicle Stim. Hormone (FSH) Ⓢ	7401	☐ Phenytoin (Dilantin) Ⓢ	3038	☐ Urinalysis (Microscopic if indicated) Ⓤ		
1818	☐ Glucose Ⓖ	1180	☐ Potassium Ⓢ	3772	☐ Urinalysis, Complete Ⓤ		
	☐ Glucose Tolerance Ⓖ	4556	☐ Pregnancy, Serum, Ql. Ⓢ				
	Indicate No. Of Tubes	53520	☐ Prenatal Profile B with HBsAG 2-L Ⓡ				

PROCEDURE 17-5 MEASURING HEMATOCRIT PERCENTAGE AFTER CENTRIFUGE

Name _____ Class _____ Date _____

Total Care Clinic
Laboratory Report Form

Patient Name _____ Medical Record # _____ Age _____ Sex _____

Address _____ Phone _____

Referring Physician _____

Laboratory Findings:

Date	Blood Test	Patient Result	Normal Value/Range

Date	Urinalysis	Patient Result	Normal Value/Range

Test completed by: _____ _____
(Print name)   (Signature)

PROCEDURE 17-6 MEASURING BLOOD GLUCOSE USING A HANDHELD GLUCOMETER

Name _____ Class _____ Date _____

Total Care Clinic
Laboratory Report Form

Patient Name _____Medical Record # _____ Age _____ Sex_____

Address _____ Phone _____

Referring Physician _____

Laboratory Findings:

Date	Blood Test	Patient Result	Normal Value/Range

Date	Urinalysis	Patient Result	Normal Value/Range

Test completed by: _____ _____
(Print name)   (Signature)

PROCEDURE 17-6 MEASURING BLOOD GLUCOSE USING A HANDHELD GLUCOMETER *(concluded)*

Name _____ Class _____ Date _____

Quality Control Daily Log

Name of Unit	Glucose Control Solution	Strip Lot No./ Exp. Date	Low Control Value 35–65 mg/dL	High Control Value 175–235 mg/dL	Analyzed By	Date	Remedial Action Taken If Control Values Abnormal	Retest After Remedial Action Taken

PROCEDURE 18-1 EDUCATING PATIENTS ABOUT DAILY WATER REQUIREMENTS

Name _____ Class _____ Date _____

Total Care Clinic
Progress Notes

Name: _____ Chart #: _____

DATE	

PROCEDURE 18-2 TEACHING PATIENTS HOW TO READ FOOD LABELS

Name _____ Class _____ Date _____

Total Care Clinic
Progress Notes

Name: _____ Chart #: _____

DATE	

Procedure 18-3 Alerting Patients with Food Allergies to the Dangers or Common Foods

Name _____ Class _____ Date _____

<table>
<tr><td colspan="2" align="center">**Total Care Clinic**
Progress Notes</td></tr>
<tr><td colspan="2">Name: _____ Chart #: _____</td></tr>
<tr><td>DATE</td><td></td></tr>
<tr><td></td><td></td></tr>
<tr><td></td><td></td></tr>
<tr><td></td><td></td></tr>
<tr><td></td><td></td></tr>
<tr><td></td><td></td></tr>
<tr><td></td><td></td></tr>
<tr><td></td><td></td></tr>
<tr><td></td><td></td></tr>
<tr><td></td><td></td></tr>
<tr><td></td><td></td></tr>
<tr><td></td><td></td></tr>
<tr><td></td><td></td></tr>
<tr><td></td><td></td></tr>
<tr><td></td><td></td></tr>
<tr><td></td><td></td></tr>
<tr><td></td><td></td></tr>
<tr><td></td><td></td></tr>
<tr><td></td><td></td></tr>
<tr><td></td><td></td></tr>
</table>

PROCEDURE 19-1 HELPING THE PHYSICIAN COMPLY WITH THE CONTROLLED SUBSTANCES ACT OF 1970

Name _____ Class _____ Date _____

Sample Only

Form-224	**APPLICATION FOR REGISTRATION** **Under the Controlled Substances Act**	APPROVED OMB NO 1117-0014 **FORM DEA-224 (10-06)** Previous editions are obsolete

INSTRUCTIONS   **Save time—apply on-line at www.deadiversion.usdoj.gov**

1. To apply by mail complete this application. Keep a copy for your records.
2. Print clearly, using black or blue ink, or use a typewriter.
3. Mail this form to the address provided in Section 7 or use enclosed envelope.
4. Include the correct payment amount. FEE IS NON-REFUNDABLE.
5. If you have any questions call 800-882-9539 prior to submitting your application.

IMPORTANT: DO NOT SEND THIS APPLICATION AND APPLY ON-LINE.

DEA OFFICIAL USE:

Do you have other DEA registration numbers?
☐ NO   ☐ YES

MAIL-TO ADDRESS   Please print mailing address changes to the right of the address in this box.

FEE FOR THREE (3) YEARS IS $551
FEE IS NON-REFUNDABLE

SECTION 1   **APPLICANT IDENTIFICATION**   ☐ **Individual Registration**   ☐ **Business Registration**

Name 1   (Last Name of individual -OR- Business or Facility Name)

Name 2   (First Name and Middle Name of individual -OR- Continuation of business name)

Street Address Line 1 (if applying for fee exemption, this must be address of the fee exempt institution)

Address Line 2

City   State   Zip Code

Business Phone Number   Point of Contact

Business Fax Number   Email Address

DEBT COLLECTION INFORMATION

Mandatory pursuant to Debt Collection Improvements Act

Social Security Number (*if registration is for individual*)

Provide **SSN** or **TIN**. See additional information note #3 on page 4.

Tax Identification Number (*if registration is for business*)

FOR Practitioner or MLP ONLY:

Professional Degree: *select from list only*

Professional School:

Year of Graduation:

National Provider Identification:

Date of Birth (*MM-DD-YYYY*):

SECTION 2   **BUSINESS ACTIVITY**

Check one business activity box only

☐ Central Fill Pharmacy
☐ Retail Pharmacy
☐ Nursing Home
☐ Automated Dispensing System

☐ Practitioner (DDS, DMD, DO, DPM, DVM, MD or PHD)
☐ Practitioner Military (DDS, DMD, DO, DPM, DVM, MD or PHD)
☐ Mid-level Practitioner (MLP) (DOM, HMD, MP, ND, NP, OD, PA, or RPH)
☐ Euthanasia Technician

☐ Ambulance Service
☐ Animal Shelter
☐ Hospital/Clinic
☐ Teaching Institution

FOR Automated Dispensing System (ADS) ONLY:

DEA Registration # of Retail Pharmacy for this ADS

An ADS is automatically fee-exempt. Skip Section 6 and Section 7 on page 2. You must attach a notorized affidavit.

SECTION 3   **DRUG SCHEDULES**

Check all that apply

☐ Schedule II Narcotic
☐ Schedule II Non-Narcotic

☐ Schedule III Narcotic
☐ Schedule III Non-Narcotic

☐ Schedule IV
☐ Schedule V

PROCEDURE 19-1 HELPING THE PHYSICIAN COMPLY WITH THE CONTROLLED SUBSTANCES ACT OF 1970 *(continued)*

Name _____ Class _____ Date _____

Sample Only

SECTION 4 **STATE LICENSE(S)** Be sure to include both state license numbers if applicable	You MUST be currently authorized to prescribe, distribute, dispense, conduct research, or otherwise handle the controlled substances in the schedules for which you are applying under the laws of the **state** or jurisdiction in which you are operating or propose to operate. State License Number (required) [ ][ ][ ][ ][ ][ ][ ][ ][ ][ ][ ][ ][ ][ ][ ] Expiration Date (required) / / MM - DD - YYYY What state was this license issued in? _____ State Controlled Substance License Number (if required) [ ][ ][ ][ ][ ][ ][ ][ ][ ][ ][ ][ ][ ][ ] Expiration Date / / MM - DD - YYYY What state was this license issued in? _____

SECTION 5

LIABILITY

IMPORTANT

All questions in this section must be answered.

1. Has the applicant ever been **convicted of a crime** in connection with controlled substance(s) under state or federal law, or is any such action pending?   YES ☐ NO ☐

   Date(s) of incident MM-DD-YYYY: [ ][ ] – [ ][ ] – [ ][ ][ ][ ]

2. Has the applicant ever surrendered (for cause) or had a **federal** controlled substance registration revoked, suspended, restricted, or denied, or is any such action pending?   YES ☐ NO ☐

   Date(s) of incident MM-DD-YYYY: [ ][ ] – [ ][ ] – [ ][ ][ ][ ]

3. Has the applicant ever surrendered (for cause) or had a **state** professional license or controlled substance registration revoked, suspended, denied, restricted, or placed on probation, or is any such action pending?   YES ☐ NO ☐

   Date(s) of incident MM-DD-YYYY: [ ][ ] – [ ][ ] – [ ][ ][ ][ ]

4. If the applicant is a **corporation** (other than a corporation whose stock is owned and traded by the public), association, partnership, or pharmacy, has any officer, partner, stockholder, or proprietor been **convicted of a crime** in connection with controlled substance(s) under state or federal law, or ever surrendered, for cause, or had a **federal** controlled substance registration revoked, suspended, restricted, denied, or ever had a **state** professional license or controlled substance registration revoked, suspended, denied, restricted or placed on probation, or is any such action pending?   YES ☐ NO ☐

   Date(s) of incident MM-DD-YYYY: [ ][ ] – [ ][ ] – [ ][ ][ ][ ]   *Note: If question 4 does not apply to you, be sure to mark 'NO'. It will slow down processing of your application if you leave it blank.*

- -

EXPLANATION OF "YES" ANSWERS

Applicants who have answered "YES" to any of the four questions above **must provide a statement to explain each "YES" answer.**

Use this space or attach a separate sheet and return with application

Liability question # _____   Location(s) of incident: _____

Nature of incident:

Disposition of incident:

SECTION 6   EXEMPTION FROM APPLICATION FEE

☐ Check this box if the applicant is a federal, state, or local government official or institution. Does not apply to contractor-operated institutions.

Business or Facility Name of Fee Exempt Institution. **Be sure to enter the address of this exempt institution in Section 1.**

[ ]

FEE EXEMPT CERTIFIER

Provide the name and phone number of the certifying official

The undersigned hereby certifies that the applicant named hereon is a federal, state or local government official or institution, and is exempt from payment of the application fee.

_____   Date
Signature of certifying official (other than applicant)

_____   _____
Print or type name and title of certifying official   Telephone No. (required for verification)

SECTION 7
METHOD OF PAYMENT

Check one form of payment only

Sign if paying by credit card

☐ Check   Make check payable to: **Drug Enforcement Administration**
See page 4 of instructions for important information.

☐ American Express ☐ Discover ☐ Master Card ☐ Visa

Credit Card Number [ ][ ][ ][ ][ ][ ][ ][ ][ ][ ][ ][ ][ ][ ][ ][ ]   Expiration Date [ ][ ] – [ ][ ]

_____
Signature of Card Holder

_____
Printed Name of Card Holder

Mail this form with payment to:

U.S. Department of Justice
Drug Enforcement Administration
P.O. Box 28083
Washington, DC 20038-8083

FEE IS NON-REFUNDABLE

SECTION 8
APPLICANTS SIGNATURE

Sign in ink

I certify that the foregoing information furnished on this application is true and correct.

_____   _____
Signature of applicant (sign in ink)   Date

_____
Print or type name and title of applicant

WARNING: Section 843(a)(4)(A) of Title 21, United States Code states that any person who knowingly or intentionally furnishes false or fraudulent information in this application is subject to imprisonment for not more than four years, a fine of not more than $30,000,00 or both.

Name _____ Class _____ Date _____

Sample Only

DEA Form-222 (Oct. 1992)	**U.S. OFFICIAL ORDER FORMS - SCHEDULES I & II** Drug Enforcement Administration **SUPPLIER'S Copy 1**

See Reverse of PURCHASER'S Copy for Instructions	No order form may be issued for Schedule I and II substances unless a completed application form has been received. (21 CFR 1305.04).	OMB APPROVAL No. 1117-0010

To: (Name of Supplier)

Street Address

Address

City   State

Date (MM-DD-YYYY)   Suppliers DEA Registration No.

To Be Filled in By **PURCHASER**   To Be Filled in By **SUPPLIER**

Line No.	No. of Packages	Size of Package	Name of Item	National Drug Code	Packages Shipped	Date Shipped
1						
2						
3						
4						
5						
6						
7						
8						
9						
10						

◀ **LAST LINE COMPLETED** *(MUST BE 10 OR LESS)*

Signature of **PURCHASER** or Attorney or Agent

Date Issued   DEA Registration No.

Schedules   Name and Address of Registrant

Registered As a

No. of This Order Form

PROCEDURE 19-1 HELPING THE PHYSICIAN COMPLY WITH THE CONTROLLED SUBSTANCES ACT OF 1970 (concluded)

Name _____ Class _____ Date _____

Sample Only

OMB Approval No. 1117-0007	U.S. Department of Justice/Drug Enforcement Administration **REGISTRANTS INVENTORY OF DRUGS SURRENDERED**	PACKAGE NO.

The following schedule is an inventory of controlled substances which is hereby surrendered to you for proper disposition.

FROM: *(Include Name, Street, City, State and ZIP Code in space provided below.)*

Signature of applicant or authorized agent

Registrant's DEA Number

Registrant's Telephone Number

NOTE: CERTIFIED MAIL (Return Receipt Requested) IS REQUIRED FOR SHIPMENTS OF DRUGS VIA U.S. POSTAL SERVICE. See instructions on reverse (page 2) of form.

NAME OF DRUG OR PREPARATION Registrants will fill in Columns 1, 2, 3, and 4 ONLY.	Number of Containers	CONTENTS (Number of grams, tablets, ounces or other units per container)	Controlled Substance Content, (Each Unit)	FOR DEA USE ONLY		
				DISPOSITION	QUANTITY	
					GMS.	MGS.
1	*2*	*3*	*4*	*5*	*6*	*7*
1						
2						
3						
4						
5						
6						
23						
24						

The controlled substances surrendered in accordance with Title 21 of the Code of Federal Regulations, Section 1307.21, have been received in _____ packages purporting to contain the drugs listed on this inventory and have been: **(1) Forwarded tape-sealed without opening; (2) Destroyed as indicated and the remainder forwarded tape-sealed after verifying contents; (3) Forwarded tape-sealed after verifying contents.

DATE _____   DESTROYED BY: _____

**Strike out lines not applicable.*   WITNESSED BY: _____

INSTRUCTIONS

1. List the name of the drug in column 1, the number of containers in column 2, the size of each container in column 3, and in column 4 the controlled substance content of each unit described in column 3; e.g., morphine sulfate tabs., 3 pkgs., 100 tabs., 1/4 gr. (16 mg.) or morphine sulfate tabs., 1 pkg., 83 tabs., 1/2 gr. (32 mg.), etc.
2. All packages included on a single line should be identical in name, content and controlled substance strength.
3. Prepare this form in quadruplicate. Mail two (2) copies of this form to the Special Agent in Charge, under separate cover. Enclose one additional copy in the shipment with the drugs. Retain one copy for your records. One copy will be returned to you as a receipt. No further receipt will be furnished to you unless specifically requested. Any further inquiries concerning these drugs should be addressed to the DEA District Office which serves your area.
4. There is no provision for payment for drugs surrendered. This is merely a service rendered to registrants enabling them to clear their stocks and records of unwanted items.
5. Drugs should be shipped tape-sealed via prepaid express or certified mail (**return receipt requested**) to Special Agent in Charge, Drug Enforcement Administration, of the DEA District Office which serves your area.

PRIVACY ACT INFORMATION

AUTHORITY: Section 307 of the Controlled Substances Act of 1970 (PL 91-513).
PURPOSE: To document the surrender of controlled substances which have been forwarded by registrants to DEA for disposal.
ROUTINE USES: This form is required by Federal Regulations for the surrender of unwanted Controlled Substances. Disclosures of information from this system are made to the following categories of users for the purposes stated.
   A. Other Federal law enforcement and regulatory agencies for law enforcement and regulatory purposes.
   B. State and local law enforcement and regulatory agencies for law enforcement and regulatory purposes.
EFFECT: Failure to document the surrender of unwanted Controlled Substances may result in prosecution for violation of the Controlled Substances Act.

Under the Paperwork Reduction Act, a person is not required to respond to a collection of information unless it displays a currently valid OMB control number. Public reporting burden for this collection of information is estimated to average 30 minutes per response, including the time for reviewing instructions, searching existing data sources, gathering and maintaining the data needed, and completing and reviewing the collection of information. Send comments regarding this burden estimate or any other aspect of this collection of information, including suggestions for reducing this burden, to the Drug Enforcement Administration, FOI and Records Management Section, Washington, D.C. 20537; and to the Office of Management and Budget, Paperwork Reduction Project no. 1117-0007, Washington, D.C. 20503.

PROCEDURE 19-2 RENEWING THE PHYSICIAN'S DEA REGISTRATION

Name _____ Class _____ Date _____

Sample Only

Completed Internet Form - NOT FOR SUBMISSION
DEA/Control Number -
Submission Date:

APPLICATION FOR REGISTRATION
UNDER CONTROLLED SUBSTANCES ACT OF 1970

Form DEA 224A

NAME: APPLICANT OR BUSINESS (LAST)

(First, MI)

TAX IDENTIFYING NUMBER   AND/OR

SOCIAL SECURITY NUMBER

THE DEBT COLLECTION IMPROVEMENT ACT OF 1996 (PL 104-134) REQUIRES THAT YOU FURNISH YOUR FEDERAL TAXPAYER IDENTIFYING NUMBER TO DEA. THIS NUMBER IS REQUIRED FOR DEBT COLLECTION PROCEDURES SHOULD YOUR FEE BECOME UNCOLLECTABLE. IF YOU DO NOT HAVE A FEDERAL TAXPAYER IDENTIFYING NUMBER, USE YOUR SOCIAL SECURITY NUMBER.

PROPOSED BUSINESS ADDRESS. (WHEN ENTERING A P.O. BOX, YOU ARE REQUIRED TO ENTER A STREET ADDRESS)

CITY

STATE   ZIP CODE

APPLICANT'S BUSINESS PHONE NUMBER

APPLICANT'S FAX NUMBER

REGISTRATION CLASSIFICATION

1. BUSINESS ACTIVITY:

2. INDICATE HERE IF YOU REQUIRE ORDER FORM BOOKS. ☐

3. Drug Schedules. (Fill in all circles that apply)

☑ Schedule II Narcotic

☑ Schedule II Non Narcotic

☑ Schedule III Narcotic

☑ Schedule III Non Narcotic

☑ Schedule IV

☑ Schedule V

Practitioner Details

National Provider ID

* Degree

* Birthdate

* Graduation Year

* Professional School

4. All Applicants must answer the following:

Are you currently authorized to prescribe, distribute, dispense, conduct research, or otherwise handle the controlled substances in the schedules for which you are applying under the laws of the state or jurisdiction in which you are operating or propose to operate?

State License No. _____ State: PA
Expire Date:

State Controlled Substance Lic. No. _____ State:
Expire Date: --

1. Has the applicant ever been **convicted of a crime** in connection with controlled substance(s) under state or federal law, or is any such action pending?

2. Has the applicant ever surrendered or had a **federal** controlled substance registration revoked, suspended, restricted or denied, or is any such action pending?

3. Has the applicant ever had a **state** professional license or controlled substance registration revoked, suspended, denied, restricted, or placed on probation, or is any such action pending?

4. If the applicant is a **corporation** (other than a corporation whose stock is owned or traded by the public), association, partnership, or pharmacy, has any officer, partner, stockholder or proprietor been **convicted of a crime** in connection with controlled substances under state or federal law, or ever surrendered, for cause, or had a **federal** controlled substance registration revoked, suspended, restricted or denied, or ever had a **state** professional license or controlled substance registration revoked, suspended, denied, restricted, or placed on probation, or is any such action pending?

PROCEDURE 19-3 RENEWING A PRESCRIPTION BY TELEPHONE

Name _____ Class _____ Date _____

Total Care Clinic
Progress Notes

Name: _____ Chart #: _____

DATE	

PROCEDURE 20-1 ADMINISTERING ORAL DRUGS

Name _____ Class _____ Date _____

MEDICATION FLOWSHEET		
Patient Name	**Allergies**	

DATE	MEDICATION	REFILLS			
Start / Stop	Dosage/Direction/Amount	Date/Amount/Initials			

PROCEDURE 20-2 ADMINISTERING BUCCAL OR SUBLINGUAL DRUGS

Name _____ Class _____ Date _____

MEDICATION FLOWSHEET						
Patient Name			Allergies			
DATE	**MEDICATION**		**REFILLS**			
Start / Stop	Dosage/Direction/Amount		Date/Amount/Initials			

PROCEDURE 20-5 GIVING AN INTRADERMAL INJECTION

Name _____ Class _____ Date _____

MEDICATION FLOWSHEET		
Patient Name		Allergies

DATE	MEDICATION	REFILLS
Start / Stop	Dosage/Direction/Amount	Date/Amount/Initials

PROCEDURE 20-6 GIVING A SUBCUTANEOUS (SUB-Q) INJECTION

Name _____ Class _____ Date _____

MEDICATION FLOWSHEET		
Patient Name	**Allergies**	

DATE	MEDICATION	REFILLS			
Start / Stop	Dosage/Direction/Amount	Date/Amount/Initials			

PROCEDURE 20-7 GIVING AN INTRAMUSCULAR INJECTION

Name _____ Class _____ Date _____

MEDICATION FLOWSHEET						
Patient Name			Allergies			
DATE	**MEDICATION**		**REFILLS**			
Start / Stop	Dosage/Direction/Amount		Date/Amount/Initials			

PROCEDURE 20-8 ADMINISTERING INHALATION THERAPY

Name _____ Class _____ Date _____

MEDICATION FLOWSHEET		
Patient Name		**Allergies**

DATE	MEDICATION	REFILLS				
Start / Stop	Dosage/Direction/Amount	Date/Amount/Initials				

PROCEDURE 20-9 ADMINISTERING AND REMOVING A TRANSDERMAL PATCH AND PROVIDING PATIENT INSTRUCTION

Name _____ Class _____ Date _____

MEDICATION FLOWSHEET						
Patient Name			Allergies			
DATE	**MEDICATION**		**REFILLS**			
Start / Stop	Dosage/Direction/Amount		Date/Amount/Initials			

PROCEDURE 20-10 ASSISTING WITH ADMINISTRATION OF AN URETHRAL DRUG

Name _____ Class _____ Date _____

MEDICATION FLOWSHEET		
Patient Name		Allergies

DATE	MEDICATION	REFILLS
Start / Stop	Dosage/Direction/Amount	Date/Amount/Initials

PROCEDURE 20-11 ADMINISTERING A VAGINAL MEDICATION

Name _____ Class _____ Date _____

MEDICATION FLOWSHEET		
Patient Name		Allergies

DATE	MEDICATION	REFILLS			
Start / Stop	Dosage/Direction/Amount	Date/Amount/Initials			

PROCEDURE 20-12 ADMINISTERING A RECTAL MEDICATION

Name _____ Class _____ Date _____

MEDICATION FLOWSHEET						
Patient Name			Allergies			
DATE	**MEDICATION**		**REFILLS**			
Start / Stop	Dosage/Direction/Amount		Date/Amount/Initials			

PROCEDURE 20-13 ADMINISTERING EYE MEDICATION

Name _____ Class _____ Date _____

MEDICATION FLOWSHEET		
Patient Name		Allergies

DATE	MEDICATION	REFILLS			
Start / Stop	Dosage/Direction/Amount	Date/Amount/Initials			

PROCEDURE 20-14 PERFORMING EYE IRRIGATION

Name _____ Class _____ Date _____

MEDICATION FLOWSHEET					
Patient Name			**Allergies**		
DATE	**MEDICATION**		**REFILLS**		
Start / Stop	Dosage/Direction/Amount		Date/Amount/Initials		

PROCEDURE 20-15 ADMINISTERING EARDROPS

Name _____ Class _____ Date _____

MEDICATION FLOWSHEET					
Patient Name			Allergies		
DATE	**MEDICATION**		**REFILLS**		
Start ⟋ Stop	Dosage/Direction/Amount		Date/Amount/Initials		

Procedure 20-16 Performing Ear Irrigation

Name _____ Class _____ Date _____

MEDICATION FLOWSHEET		
Patient Name		**Allergies**

DATE	MEDICATION	REFILLS			
Start / Stop	Dosage/Direction/Amount	Date/Amount/Initials			

PROCEDURE 21-1 OBTAINING AN ECG

Name _____ Class _____ Date _____

Total Care Clinic
Progress Notes

Name: _____ Chart #: _____

DATE	

PROCEDURE 21-2 HOLTER MONITORING

Name _____ Class _____ Date _____

Total Care Clinic
Progress Notes

Name: _____ Chart #: _____

DATE	

PROCEDURE 21-3 MEASURING FORCED VITAL CAPACITY USING SPIROMETRY

Name _____ Class _____ Date _____

Total Care Clinic
Progress Notes

Name: _____ Chart #: _____

DATE	

Procedure 21-4 Obtaining a Peak Expiratory Flow Rate

Name _____ Class _____ Date _____

Total Care Clinic
Progress Notes

Name: _____ Chart #: _____

DATE	

PROCEDURE 21-5 OBTAINING A PULSE OXIMETRY READING

Name _____ Class _____ Date _____

Name _____ DOB _____ Date _____

ALLERGIES: _____

Note

Review of Systems

Systems	NL	Note	Systems	NL	Note
Constitutional			Musculoskeletal		
Eyes			Skin/breasts		
ENT/mouth			Neurologic		
Cardiovascular			Psychiatric		
Respiratory			Endocrine		
GI			Hem/lymph		
GU			Allergy/immun		

Current Medicines	Date	Current Diagnosis

H: _____ W: _____ T: _____ P: _____ R: _____

B/P Sitting _____ or Standing _____ Supine _____

Last Tetanus _____

L.M.P. _____

O2 Sat: _____ Pain Scale: _____

Social Habits Yes No

Tobacco ___ ___

Alcohol ___ ___

Rec. Drugs ___ ___

CC:

HPI:

Name _____ DOB _____ Date _____

ALLERGIES: _____

Note

Review of Systems

Systems	NL	Note	Systems	NL	Note
Constitutional			Musculoskeletal		
Eyes			Skin/breasts		
ENT/mouth			Neurologic		
Cardiovascular			Psychiatric		
Respiratory			Endocrine		
GI			Hem/lymph		
GU			Allergy/immun		

Current Medicines	Date	Current Diagnosis

H: _____ W: _____ T: _____ P: _____ R: _____

B/P Sitting _____ or Standing _____ Supine _____

Last Tetanus _____

L.M.P. _____

O2 Sat: _____ Pain Scale: _____

Social Habits Yes No

Tobacco ___ ___

Alcohol ___ ___

Rec. Drugs ___ ___

CC:

HPI:

PROCEDURE 22-1 ASSISTING WITH AN X-RAY EXAMINATION

Name _____ Class _____ Date _____

Total Care Clinic
Progress Notes

Name: _____ Chart #:_____

DATE	

PROCEDURE 22-2 DOCUMENTATION AND FILING TECHNIQUES FOR X-RAYS

Name _____ Class _____ Date _____

X-RAY EXAMINATIONS RECORD

Patient	Date	Type X-Ray	No. Taken	Referring Doctor	Comments

Work Product Documentation/Forms

Use these forms to complete application activities from the textbook or the workbook. Make additional copies for extra practice.

APPLICATION ACTIVITY FORMS

Budget Example

Example:

Expense	Monthly Amount	Annual
Rent	500.00	6000.00
Car payment and insurance	300.00	3600.00
Food	200.00	2400.00
Utilities	200.00	2400.00
Student loan	80.00	960.00
Credit cards	100.00	1200.00
Clothing	100.00	1200.00
Child care	400.00	4800.00
Other	100.00	1200.00
TOTAL	1980.00	23,760.00

Your budget:

Expense	Monthly Amount	Annual
Rent or mortgage		
Car payment and insurance		
Food		
Utilities		
Student loan		
Credit cards		
Clothing		
Child care		
Other		
TOTAL		

CHARTING FORM

Name of Patient: _____   Date: _____

Physician: _____

EMERGENCY PREPAREDNESS WORKSHEET
PREPARING FOR AN EMERGENCY – HAZARD ANALYSIS AND PLAN

1. What types of emergency situations have occurred in your community during the last five years?

2. Did any of these situations result in an emergency or disaster declaration? If you do not know, contact your local emergency management office or Red Cross. If a disaster declaration has occurred, describe briefly.

3. Select the five most likely hazards that your community has the highest probability of facing now and in the future.

Natural	Technological	Intentional
Floods	HazMat Spill	Terrorism
Winds	Power Grid Failure	Civil Distrubance
Wild Land Fires	Explosives	WMD (weapons of mass destruction)
Lightning Fires	Chemical Fire	Strikes
Tsunami	Pipeline	Riots
Tornado	Utility Services Failure	Nuclear Attack
Earthquake	Poisons	Nuclear Attack Fallout
Volcanic Eruptions	Radioactive Materials	
Pandemics	Chemical Waste	

4. For each of the five hazards you selected describe what your role as a Medical Assistant will be if the hazard/emergency occurs in your community.

5. Create a list of local community resources that would be utilized if a hazard or emergency occurred in your area.

EQUIPMENT CHECKLIST

Equipment Description	Shannon Photocopier	Model No. 123A9
Serial Number: 56AC90-001L		
Date:	**Action/Comments**	**Initials**
9/17/XX	Machine checked	SM, CMA (AAMA)

GROWTH CHART (2–20 YEARS BOYS)

2 to 20 years: Boys
Stature-for-age and Weight-for-age percentiles

NAME _____

RECORD # _____

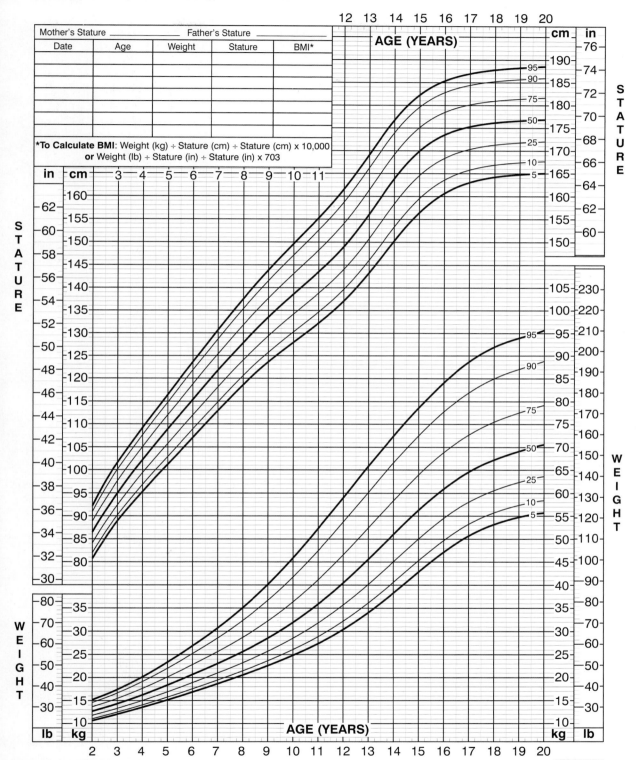

*To Calculate BMI: Weight (kg) ÷ Stature (cm) ÷ Stature (cm) x 10,000
or Weight (lb) ÷ Stature (in) ÷ Stature (in) x 703

Published May 30, 2000 (modified 11/21/00).
SOURCE: Developed by the National Center for Health Statistics in collaboration with
the National Center for Chronic Disease Prevention and Health Promotion (2000).
http://www.cdc.gov/growthcharts

CDC
SAFER · HEALTHIER · PEOPLE™

GROWTH CHART (2–20 YEARS GIRLS)

2 to 20 years: Girls
Stature-for-age and Weight-for-age percentiles

NAME _____

RECORD # _____

Mother's Stature _____		Father's Stature _____		
Date	Age	Weight	Stature	BMI*

***To Calculate BMI:** Weight (kg) ÷ Stature (cm) ÷ Stature (cm) x 10,000
or Weight (lb) ÷ Stature (in) ÷ Stature (in) x 703

AGE (YEARS)

12 13 14 15 16 17 18 19 20

STATURE

95
90
75
50
25
10
5

WEIGHT

95
90
75
50
25
10
5

AGE (YEARS)

2 3 4 5 6 7 8 9 10 11 12 13 14 15 16 17 18 19 20

lb kg kg lb

Published May 30, 2000 (modified 11/21/00).
SOURCE: Developed by the National Center for Health Statistics in collaboration with
the National Center for Chronic Disease Prevention and Health Promotion (2000).
http://www.cdc.gov/growthcharts

CDC
SAFER · HEALTHIER · PEOPLE™

GROWTH CHART (BIRTH–36 MONTHS BOYS)

Birth to 36 months: Boys
Length-for-age and Weight-for-age percentiles

NAME _____

RECORD # _____

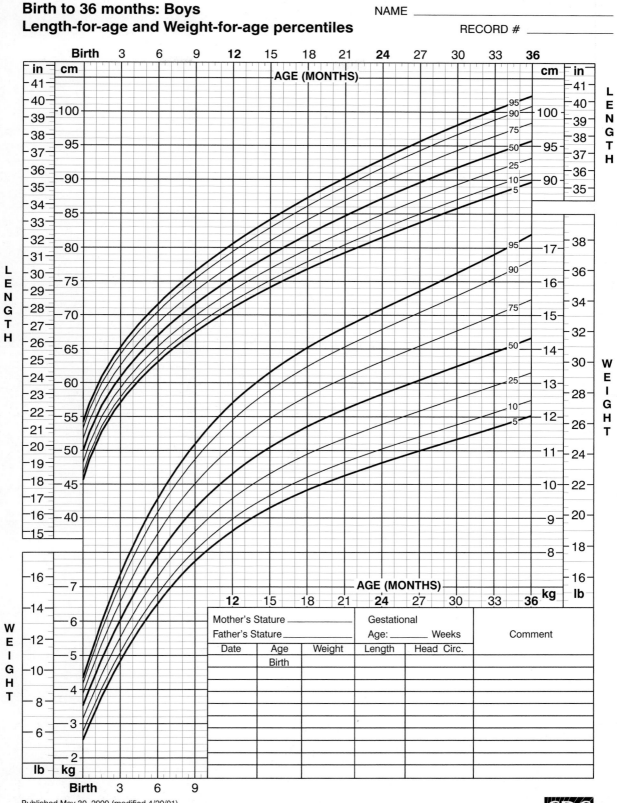

Published May 30, 2000 (modified 4/20/01).
SOURCE: Developed by the National Center for Health Statistics in collaboration with
the National Center for Chronic Disease Prevention and Health Promotion (2000).
http://www.cdc.gov/growthcharts

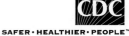

SAFER · HEALTHIER · PEOPLE™

Growth Chart (Birth–36 months Girls)

Birth to 36 months: Girls
Length-for-age and Weight-for-age percentiles

NAME _____

RECORD # _____

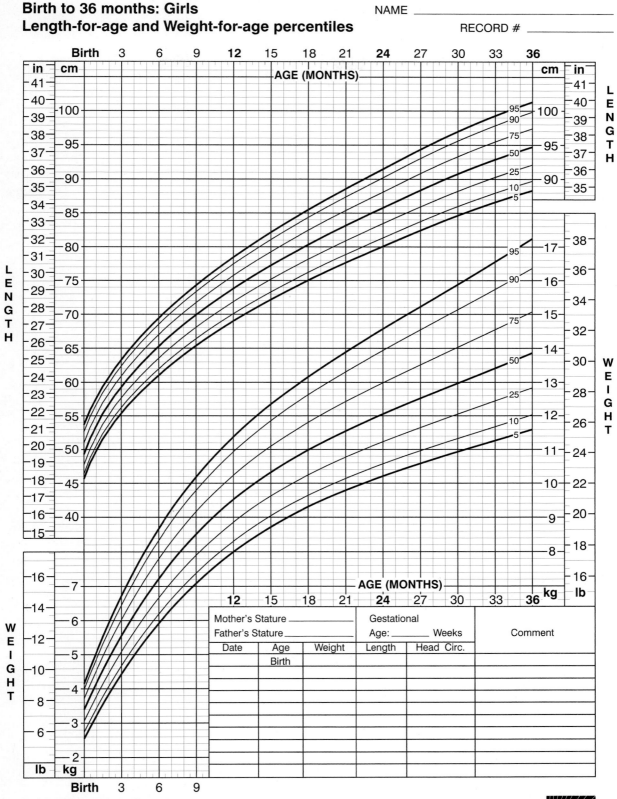

Published May 30, 2000 (modified 4/20/01).
SOURCE: Developed by the National Center for Health Statistics in collaboration with
the National Center for Chronic Disease Prevention and Health Promotion (2000).
http://www.cdc.gov/growthcharts

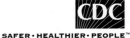

SAFER · HEALTHIER · PEOPLE™

HEALTH HISTORY FORM

HEALTH HISTORY
(Confidential)

Name_____ Today's Date_____

Age_____ Birthdate_____ Date of last physical examination_____

What is your reason for visit?_____

SYMPTOMS Check (✓) symptoms you currently have or have had in the past year.

GENERAL
- ☐ Chills
- ☐ Depression
- ☐ Dizziness
- ☐ Fainting
- ☐ Fever
- ☐ Forgetfulness
- ☐ Headache
- ☐ Loss of sleep
- ☐ Loss of weight
- ☐ Nervousness
- ☐ Numbness
- ☐ Sweats

MUSCLE/JOINT/BONE
Pain, weakness, numbness in:
- ☐ Arms
- ☐ Back
- ☐ Feet
- ☐ Hands
- ☐ Hips
- ☐ Legs
- ☐ Neck
- ☐ Shoulders

GENITO-URINARY
- ☐ Blood in urine
- ☐ Frequent urination
- ☐ Lack of bladder control
- ☐ Painful urination

GASTROINTESTINAL
- ☐ Appetite poor
- ☐ Bloating
- ☐ Bowel changes
- ☐ Constipation
- ☐ Diarrhea
- ☐ Excessive hunger
- ☐ Excessive thirst
- ☐ Gas
- ☐ Hemorrhoids
- ☐ Indigestion
- ☐ Nausea
- ☐ Rectal bleeding
- ☐ Stomach pain
- ☐ Vomiting
- ☐ Vomiting blood

CARDIOVASCULAR
- ☐ Chest pain
- ☐ High blood pressure
- ☐ Irregular heart beat
- ☐ Low blood pressure
- ☐ Poor circulation
- ☐ Rapid heart beat
- ☐ Swelling of ankles
- ☐ Varicose veins

EYE, EAR, NOSE, THROAT
- ☐ Bleeding gums
- ☐ Blurred vision
- ☐ Crossed eyes
- ☐ Difficulty swallowing
- ☐ Double vision
- ☐ Earache
- ☐ Ear discharge
- ☐ Hay fever
- ☐ Hoarseness
- ☐ Loss of hearing
- ☐ Nosebleeds
- ☐ Persistent cough
- ☐ Ringing in ears
- ☐ Sinus problems
- ☐ Vision – Flashes
- ☐ Vision – Halos

SKIN
- ☐ Bruise easily
- ☐ Hives
- ☐ Itching
- ☐ Change in moles
- ☐ Rash
- ☐ Scars
- ☐ Sore that won't heal

MEN only
- ☐ Breast lump
- ☐ Erection difficulties
- ☐ Lump in testicles
- ☐ Penis discharge
- ☐ Sore on penis
- ☐ Other

WOMEN only
- ☐ Abnormal Pap smear
- ☐ Bleeding between periods
- ☐ Breast lump
- ☐ Extreme menstrual pain
- ☐ Hot flashes
- ☐ Nipple discharge
- ☐ Painful intercourse
- ☐ Vaginal discharge
- ☐ Other

Date of last
menstrual period_____

Date of last
Pap smear_____

Have you had
a mammogram?_____

Are you pregnant?_____

Number of children_____

CONDITIONS Check (✓) conditions you have or have had in the past.

- ☐ AIDS
- ☐ Alcoholism
- ☐ Anemia
- ☐ Anorexia
- ☐ Appendicitis
- ☐ Arthritis
- ☐ Asthma
- ☐ Bleeding Disorders
- ☐ Breast Lump
- ☐ Bronchitis
- ☐ Bulimia
- ☐ Cancer
- ☐ Cataracts

- ☐ Chemical Dependency
- ☐ Chicken Pox
- ☐ Diabetes
- ☐ Emphysema
- ☐ Epilepsy
- ☐ Glaucoma
- ☐ Goiter
- ☐ Gonorrhea
- ☐ Gout
- ☐ Heart Disease
- ☐ Hepatitis
- ☐ Hernia
- ☐ Herpes

- ☐ High Cholesterol
- ☐ HIV Positive
- ☐ Kidney Disease
- ☐ Liver Disease
- ☐ Measles
- ☐ Migraine Headaches
- ☐ Miscarriage
- ☐ Mononucleosis
- ☐ Multiple Sclerosis
- ☐ Mumps
- ☐ Pacemaker
- ☐ Pneumonia
- ☐ Polio

- ☐ Prostate Problem
- ☐ Psychiatric Care
- ☐ Rheumatic Fever
- ☐ Scarlet Fever
- ☐ Stroke
- ☐ Suicide Attempt
- ☐ Thyroid Problems
- ☐ Tonsillitis
- ☐ Tuberculosis
- ☐ Typhoid Fever
- ☐ Ulcers
- ☐ Vaginal Infections
- ☐ Venereal Disease

MEDICATIONS List medications you are currently taking | **ALLERGIES** To medications or substances

Pharmacy Name_____ Phone_____

HEALTH HISTORY FORM *(concluded)*

(All information is strictly confidential)

FAMILY HISTORY Fill in health information about your family.

Relation	Age	State of Health	Age at Death	Cause of Death	Check (✓) if your blood relatives had any of the following: Disease	Relationship to you
Father					Arthritis, Gout	
Mother					Asthma, Hay Fever	
Brothers					Cancer	
					Chemical Dependency	
					Diabetes	
					Heart Disease, Strokes	
Sisters					High Blood Pressure	
					Kidney Disease	
					Tuberculosis	
					Other	

HOSPITALIZATIONS

Year	Hospital	Reason for Hospitalization and Outcome

PREGNANCY HISTORY

Year of Birth	Sex of Birth	Complications if any

HEALTH HABITS Check (✓) which substances you use and describe how much you use.

Caffeine	
Tobacco	
Drugs	
Other	

Have you ever had a blood transfusion? ☐ Yes ☐ No
If yes, please give approximate dates._____

SERIOUS ILLNESS/INJURIES	DATE	OUTCOME

OCCUPATIONAL CONCERNS
Check (✓) if your work exposes you to the following:

Stress	
Hazardous Substances	
Heavy Lifting	
Other	

Your occupation:

I certify that the above information is correct to the best of my knowledge. I will not hold my doctor or any members of his/her staff responsible for any errors or omissions that I may have made in the completion of this form.

_____   _____
Signature   Date

_____   _____
Reviewed By   Date

INVENTORY WORKSHEET

Medical Office Supply Inventory

Description	Quantity	On-Hand	Needed	Notes
Batteries	4	0	2	*Check expiration dates*

LABORATORY REPORT FORM

Total Care Clinic
Laboratory Report Form

Patient Name _____ Medical Record # _____ Age _____ Sex _____

Address _____ Phone _____

Referring Physician _____

Laboratory Findings:

Date	Blood Test	Patient Result	Normal Value/Range

Date	Urinalysis	Patient Result	Normal Value/Range

Test completed by: _____ _____
                            (Print name)   (Signature)

LABORATORY REQUISITION FORM

Name _____ Class _____ Date _____

70Y

Account No.

Specimen Date Mo Day Yr	Specimen Time Hr Min	Patient Name (Last)	(First, MI)	Sex	Date of Birth Mo Day Yr	Age Yrs Mos

50 8649 9000 4

Patient I.D. #   Physician I.D.   Patient/Resp. Party's Phone #

* I certify that I have read the informed consent on the back and understand its content.

Responsible Party or Insured's Name (Last, First)   Patient's SS #

Patient's Signature

Address   City   State   Zip Code

Resp. Party's Employer   Medicaid Number/HMO #   Medicare #

Physician Name   UPIN #   Physician's Signature   Provider #

Diagnosis Code (ICD-9)   Insurance Code or Company Name and Address   Insurance I.D. #   Workers Comp. Yes No

Group # or Name   Relationship to Insured (Circle One) 1-Self 2-Spouse 3-Other

REV. 6/95

Urine Random   † Ⓤ Total 24hr. Vol. _____ Ht. _____ Wt. _____

| ✸ = EDTA Plasma | Ⓢ = Serum | Ⓡ = Red | Ⓖ = Gray | Ⓑ = Light Blue |
| AF = Amniotic Fluid | Ⓕ = Frozen Specimen | Ⓛ = Lavender | GN = Green | RB = Royal Blue |

Apply Labels to Patient Specimens Only Patient Control No. ➡

50 8649 9000 4

50 8649 9000 4   50 8649 9000 4   50 8649 9000 4

50 8649 9000 4   50 8649 9000 4   50 8649 9000 4

CHEMISTRY REQUEST

#	Test		#	Test		#	Test	
58867	☐ Basic Chemistry	Ⓢ	1693	☐ Glycohemoglobin, Total	Ⓛ	4465	☐ Prolactin	Ⓢ
1396	☐ Amylase, Serum	Ⓢ	4416	☐ HCG, Beta Chain, Quant	Ⓢ	4747	☐ Prostatic Acid Phosphatase (EIA)	Ⓢ
6254	☐ Antinuclear Antibody (ANA), Qnt.	Ⓢ	1453	☐ Hemoglobin A1C	Ⓛ	10322	☐ Prostate-Specific Antigen (PSA)	Ⓢ
1040	☐ BUN	Ⓢ	6510	☐ Hepatitis B Surf Antigen (HBsAg)	Ⓢ	5199	☐ Prothrombin Time	Ⓑ
7419	☐ Carbamazepine (Tegretol)	Ⓢ	6395	☐ Hepatitis B Surf Antibody (Anti HBs)	Ⓢ	6502	☐ Ra Latex Screen	Ⓢ
5009	☐ CBC With Differential	Ⓛ	58560	☐ Hepatitis Profile I (Diagnostic)	Ⓢ	5215	☐ Sedimentation Rate	Ⓛ
2139	☐ CEA-EIA Roche	△ ✸	46938	☐ Hepatitis Profile II (Follow up)	Ⓢ	6072	☐ STS	Ⓢ
98012	☐ Chlamydia by DNA Probe	△	58552	☐ Hepatitis Profile VII (A and B)	Ⓢ	1149	☐ T₄ (Thyroxine)	Ⓢ
96479	☐ Chlamydia/GC, DNA Probe	△	83824	☐ HIV-1 ABS-EIA	Ⓢ	7336	☐ Theophylline (Theo-Dur)	Ⓢ
1065	☐ Cholesterol, Total	Ⓢ	7625	☐ Lead, Blood	RB	620	☐ Thyroid Profile I	Ⓢ
1370	☐ Creatinine, Serum	Ⓢ	235002	☐ Lipid Profile I (Lipoprotein Analysis)	Ⓢ	27011	☐ Thyroid Profile II	Ⓢ
7385	☐ Digoxin (Lanoxin)	Ⓢ	235028	☐ Lipid Profile III (incl Apolipoproteins)	Ⓢ	4259	☐ TSH, 3rd Generation	Ⓢ
604	☐ Electrolytes (Na, K, Cl)	Ⓢ	7708	☐ Lithium	Ⓢ	810	☐ Vitamin B-12 and Folate	Ⓢ
4598	☐ Ferritin	Ⓢ	505	☐ Liver Profile A	Ⓢ			
4309	☐ Follicle Stim. Hormone (FSH)	Ⓢ	7401	☐ Phenytoin (Dilantin)	Ⓢ		**URINE CHEMISTRY**	
1818	☐ Glucose	Ⓖ	1180	☐ Potassium	Ⓢ	3038	☐ Urinalysis (Microscopic if indicated)	Ⓤ
	☐ Glucose Tolerance	Ⓖ	4556	☐ Pregnancy, Serum, Ql.	Ⓢ	3772	☐ Urinalysis, Complete	Ⓤ
	Indicate No. Of Tubes _____		53520	☐ Prenatal Profile B with HBsAG	2-L Ⓡ			

ADDITIONAL TESTS

Test #	Name
☐ 1375	24 Hr Urine for Protein Ⓤ
☐ 4550	Pregnancy, Urine, Qul Ⓤ

Medical History Form

Total Care Clinic
Medical History

Name _____ Age _____ Sex _____ S M W D
Address _____ Phone _____ Date _____

Occupation _____ Ref. by _____
Chief Complaint _____

Present Illness _____
_____
_____
_____
_____

History —Military _____
        —Social _____
        —Family _____
        —Marital _____
        —Menstrual _____ Menarche _____ Para. _____ LMP _____
        —Illness Measles Pert. Var. Pneu. Pleur. Typh. Mal. Rh. Fev. Sc. Fev. Diphth. Other
        —Surgery _____
        —Allergies _____
        —Current Medications _____

Physical Examination

Temp. _____ Pulse _____ Resp. _____ BP _____ Ht. _____ Wt. _____
General Appearance _____ Skin _____ Mucous Membrane _____
Eyes: _____ Vision _____ Pupil _____ Fundus _____
Ears: _____
Nose: _____
Throat: _____ Pharynx _____ Tonsils _____
Chest: _____ Breasts _____
Heart: _____
Lungs: _____
Abdomen: _____
Genitalia: _____
Rectum: _____
Pelvic: _____
Extremities: _____ Pulses: _____
Lymph Nodes: _____ Neck _____ Axilla _____ Inguinal _____ Abdominal _____
Neurological: _____
Diagnosis: _____
_____
_____

Treatment: _____
_____
_____

Laboratory Findings: _____
Date _____ Blood _____
_____
_____

Date _____ Urine _____
_____
_____
_____
_____

MEDICAL RECORD (VITAL SIGNS)

TOTAL CARE CLINIC

Facility _____

DATE	TIME	T	P	R	BP		DATE	TIME	T	P	R	BP	

Patient Name:	Last:	First:	Middle:	Physician:

VITAL SIGN CHART # _____

MEDICAL RECORD (HEIGHT AND WEIGHT)

TOTAL CARE CLINIC

Facility _____

MONTH: _____ YEAR: _____

DATE	WEIGHT	HEIGHT

MONTH: _____ YEAR: _____

DATE	WEIGHT	HEIGHT

MONTH: _____ YEAR: _____

DATE	WEIGHT	HEIGHT

MONTH: _____ YEAR: _____

DATE	WEIGHT	HEIGHT

MONTH: _____ YEAR: _____

DATE	WEIGHT	HEIGHT

MONTH: _____ YEAR: _____

DATE	WEIGHT	HEIGHT

MONTH: _____ YEAR: _____

DATE	WEIGHT	HEIGHT

MONTH: _____ YEAR: _____

DATE	WEIGHT	HEIGHT

MONTH: _____ YEAR: _____

DATE	WEIGHT	HEIGHT

MONTH: _____ YEAR: _____

DATE	WEIGHT	HEIGHT

MONTH: _____ YEAR: _____

DATE	WEIGHT	HEIGHT

MONTH: _____ YEAR: _____

DATE	WEIGHT	HEIGHT

Patient Name:	Last:	First:	Middle:	Admin. Number:
Physician:				

WEIGHT RECORD

MEDICATION FLOWSHEET

MEDICATION FLOWSHEET		
Patient Name	**Allergies**	

DATE	MEDICATION	REFILLS				
Start / Stop	Dosage/Direction/Amount	Date/Amount/Initials				

PATIENT REGISTRATION FORM

Community Health Center • 6508 South Street • Kokomo, IN 46902
(317) 555-1234 • Fax: (317) 555-1245

Patient Registration
Patient Information

Name: _____ Today's Date: _____

Address: _____

City: _____ State: _____ Zip Code: _____

Telephone (Home): _____ (Work): _____ (Cell): _____

Birthdate: _____ Age: _____ Sex: M F   No. of Children _____ Marital Status: M S W D

Social Security Number: _____ Employer: _____ Occupation: _____

Primary Physician: _____

Referred by: _____

Person to Contact in Emergency: _____

Emergency Telephone: _____

Special Needs: _____

Responsible Party

Party Responsible for Payment: Self   Spouse   Parent   Other

Name (If Other Than Self): _____

Address: _____

City: _____ State: _____ Zip Code: _____

Primary Insurance

Primary Medical Insurance: _____

Insured party: Self   Spouse   Parent   Other

ID#/Social Security No.: _____ Group/Plan No.: _____

Name (If Other Than Self): _____

Address: _____

City: _____ State: _____ Zip Code: _____

Secondary Insurance

Secondary Medical Insurance: _____

Insured party: Self   Spouse   Parent   Other

ID#/Social Security No.: _____ Group/Plan No.: _____

Name (If Other Than Self): _____

Address: _____

City: _____ State: _____ Zip Code: _____

PROGRESS NOTES

Total Care Clinic
Progress Notes

Name: _____ Chart #: _____

DATE	